MEDICAL RADIOLOGY
Diagnostic Imaging

Editors:
A. L. Baert, Leuven
K. Sartor, Heidelberg

Springer

Berlin
Heidelberg
New York
Hong Kong
London
Milan
Paris
Tokyo

A. M. Davies · J. Hodler (Eds.)

Imaging of the Shoulder

Techniques and Applications

With Contributions by

V. Baudrez · P. W. P. Bearcroft · T. H. Berquist · S. Bianchi · A. Blum · Y. Carrillon
V. N. Cassar-Pullicino · C. B. Chung · A. M. Davies · L. E. Derchi · J. Fasel
M. A. M. Feldberg · J. F. Garcia · J. Hodler · K. Johnson · A. Keller · P. Lang · N. Lektrakul
C. Martinoli · L. Neumann · W. Peh · N. Prato · B. J. Preston · S.-T. Quek · J.-J. Railhac
D. Resnick · B. Roger · A. Stäbler · T. Tavernier · N. Teodorovic · B. Tins · B. C. Vande Berg
D. Vanel · H. Wouter van Es · D. Weishaupt · S. Wildermuth · T. D. Witkamp · B. Wollman
H. Yoshioka · M. Zanetti · M. B. Zlatkin

Foreword by

A. L. Baert

With 299 Figures in 596 Separate Illustrations, 27 in Color and 11 Tables

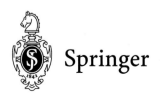

Springer

A. Mark Davies, MD
Consultant Radiologist
The MRI Centre
Royal Orthopaedic Hospital
Birmingham B31 2AP
UK

Jürg Hodler, MD, MBA
Department of Radiolgy
Orthopedic University Hosptal Balgrist
Forchstrasse 340
8008 Zurich
Switzerland

Medical Radiology · Diagnostic Imaging and Radiation Oncology
Series Editors: A. L. Baert · L. W. Brady · H.-P. Heilmann · M. Molls · K. Sartor

Continuation of
Handbuch der medizinischen Radiologie
Encyclopedia of Medical Radiology

ISBN 3-540-67293-1 Springer-Verlag Berlin Heidelberg New York

Library of Congress Cataloging-in-Publication Data

Imaging of the shoulder : techniques and applications / A. M. Davies, J. Hodler (eds) ; with
  contributions by V. Baudrez ... [et al.] ; foreword by A. L. Baert.
    p. ; cm. -- (Medical radiology)
    Includes bibliographical references and index
    ISBN 3-540-67293-1 (hard: alk. paper)
    1. Shoulder--Imaging. 2. Shoulder--Radiography. I. Davies, A. M. (Arthur Mark),
  1954- II. Hodler, Jürg. III. Series.
    [DNLM: 1. Shoulder--radiography. 2. Radiography--methods. WE 810 I31 2004]
  RC939.I435 2004
  617.5'720754--dc21   2003041570

Springer-Verlag Berlin Heidelberg New York
a member of BertelsmannSpringer Science+Business Media GmbH

http//www. springer.de
© Springer-Verlag Berlin Heidelberg 2004
Printed in Germany

Cover-Design and Typesetting: Verlagsservice Teichmann, 69256 Mauer

21/3150xq – 5 4 3 2 1 0 – Printed on acid-free paper

Foreword

It is my great pleasure and privilege to introduce another volume on modern musculo-skeletal imaging edited by A. M. Davies and J. Hodler following two already published, superb and highly successful volumes on imaging of the knee, edited by A.M. Davies and V. N. Cassar-Pullicino, and imaging of the foot and ankle, edited by A. M. Davies, R. W. Whitehouse and J.P.R. Jenkins.

The concept of these volumes is based on comprehensive coverage both of the imaging modalities and of the applications of all these techniques to a specific anatomical area and all the pathological conditions related to it.

The short "gestational" period of this volume – less than 18 months between the beginning of the project and final manuscript delivery to the publisher – ensures, as in the two foregoing volumes, that the most recent advances in shoulder imaging and radiological management are covered.

I am greatly indebted to Dr. Davies and Dr. Hodler for their brilliant editorial work and personal contributions. I congratulate them on their judicious choice of contributing authors, all well-known experts in the field.

I am convinced that this excellent volume will be of great interest for both radiologists in training and certified radiologists, and also for orthopaedic surgeons and rheumatologists. It is my sincere wish that this work meet with the same success as so many previous volumes in the series Medical Radiology – Diagnostic Imaging.

Leuven   ALBERT L. BAERT

Preface

As our understanding of the disease processes and the biomechanics of shoulder disorders improves, there is a need to continuously update radiologists, orthopaedic surgeons and other professionals working in this field. Several recent texts on the shoulder have concentrated on a single imaging technique such as MR imaging. This book, in common with several others published in this series, takes a dual approach to the subject.

The first section acquaints the reader with the full range of techniques available for imaging shoulder pathology, emphasising the indications and contraindications. The six chapters include contributions on radiography, computed tomography and CT arthrography, magnetic resonance imaging and MR arthrography, ultrasound and interventional techniques. The remaining 13 chapters discuss the optimal application of these techniques to specific pathologies, highlighting practical solutions to both common and uncommon clinical problems.

The discerning reader may note a few minor contradications in the text (recommended gauge of needle, volume of contrast medium, use or not of local anaesthetics for arthrography, etc.), reflecting the different practises of the authors. The editors have deliberately not edited out these inconsistencies, thereby allowing the reader to appreciate that, even between centres of excellence, practises can and will vary.

The editors are grateful to the international panel of authors for their contributions to this book, which aims to provide a comprehensive overview of current imaging of the shoulder.

Birmingham

Zurich

A. Mark Davies

Jürg Hodler

Contents

Imaging Techniques

1 Shoulder Radiography

S. Bianchi, N. Prato, C. Martinoli, L. E. Derchi

CONTENTS

Although in recent years US, CT and MRI, together with CT and MR arthrography, have gained wide popularity in the evaluation of shoulder diseases, standard radiography (SR) still remains the most often performed imaging examination of this anatomical region. The main advantages of SR are the easy accessibility, low cost, panoramic view and short time of examination. Additionally, the basic findings provided by radiography are well known and familiar both to radiologists and clinicians.

Disadvantages of SR include the low capability to assess soft tissues lesions (with the exclusion of

S. Bianchi, MD
Division of Radiodiagnosis and Interventional Radiology, Hopital Cantonal Universitaire, 24 rue Micheli-du-Crest, 1211 Geneva, Switzerland
N. Prato, MD
Division of Radiodiagnosis, Ospedale San Carlo, Piazzale Gianasso, 16158 Genoa, Italy
C. Martinoli, MD
Istituto di Radiologia, Università di Genova, Largo R Benzi 8, 16100 Genoa, Italy
L. E. Derchi, MD
Istituto di Radiologia, Università di Genova, Largo R Benzi 8, 16100 Genoa, Italy

tendon calcifications), presence of localised alterations of the articular cartilages, or of intraarticular and bursal effusion, and the inability to image the glenoid labrum and the bone marrow. As in many other joints, however, SR is the first technique to be used if an imaging modality is needed; others are then performed on the basis of the clinical findings, the structure to be evaluated and the results of SR.

The aims of this chapter are to illustrate the current techniques of shoulder SR, including a survey of the different views, to describe the normal radiographic anatomy and to propose a practical approach to the choice of views to be obtained in different clinical situations.

1.1
Examination Technique and Shoulder Views

1.1.1
AP View of the Shoulder Region

The anteroposterior (AP) view (Fig. 1.1) is the most commonly obtained view of the shoulder and the easiest to perform by the technologist, particularly in severely traumatised patients. The patient can be examined either standing or supine with the trunk not rotated. The X-ray beam is centred medial to the glenohumeral joint. A large cassette (30×40 cm) allows visualisation of the scapula, the proximal portion of the humerus and the lateral chest wall. Since the scapula is not oriented in a true coronal plane, but lies in a coronal oblique plane (40°), this view is not perpendicular to the scapula and is not tangential to the glenohumeral joint space. Then, the obliquity of the beam with respect to the axis of the scapula results in an elliptical appearance of the glenoid cavity. The anterior rim of the glenoid fossa projects medially while the posterior rim projects laterally. Since the humeral head overlies the glenoid, assessment of the glenohumeral space is suboptimal in this view. The arm is usually held in neutral rotation.

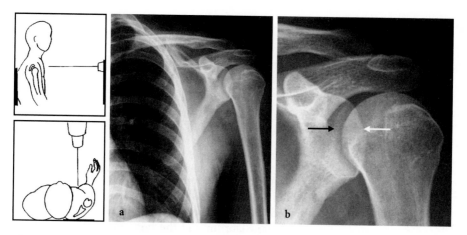

Fig. 1.1a, b. AP view of the shoulder region and examination technique with corresponding radiographs. The radiograph is obtained utilising a horizontal beam and without rotation of the trunk of the patient. **a** Since the beam is not tangential to the glenohumeral joint, the glenoid cavity appears as an ellipse that superposes to the medial aspect of the humeral head. Assessment of the glenohumeral space is suboptimal. The arm is in neutral rotation. Employment of a large cassette allows good visualisation of the scapula, proximal portion of the humerus and of the chest wall. **b** Enlargement of (**a**) shows the glenoid fossa as an elliptical structure. *White arrow,* posterior glenoid rim; *black arrow,* anterior glenoid rim

1.1.2
AP Tangential View

When obtaining an AP tangential view (Fig. 1.2) (also known as the subacromial view), the X-ray beam is directed tangential to the glenohumeral joint and to the subacromial space. The patient is standing in a 40° posterior oblique position with the shoulder to be examined in contact with the examining table. In this position the scapula lies parallel to the cassette and allows an optimal tangential view of the gleno-humeral joint. The articular surface of the glenoid cavity is seen in profile and, in normal conditions, no overlap of the glenoid cavity and humeral head is observed. Additional craniocaudal angulation (10–20°) of the beam leads to excellent visualisa-tion of the subacromial space. Since the orientation of the scapula, as well as the obliquity of the acro-mial arch, can vary in patients, fluoroscopic control can be used to achieve accurate positioning of the patient and correct tilting of the X-ray beam. Three radiographs are obtained with the arm in different rotations (neutral, internal and external). After each rotation of the humerus the obliquity of the patient, as well as the correct visualisation of the subacromial space, must be checked since changes in the rotation of the arm are frequently associated with changes in the position of the patient. The coracoid process overlies the medial aspect of the humeral head. Due to the orientation of the beam, the inferior surface of the acromion appears as a regular cortical line. The different rotations of the arm allow good evaluation of the humeral head structures. The internal rota-

tion visualises the lesser tuberosity (LT) in profile. The LT appears as a triangular structure seen in the most medial aspect of the head that projects over the glenoid cavity. Due to the larger size of the greater tuberosity (GT) the anterior two thirds of it are imaged face-on while the posterior third is seen in profile. In neutral rotation the LT is visualised „en face" while the middle portion of the GT is seen „en profile". External rotation allows profile visualisation of the LT and of the anterior portion of the GT. The biceps sulcus lies between the two tuberosities and can be examined in profile both in maximal external and internal rotation and „en face" in neutral rota-tion. Due to tangential orientation of the beam, the anterior and posterior rims of the glenoid fossa are superimposed. The glenohumeral joint space width can be accurately evaluated and reflects the thick-ness of both the humeral and glenoid cartilages. A thin curvilinear radiolucency extending from the undersurface of the acromion to the GT and located deep to the deltoid muscle can be frequently imaged in AP projection, especially if this is obtained with internal rotation of the arm (MITCHELL et al. 1988). The finding corresponds to the fat located on either side of the subacromial synovial bursa. A radiolucent area in the lateral aspect of humeral head is some-times apparent in the AP views. This finding, known as „the humeral pseudocyst", is a normal variant and must be differentiated from different diseases such as a chondroblastoma, a giant cell tumor or a metas-tasis (HELMS 1978). In an attempt to elucidate the nature of the pseudocyst, RESNICK and CONE (1983) examined a large number of macerated specimens

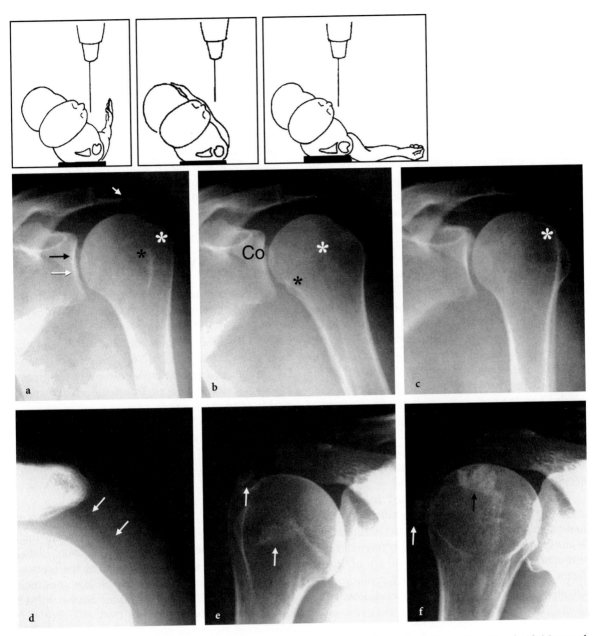

Fig. 1.2a–f. AP tangential view and examination technique with corresponding radiographs. Radiographs obtained with (a) neutral, (b) internal and (c) external rotation of the arm. The views allow optimal assessment of the glenohumeral joint and subacromial space. Note superposition of the anterior and posterior glenoid rim (*arrows*) and the sharply defined cortical line corresponding to the inferior surface of the acromion (*small arrow*). The coracoid process overly the medial aspect of the humeral head (*Co*). The different rotations of the arm lead to *en face* and *en profile* view of the greater tuberosity (GT) (*asterisk*) and lesser tuberosity (*small asterisk*). **d** Peribursal fat. A thin curvilinear radiolucency (*arrows*) extending from the undersurface of the acromion to the GT corresponds to the fat located at each side of the subacromiodeltoideal bursa. **e, f** Rotator cuff calcifications. External (**e**) and internal (**f**) rotation projections disclose calcifications inside the supraspinatus (*black arrow*) and infraspinatus (*white arrow*) tendons. With internal rotation the calcification located inside the posterior infraspinatus tendon moves laterally

and concluded that the image is due to the difference of density between the abundant spongiosa in the medial metaphysis and the more porous spongiosa in the GT region, laterally. The more abundant metaphyseal spongiosa explains why the pseudocyst is more apparent in young individuals. In the rare cases in which the image is doubtful, examination of the contralateral shoulder performed with the identical angulation of the X-ray beam and the same rotation of the arm, shows a similar finding.

1.1.3
Outlet View

This view (Fig. 1.3 is also known as the Y, mercedes-benz or scapular axial view. The patient is standing, positioned in an anterior oblique position with the anterior aspect of the examined shoulder in contact with the cassette. The arm is in neutral rotation. The beam, centred on the posterior aspect of the shoulder, has a slight craniocaudal inclination (10°) tangential to the scapula. The correct positioning of the patient and orientation of the beam can be obtained by performing the examination under fluoroscopic control. This makes it possible to tilt the X-ray beam and to rotate the patient in such a way as to reach optimal tangential view of both the subacromial space and the scapula. In severe trauma, an anterior oblique position of the horizontal patient with the beam centred on the anterior aspect of the shoulder can also be obtained, although magnification of the image, due to the increased distance between the shoulder and the cassette, is evident (DE SMET 1980b). The scapula is imaged as a Y, formed by the coracoid (anteriorly), the body of the scapula (inferiorly) and the acromion (posteriorly). In normal conditions the humeral head appears centred on the Y. The subacromial space and the scapulothoracic spaces are seen tangentially. The LT is imaged between the scapula and the chest wall. The GT is seen „en face".

The acromion is well visualised in this view. Its shape can be assessed and classified into three main types: flat, curved and hooked (BIGLIANI and MORRISON 1986). More recently, the anterior tilt of the acromion has been analyzed as an additional factor affecting anterior impingement syndrome and secondary rotator cuff tears (PRATO et al. 1998).

1.1.4
Leclercq Test

The Leclercq test was introduced in 1950 as a radiological indirect evaluation of the supraspinatus tendon (Fig. 1.4) (LECLERCQ 1950). The patient is standing in a slight posterior oblique position. First, a reference radiograph is obtained with the arm hanging against the patient's side. Then, to obtain an actively resisted abduction, the patient is asked to apply pressure to the handle of the radiographic table with the distal part of the forearm. The manoeuvre is performed at 30° of abduction. The test is considered to be positive when the distance between the

humeral head and the lower surface of the acromion decreases by more than 2 mm as compared to the reference radiograph (PRATO et al. 1991). A similar projection, with an abduction of 90° or to the maximum extent, has been described more recently in the English radiological literature (BLOOM 1991). In positive tests, the superior displacement of the humeral head can be explained by the lack of action of the supraspinatus tendon, which normally depresses the humeral head and fixes it against the glenoid to provide a fulcrum for abduction of the arm (VAN LING and MULDER 1963).

1.1.5
Bicipital Groove View

This view is obtained with the patient supine and the x-ray beam directed cranially with a medial angulation of 15–25° (Fig. 1.5). The projection allows a nearly tangential view of the anterior face of the humeral head (CONE et al. 1983). The bicipital sulcus, GT and LT are demonstrated. Erosions of the groove as well as spurs are imaged. Due to the relatively poor quality of the radiographic findings, when accurate evaluation of the bicipital groove is warranted, CT scan is nowadays the technique of choice.

1.1.6
Axillary View

The axillary projection provides a view orthogonal to that obtained with the AP view (DE SMET 1980a) (Fig. 1.6). The view can be obtained in the erect or horizontal positions, depending on the condition of the patient. Different techniques can be utilised (KREEL and PARIS 1979; NEER 1990). A curvilinear cassette can be placed under the patient's axilla and the beam can be oriented on the upper face of the shoulder. Alternatively, the beam can also be centred to the axilla and the cassette placed over the shoulder. An abduction of at least 30–40° is usually necessary to obtain diagnostic radiographs. The main utility of this view is its possibility to image the anterior and posterior aspects of the glenoid fossa and to assess glenohumeral relations. The projection can be obtained with external or internal rotation of the arm, although appreciation of different humeral head faces can be easily obtained by the AP projection performed in different rotation. The anterior part of the coracoid process as well as the acromioclavicular joint are well imaged.

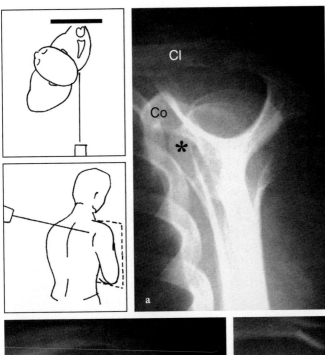

Fig. 1.3a–d. Outlet view and examination technique with corresponding radiographs. **a** The scapula is imaged in the axial plane. The beam is tangential to the scapulothoracic joint and the subacromial space allowing their optimal evaluation. The humeral head is centred on the Y formed by the coracoid, the body of the scapula and the acromion. *Acr*, acromion; *Cl*, lateral epiphysis of the clavicle; *Co*, coracoid; *asterisk*, small tuberosity. **b–d** Acromion morphology. **b** Type 1: flat acromion; **c** type 2: curved acromion; **d** type 3: hooked acromion. **e** Rotator cuff calcifications. Calcifications of the supraspinatus (*black arrow*) and infraspinatus (*white arrow*) tendons are evident

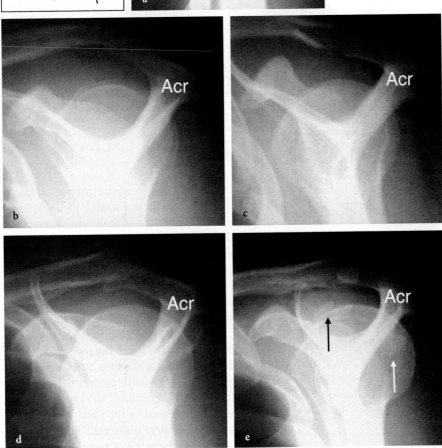

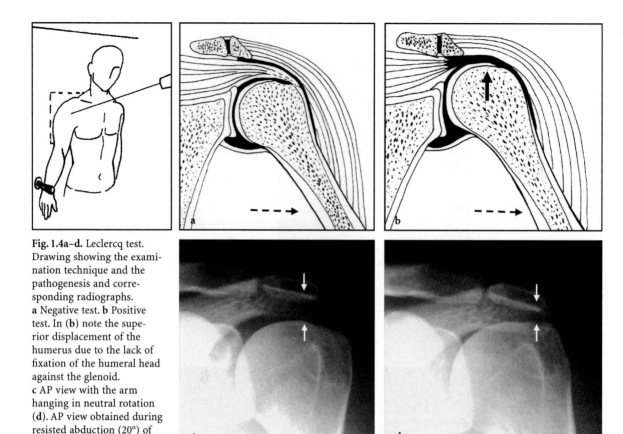

Fig. 1.4a–d. Leclercq test. Drawing showing the examination technique and the pathogenesis and corresponding radiographs.
a Negative test. **b** Positive test. In (**b**) note the superior displacement of the humerus due to the lack of fixation of the humeral head against the glenoid.
c AP view with the arm hanging in neutral rotation (**d**). AP view obtained during resisted abduction (20°) of the arm. Positive test

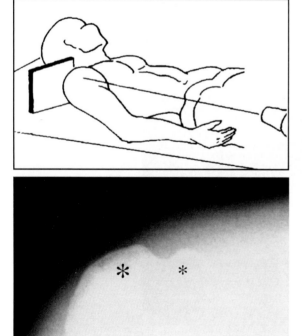

Fig. 1.5. Bicipital groove view and examination technique with corresponding radiographs. Radiograph shows the greater (*large asterisk*) and lesser (*small asterisk*) tuberosities as well as the bicipital groove

1.1.7
Apical Oblique View

In order to obtain this view, the patient is examined, either standing or horizontal, in a posterior oblique position (45°) relative to the X-ray tube (Fig. 1.7. This can be easily obtained by rotating the unexamined shoulder away from the cassette. The X-ray beam is tilted at approximately 45° of caudal angulation and centred on the glenohumeral space (GARTH et al. 1984). Although the apical oblique projection is not a true axial view like the axillary view, it is useful in estimating the relationship between the humeral head and the glenoid fossa. In normal cases the humeral head is at the same level of the glenoid fossa. Because of the cranio-caudal and anteroposterior direction of the incident beam, displacement of the head in the axial plane can be diagnosed. A posteriorly dislocated humeral head projects superior to the glenoid cavity, while in anterior dislocation it projects inferior to it (SLOTH and JUST 1989). This projection effectively images the anteroinferior aspect of the anterior glenoid rim as well as the posterocranial segment of the humeral head. Both areas are commonly injured in anterior dislocation of the shoulder.

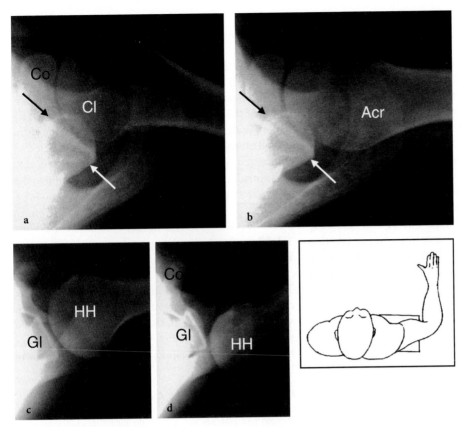

Fig. 1.6a–d. Axillary view. Drawing showing the examination technique and corresponding radiographs. **a, b** Internal (**a**) and external (**b**) rotation axillary views allow tangential demonstration of the anterior and posterior aspect of the glenoid fossa and scapular neck. Accurate assessment of the glenohumeral relations and of the acromioclavicular joint is also obtained. White arrow = posterior glenoid rim, black arrow = anterior glenoid rim. *Acr*, acromion; *Cl*, lateral epiphysis of the clavicle; *Co*, coracoid. **c, d** Axillary views in a patient with voluntary shoulder instability obtained before (**c**) and after (**d**) dislocation confirm posterior subluxation of the humeral head. *Gl*, glenoid cavity; *HH*, humeral head

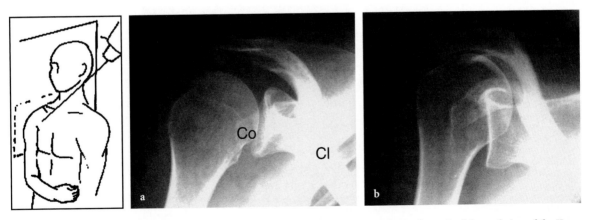

Fig. 1.7a, b. Apical oblique view and examination technique with corresponding radiographs. **a** Caudal angulation of the X-ray beam results in an elongated appearance of the humeral head. The clavicle appears shorter because of the posterior oblique position of the patients. The posterosuperior aspect of the humeral head and the inferior aspect of the anterior glenoid rim are well visualised. *Co*, coracoid process; *Cl*, clavicle. **b** In a patient with posterior dislocation of the shoulder note superior displacement of the humerus and superposition of glenoid fossa and humeral head

1.1.8
Bernageau View

The Bernageau view was introduced in 1966 to obtain an optimal visualisation of the anteroinferior segment of the glenoid rim in patients with anterior instability (BERNAGEAU et al. 1966) (Fig. 1.8). Because of the curvilinear shape of the rim, its inferior portion superimposes on the superior segment when imaged in the axillary view (that is tangential to the middle third). Since the inferior portion of the rim is more frequently damaged in anterior shoulder dislocation, the authors introduced this projection to allow its true tangential view and accurate assessment. The patient (standing or seated) is examined in anterior oblique position with the arm abducted at 135° and the hand resting on the head. The beam is directed on the posterior aspect of the shoulder. A 30° caudal tilt of the X-ray beam is utilised. Optimal angulation of the beam and rotation of the patient can be obtained under fluoroscopic guide. Bilateral examination has been suggested for evaluation of subtle changes (BERNAGEAU and PATTE 1984)

1.1.9
Stryker View

This projection, also known as the „notch" view, was reported in 1959 as a useful means for detecting humeral head fractures associated with anterior dislocation of the shoulder (HALL et al. 1959) (Fig. 1.9. The patient is supine with his/her arm flexed and the palm placed on the top of the head. The beam is directed to the coracoid process, 10° cephalad. This view is also performed in a standing patient. Furthermore, the view allows a good assessment of the AC joint.

1.1.10
West Point View

The West Point view was introduced to evaluate bone changes secondary to anterior dislocations of the shoulder (ROKOUS et al. 1972). The patient lies prone with the arm abducted at 90° and the forearm hanging over the lateral aspect of the table. The cassette

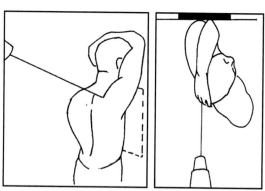

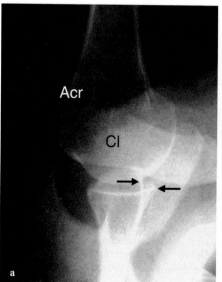

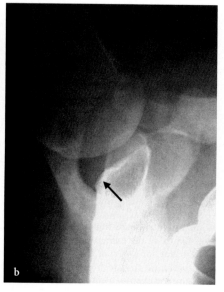

Fig. 1.8a, b. Bernageau view and examination technique with corresponding radiographs. a The inferior segment of anterior glenoid rim appears as a triangular structure (black arrows), the superior segment appears as a cortical line (white arrow). Acr, acromion; Cl, clavicle. b In a patient with posterior instability of the shoulder the Bernageau projection shows hypoplasia of the posterior rim of the glenoid (black arrow)

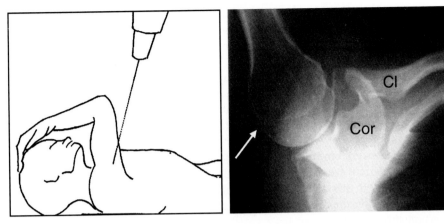

Fig. 1.9. Stryker view and examination technique with corresponding radiographs. Radiograph shows the postero-superior portion of the humeral head (*white arrow*). The coracoid including its base is well demonstrated. *Cor,* coracoid process

is positioned on the superior aspect of the shoulder, perpendicular to the table. The ray beam is directed to the axilla and is angled 25° in a cephalad direction and 25° in a lateral to medial direction.

1.1.11
AC Views

The AC joint is imaged in almost all the shoulder views but superimposition of other structures usually limits the correct interpretation of the radiological findings (Fig. 1.10). Optimal visualisation of the joint can be obtained in an AP view with a 15° cephalic tilt of the beam. Utilisation of equalisation silicone filters is useful since they avoid peripheral over-penetration and allow a better assessment of both the AC joint and the subacromial space.

Stress AP radiographs are performed by asking the patient to hold a 5 kg weight in both hands. The traction on the upper arms allows good visualisa-

tion of AC instability, particularly in patients with mild subluxation. Imaging of both joints in a single cassette provides comparison with the contralateral joint and allows demonstration of subtle findings.

1.1.12
Sternoclavicular Views

Although different views have been described to evaluate the sternoclavicular joint, all lead to poor results because of the impossibility of imaging the joint in the axial plane.

1.2
Clinical Application

A radiograph of the shoulder can be performed basically in two situations: As a part of a radiographic

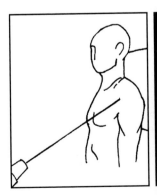
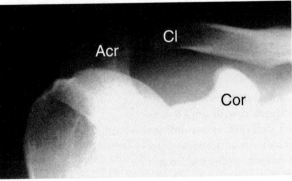

Fig. 1.10. AC view and examination technique with corresponding radiographs. Cranial oriented X-ray beam shows the acromioclavicular joint. *Acr,* acromion; *Cl,* clavicle; *Cor,* coracoid process

evaluation of an acute post-traumatic patient, to rule out the possibility of a fracture or a dislocation, or as a part of an imaging evaluation when a shoulder problem is clinically suspected.

1.2.1
Acute Post-traumatic Examination

The most common questions to be answered in the radiographic evaluation of the acute patient are two: Is there a fracture? Is there a dislocation? In this clinical setting, the smaller number of views in the most comfortable patient positions must be obtained.

If the patient cannot stand up and lies supine, the shoulder can be imaged in the anteroposterior view with a 35×43 cm cassette. The use of a wider cassette allows panoramic evaluation of the shoulder joint, proximal humerus, scapula, clavicle and upper ribs. Additional radiographic views are usually delayed in these patients after assessment of potential associated thoracic or abdominal lesions. CT can be obtained if the SR is equivocal or if there is a strong clinical suspicion of lesions that are not demonstrated by the SR. Typical indications of CT include a suspicion of posterior shoulder dislocation or dislocation of the medial head of the clavicle with possible vascular compression.

In the traumatised patient that can be examined in the upright position, two views are always required. First, an anteroposterior view, then, a second view which depends on the condition of the patient, i.e. on the possibility to achieve abduction of the humerus. If pain doesn't limit abduction over 45° a good quality axillary view can be obtained and may be the most informative projection. If abduction is limited, an apical oblique or an outlet view can be performed. Both projections can be obtained technically without asking the patient to move the arm and can evaluate the glenohumeral relationships.

1.2.2
Standard Examination

Evaluation of inflammatory and degenerative disorders can be effectively performed with an AP tangential view obtained with different arm rotations (i.e. neutral, internal, external). An outlet view must be added in the study of patients suffering from a rotator cuff pathology since this can demonstrate the presence and site of calcifications, the shape of the acromion, as well as calcifications and spurs of the coracoacromial ligament. In patients with a history of previous shoulder instability, the Bernageau projection allows optimal visualisation of the anteroinferior segment of the glenoid rim. The Hill-Sachs lesion can be well imaged in a variety of views including the apical oblique view, the AP view obtained with maximal internal rotation, the Stryker view and the West Point view (SARTORIS and RESNICK 1995).

Acknowledgements. The authors thank Miss. Mariella Ferrando RDT and Mr. Alessandro Franconeri RDT for their help in preparing the schematic drawings and the illustrations

References

Bernageau J, Faguer B, Debeyre G (1966) Etude arthropneumotomographique d'une luxation récidivante de l'épaule. Rev Rhum 33:135–137

Bernageau J, Patte D (1984) Le profil glenoidien. J Traumatol Sport 1:15–19

Bigliani LU, Morrison DS (1986) The morphology of the acromion and its relationship to rotator cuff tear. Orthop Trans 11:234–240

Bloom RA (1991) The active abduction view: a new maneuvre in the diagnosis of rotator cuff tears. Skeletal Radiol 20: 255–258

Kreel L, Paris A (1979) Humerus and shoulder girdle. In: Kreel L, Paris A (eds) Clark's positioning in radiography, 10th edn. Heinemann Medical Books

Cone RO, Danzig L, Resnick D et al (1983) The bicipital groove: radiographic, anatomic and pathologic study. AJR 141:781–788

De Smet AA (1980a) Axillary projection in radiography of the nontraumatized shoulder. AJR 134:511–514

De Smet AA (1980b) Anterior oblique projection in radiography of the traumatized shoulder. AJR 134:515–518

Garth WP, Slappey CE, Ochs CW (1984) Roentgenographic demonstration of instability of the shoulder: the apical oblique projection. J Bone J Surg Am 66:1450–1453

Hall RH, Isaac F, Booth CR (1959) Dislocations of the shoulder with special reference to accompanying small fractures. J Bone J Surg Am 41:489–494

Helms CA (1978) Pseudocysts of the humerus. AJR 11:287–288

Leclercq R (1950) Diagnostic de la rupture du sus-epineux. Rev Rhum 10:510–515

Mitchell MJ, Causey G, Berthoty DP et al (1988) Peribursal fat plane of the shoulder: anatomic study and clinical experience. Radiology 168:699–704

Neer CS II (1990) Anatomy of shoulder reconstruction. In: Neer CS II (ed) Shoulder reconstruction. Saunders, Philadelphia, pp 1–35

Prato N, Bianchi S, Schiaffini E et al (1991) The Leclercq test in diagnosis of tear in the rotator cuff. Chir Organi Mov 76:73–76

Prato N, Peloso D, Franconeri A et al (1998) The anterior tilt of the acromion: radiographic evaluation and correlation with shoulder diseases. Eur Radiol 8:1639–1646

Resnick D, Cone III RO (1983) The nature of humeral pseudo-cyst. Radiology 150:27–28

Rokous JR, Feagin JA, Abbott HG (1972) Modified axillary roentgenogram: a useful adjunct in the diagnosis of recurrent instability of the shoulder. Clin Orthop 82:84–86

Sartoris DJ, Resnick D (1995) Plain film radiography: routine and specialized techniques and projections. In: Resnick D (ed) Diagnosis of bone and joint disorders. Saunders, Philadelphia, pp1–40

Sloth C, Just SL (1989) The apical oblique radiograph in examination of acute shoulder trauma. Eur J Radiol 9:147–151

Van Ling B, Mulder JD (1963) Function of the supraspinatus muscle and its relation to the supraspinatus syndrome. J Bone Joint Surg (Br) 45:750

2 Arthrography and Bursography

B. Tins and V. N. Cassar-Pullicino

CONTENTS

2.1
Introduction

Shoulder arthrography dates back to the 1930s when air (Oberholzer 1933) and iodinated contrast medium (Lindblom and Palmer 1939) were used for the assessment of habitual shoulder joint dislocation and tendon injuries. Shoulder arthrography found broader use in the 1970s especially with the advent of double contrast arthrography. In combination with conventional tomography, the rotator cuff (Kilcoyne and Matsen 1983) and glenoid labrum could be assessed. In the 1980s, computed tomography (CT) arthrography supplemented conventional arthrography. Magnetic resonance imaging (MRI) with and without arthrography techniques and ultrasound began to be used in the 1990s for the assessment of the shoulder joint. Currently there are few indications left for conventional arthrography of the shoulder joint in isolation as this is combined with either CT or MRI (Peh and Cassar-Pullicino

B. Tins, MD
Department of Radiology, The Robert Jones and Agnes Hunt Orthopaedic Hospital, Oswestry, Shropshire, SY10 7AG, UK
V. N. Cassar-Pullicino, MD, FRCR
Department of Radiology, The Robert Jones and Agnes Hunt Orthopaedic Hospital, Oswestry, Shropshire, SY10 7AG, UK

2001). Arthrography of the acromioclavicular joint and bursography of the subdeltoid/subacromial bursa never found widespread application and are almost obsolete today, although therapeutic injections are administered to these sites by clinicians.

2.2
Shoulder Arthrography

Standard radiographic views of the shoulder should be reviewed before arthrography. Antero-posterior (AP), axial and bicipital views are recommended (Kaye and Schneider 1979; Rafii and Minkoff 1998); the AP view should be taken in internal and external rotation.

2.2.1
Joint Puncture

Although an anterior approach is commonly employed, Neviaser (1980) introduced a posterior approach, while Lindblom and Palmer (1939) originally used a superior approach through the rotator cuff using a skull unit without fluoroscopy. Currently there are two approaches for joint puncture, a posterior and the far more popular anterior approach. The anterior approach can be performed blindly, with ultrasound guidance or under fluoroscopy. Fluoroscopy allows exact needle placement and observation of contrast medium entering the joint as well as abnormal communications. Arthrography is an invasive procedure with rare but potentially severe adverse effects and the patient's consent should be obtained and documented. All procedures should be performed using aseptic technique.

For an anterior joint puncture the patient is positioned supine on a X-ray table, the fluoroscopic beam perpendicular to the table. External rotation of the arm and fixation of the hand with a sandbag aids the procedure. The puncture site is located with fluoroscopy and marked. The skin is disinfected and local anaesthesia (e.g. 1% lidocaine) can be applied. Typically a 22 G spinal needle with an obturator is used. Larger bore needles (18–20 G) with an increased length of 12 cm can be used in larger patients (FARMER and HUGHES 2002; KAYE and SCHNEIDER 1979; RAFII and MINKOFF 1998; RESNICK 1995). The needle is advanced parallel to the X-ray beam and aimed at the junction of the middle and caudal third of the glenohumeral joint, slightly more to the humeral side of the joint space (Fig. 2.1a). The needle should be advanced till increased resistance is felt. The obturator is removed and contrast medium injected. This should flow freely from the needle tip and outline the glenohumeral joint (Fig. 2.1a). If contrast medium pools around the needle tip it is positioned incorrectly. Sometimes initial high resistance to the injection is encountered; this can occur when the needle opening is pressed against and occluded by an adjacent structure. Rotation of the needle by 90° or so is often sufficient to achieve easier flow.

In the supine position the articular surfaces of the glenohumeral joint overlap at fluoroscopy. Therefore, it is important to identify the anterior (more medially located) from the posterior rim of the bony glenoid and target the needle lateral to it for joint puncture. In some institutions the patient lies in the supine oblique position, elevating the contralateral shoulder 30–40° which results in a profile appearance of the glenohumeral joint as the anterior and posterior rims of the bony glenoid are superimposed. However, in this position the glenoid labrum overlies the joint space and usually acts as an obstacle to entering the joint space. The needle is therefore targeted lateral to the joint space over and towards the humeral head. The arm is externally rotated as much as possible with a mild degree of abduction. This creates maximum exposure of the capsule to the needle puncture, increasing the humeral articular surface available. The point of entry of the needle should be in the lower half of the joint space. It is essential to avoid the tip of the coracoid process as this can overlie the

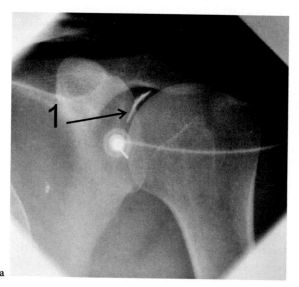

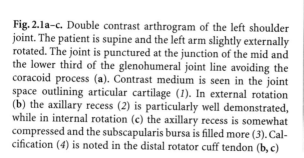

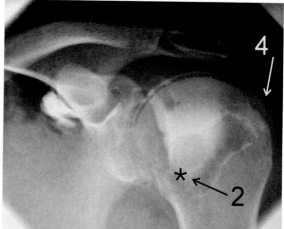

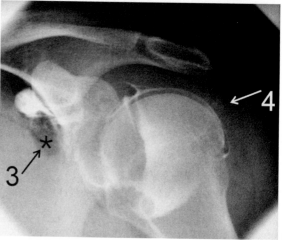

Fig. 2.1a–c. Double contrast arthrogram of the left shoulder joint. The patient is supine and the left arm slightly externally rotated. The joint is punctured at the junction of the mid and the lower third of the glenohumeral joint line avoiding the coracoid process (a). Contrast medium is seen in the joint space outlining articular cartilage (1). In external rotation (b) the axillary recess (2) is particularly well demonstrated, while in internal rotation (c) the axillary recess is somewhat compressed and the subscapularis bursa is filled more (3). Calcification (4) is noted in the distal rotator cuff tendon (b, c)

superior part of the joint space, especially in this supine oblique position.

A posterior approach has been described mainly to avoid inadvertent contamination of anterior structures with contrast medium. The patient is positioned prone oblique, the symptomatic shoulder raised rendering the glenoid parallel to the fluoroscopy beam. A 21 G needle is aimed at the inferomedial quadrant of the humerus (FARMER and HUGHES 2002).

2.2.2
Contrast Media

Arthrography of the shoulder joint can be performed utilising single and double contrast techniques.

Single contrast media are either negative (air) or positive (iodinated contrast), the latter being more common. A total of 10–15 ml of contrast medium is injected, more in lax joints. Using low osmolar preparations avoids additional influx of water into

the joint. The pre-contrast series of films consisting of AP views in internal and external rotation, axial and bicipital views are repeated after gentle exercise (Figs. 2.1, 2.2). Single contrast air arthrograms are usually part of a CT arthrogram for evaluation of loose bodies and of limited value on their own. TOTTY and MURPHY (1984) satisfactorily demonstrated the rotator cuff by air in a patient allergic to contrast media.

Several studies have shown that non-ionic media when compared with ionic media produce a lower morbidity if the examination is prolonged (HALL et al. 1985; TALLROTH and VANKKA 1985; WELLINGS et al. 1994). Double contrast studies are also associated with less morbidity than single contrast studies, while sodium containing media and use of intra-articular adrenaline to delay the dilution of hyperosmolar ionic media are associated with increased morbidity. However intra-articular adrenaline does hinder contrast medium resorption from and water influx into the joint, thus maintaining sharper tissue

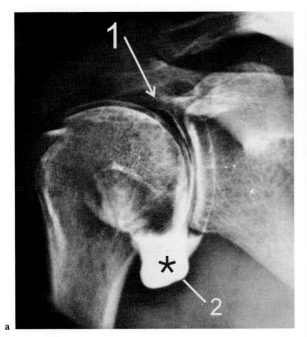

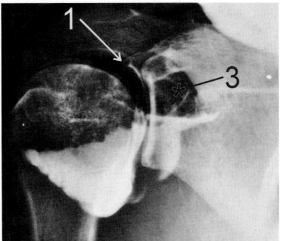

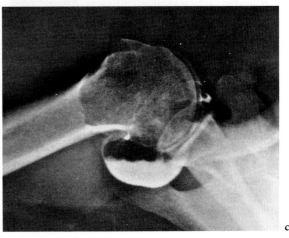

Fig. 2.2a–c. Double contrast shoulder arthrogram. Patient erect. External (**a**) and internal (**b**) rotation, axial view (**c**). Note the long head of the biceps tendon arising from the superior labrum (*1*) and the change of size and shape of the axillary recess (*2*) and subscapularis bursa (*3*) in internal and external rotation

outlines for longer (LINKOUS and GILULA 1998; WELLINGS et al. 1994).

The amount of injected contrast media has varied in previous publications. LINDBLOM and PALMER (1939) injected 6 ml of Abrodil (oil medium) mixed with Novocain, while NEVIASER (1980) used a mixture of 12 ml of single contrast medium with 4 ml of 1% lidocaine. KAYE and SCHNEIDER (1979) recommended 10–12 ml of contrast medium, while RESNICK (1981) used 10–15 ml of contrast medium with 2–3 ml of local anaesthetic. TIRMAN et al. (1981) insisted that no more than 12 ml of contrast medium should be injected intra-articularly. Both single and double contrast examinations readily depict the completely torn rotator cuff (AHOVUO 1984) by demonstrating the abnormal communication with the subacromial bursa. However, the definition of the capsule, the rotator cuff, its torn margins and its internal structure are better visualised using a double contrast technique (GOLDMAN 1979).

At double contrast arthrography of the shoulder a small amount (<4 ml) of iodinated contrast medium with 10–15 ml of air are injected into the shoulder joint. The first series of images is taken as in a single contrast technique. In the erect position the patient then exercises again, and a weight is suspended from the wrist to distract the shoulder joint. The AP internal/external rotation views are repeated. GARCIA (1984) showed that the rotator cuff defect is widened and its margins are optimally assessed using this technique. Carrying hand-held weights on the contrary elevates the humeral head and approximates the edges of the tear. MINK et al. (1985) showed that conventional double contrast shoulder arthrography in the erect position is a reliable predictor of the size and quality of the edges of the torn cuff. The double contrast technique is superior if used by experienced examiners, especially in demonstrating partial under-surface rotator cuff tears. AP and lateral tomograms in the erect position estimate optimally the size of the tear and the state of the cuff for repair assessment (KILCOYNE and MATSEN 1983).

2.2.3
Radiographic Assessment

The immediate post-arthrographic assessment described previously can be summarised as follows. A single film is taken with the needle in situ after completion of the injection. After removal of the needle, the shoulder is passively manipulated to ensure uniform distribution of the contrast medium.

With the patient supine, AP exposures with the shoulder in neutral position, external rotation with abduction, and internal rotation and adduction are obtained. These views can be repeated at double contrast arthrography with the patient in the erect position for assessment of the rotator cuff. Prone and supine axial views are indicated to assess the glenoid labrum, while bicipital groove views can also be obtained if indicated.

In normal arthrograms contrast medium is seen between the humeral head and the glenoid. An axillary and a sub-scapular recess are seen with a notch between them (Figs. 2.1, 2.2). Contrast medium can be seen around the long head of the biceps tendon and some can leak into the biceps or subscapularis muscle. There is no normal communication with the subdeltoid/subacromial bursa and contrast medium seen cranio-lateral to the greater tuberosity is abnormal indicating the presence of a full thickness tear of the rotator cuff (Figs. 2.3, 2.4, 2.5). The amount of contrast medium in the subacromial bursa has no direct correlation with the size of the complete rotator cuff tear. The more inflamed the synovium of the bursa, the lesser the amount of visible contrast medium.

2.2.4
Arthro-tomography

Single and double contrast techniques can be supplemented by conventional tomography (hypocycloidal in particular) to demonstrate the rotator cuff (see above). Meticulous patient positioning and radiographic technique are necessary and this technique has been superseded by CT and MRI with or without arthrography.

EL-KHOURY et al. (1986) utilised arthro-tomography for glenoid labral visualisation. At double contrast arthrography, the patient is placed in the decubitus position on the affected side with the scapula perpendicular to the fluoroscopy table. Fine section hypocycloidal tomography provides optimal visualisation of anterior labral margins and bony integrity (Fig. 2.6).

2.2.5
Pitfalls

Inadvertent contrast medium injection of the subdeltoid bursa instead of the shoulder joint can occur especially when the bursa is fluid-filled (Fig. 2.7). On

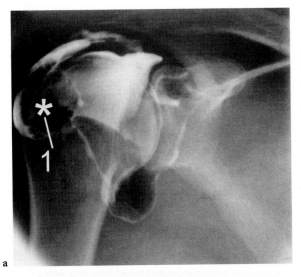
a

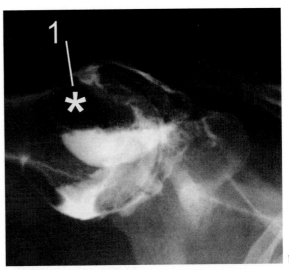
b

Fig. 2.3. Double contrast shoulder arthrogram imaged in external rotation (a) and abduction (b). A large amount of contrast medium is seen in the subacromial/subdeltoid bursa (1) indicating rotator cuff tear. Note the position of the subdeltoid bursa in the two projections. There should be no contrast medium overlying the greater tuberosity in a normal arthrogram

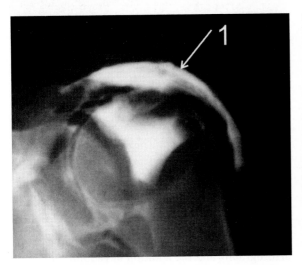

Fig. 2.4. Double contrast shoulder arthrogram. Rotator cuff tear with contrast medium in the subacromial/subdeltoid bursa (1) outlining the undersurface of the deltoid muscle. Note the extension of contrast medium lateral and distal to the greater tuberosity

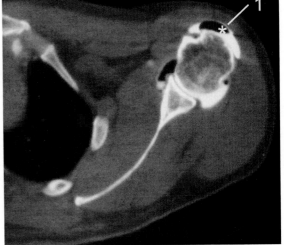

Fig. 2.5. Double contrast CT arthrogram of the left shoulder joint. Contrast medium is seen anterolateral to the greater tuberosity (1) indicating abnormal communication of the joint with the subdeltoid bursa indicating rotator cuff tear

cursory observation the findings mimic a rotator cuff tear. However, at no time is contrast medium seen in the glenohumeral joint space if the cuff is intact and this allows the proper distinction.

Inadequate needle position is easily recognised by pooling of contrast around the needle tip. If this happens during an anterior needle approach it may reduce acquisition of optimum image detail making interpretation difficult with respect to the capsulo-labral complex.

2.2.6
Complications

Allergic reactions to contrast media or local anaesthetic can rarely occur. There is a low risk of infection. Mild synovitis for up to 48 h after injection is not infrequent. In patients with bleeding disorders there is a slightly increased risk of haemorrhage. Overall significant complications are very rare (KAYE and SCHNEIDER 1979; RAFII and MINKOFF 1998).

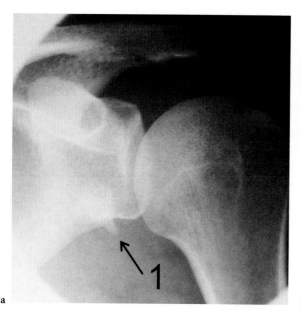

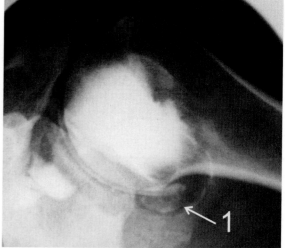

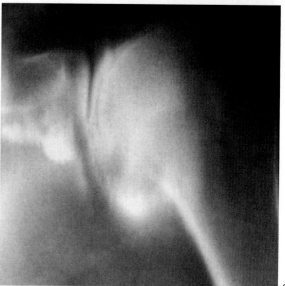

Fig. 2.6. Double contrast shoulder arthrogram after shoulder injury. On the plain radiograph (**a**) a bony fragment is noted (*1*). This becomes more apparent on the double contrast arthrogram (**b**). Tomograms for the assessment of the labral complex were performed (**c**)

2.2.7
Indications and Findings

The main indications for shoulder joint arthrography are the assessment of rotator cuff integrity, the assessment of instability of the glenohumeral joint, and diagnosis of adhesive capsulitis.

2.2.7.1
Rotator Cuff Disease

Rotator cuff disease can be diagnosed by conventional single and double contrast arthrography alone. However, an extensive review of the literature on imaging of the shoulder joint for internal derangement found limited effectiveness for conventional arthrography of the shoulder in comparison with MRI and MR

arthrography and the addition of gadolinium to any arthrography has the advantage of making it possible to perform an MR arthrogram immediately afterwards if conventional arthrography is inconclusive (HAHN OH et al. 1999). CT arthrography and ultrasound are insufficient for the complete assessment of every area of the shoulder joint. Assessment of the rotator cuff with ultrasound is operator-dependent and a recent study suggests that even in experienced hands small tears are difficult to diagnose (FERRARI et al. 2002). For the assessment of only the rotator cuff conventional arthrography may however be adequate. With an accuracy rate of over 90%, conventional arthrography compares very favourably in assessing the integrity of the rotator cuff (STILES and OTTE 1993). From a patient's point of view the discomfort of a shoulder arthrogram is less or a least

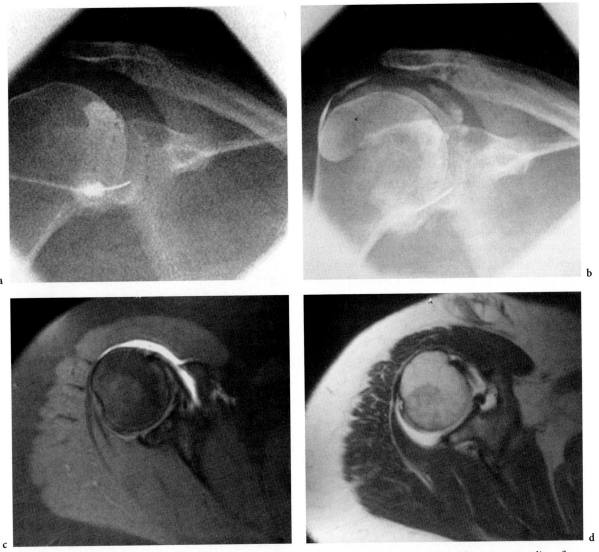

Fig. 2.7a–d. MR arthrogram to exclude rotator cuff tear and internal derangement. On arthrography contrast medium flows freely from the needle tip but does not outline the joint line (**a**). The fluoroscopic appearance is reminiscent of a rotator cuff tear with contrast medium in the subdeltoid bursa (**b**); these are features of inadvertent injection of the subcoracoid/subdeltoid bursa. On MRI no contrast medium is seen in the joint space (**c**) compared with the appearance of a successful repeat MR arthrogram a few weeks later (**d**)

no worse than the discomfort associated with an MRI examination (BINKERT et al. 2001).

Post-operative assessment of the rotator cuff after repair can show a persistent leak into the subacromial bursa in 90% of patients (CALVERT et al. 1986) most of whom are asymptomatic. In the absence of clinical symptoms communication of the joint space with the subacromial bursa is not considered to be clinically relevant.

While double contrast arthrography is potentially more informative it is also more difficult to interpret and requires considerable experience (RESNICK 1995) and cannot be combined with MR arthrogra-phy. It may however be combined with CT arthrography. For the assessment of rotator cuff disease sagittal CT arthrography with the patient's upper body erect should be performed (BELTRAN et al. 1986).

Full thickness tears of the rotator cuff are recognised by contrast medium in the subdeltoid bursa (Figs. 2.3–2.5). In incomplete tears there is imbibition of contrast medium into the rotator cuff only. Exercise of the shoulder and a repeat examination are of particular importance in these cases since a fibrinous plug in a complete tear can prevent passage of contrast medium and create a false negative examination result.

2.2.7.2
Instability of the Glenohumeral Joint

Instability of the glenohumeral joint used to be a major indication for conventional double contrast arthrography (Fig. 2.8). It has been superseded by CT arthrography and in particular MR arthrography, although ultrasound is also used (HAMMAR et al. 2001). As with all double contrast techniques accurate positioning and experience are very important for a meaningful examination. This also applies to the conventional arthrographic technique with and without tomography, as well as to CT arthrography where prone oblique positioning with the examined shoulder raised is advised (TURNER et al. 1994). Glenohumeral alignment, the labroligamentous complex, the joint capsule, bony injuries and the rotator cuff and associated tendons can be assessed.

2.2.7.3
Adhesive Capsulitis

Adhesive capsulitis requires arthrography for its diagnosis. The normal joint easily accommodates 25 ml of air/contrast medium without resistance. Resistance to intra-articular injection of lesser amounts suggests capsular fibrosis. Indeed, the only remaining absolute indication for conventional arthrography is the assessment of adhesive capsulitis. This condition is diagnosed when there is generalised marked reduction in joint space volume (≤5 ml) with partly irregular capsular outlines (Figs. 2.9, 2.10). The syringe plunger

returns in reverse when normal applied pressure is released. There is often contrast medium extravasation along the needle tract preceded by severe pain. A therapeutic trial of forceful injection of fluid to expand the joint capsule can be undertaken. The administration of a local anaesthetic reduces discomfort and corticosteroid administration has also been advised. However, this procedure has largely been abandoned in favour of arthroscopy (RAFII and MINKOFF 1998; RESNICK 1995). Features of adhesive capsulitis include a small capacity joint capsule, obliteration of the axillary recess, non-visualisation of the biceps tendon, irregular capsular outlines and non-communication with the subscapularis bursa.

2.3
Acromioclavicular Joint Arthrography

Arthrography of the acromioclavicular joint is easily achieved by direct puncture from a superior approach in a supine patient. Up to 1 ml of contrast medium can normally be injected. If normal an L-shaped joint cavity is seen with extension of the horizontal limb beneath the clavicle (RESNICK 1995).

This technique was occasionally used in the past to assess inflammatory and synovial disease of this joint. Today there is no longer a role for this technique. Communication of the acromioclavicular joint with the subacromial bursa is seen not infrequently in severe cases of rotator cuff rupture or severe inflam-

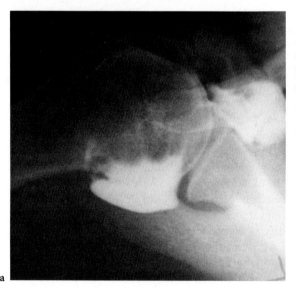
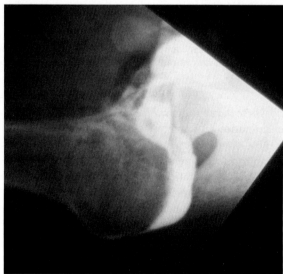

a   b

Fig. 2.8a, b. Double contrast shoulder arthrogram in a patient with recurrent shoulder dislocation. Normal alignment (**a**) and posterior dislocation (**b**) are demonstrated

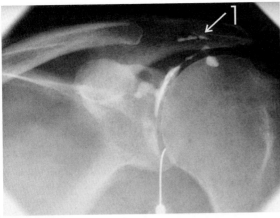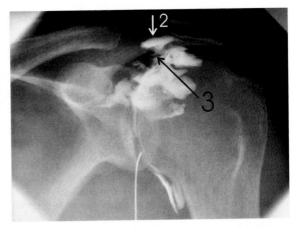

a

b

Fig. 2.9a, b. Single contrast shoulder arthrogram. The distal clavicle has been surgically removed. Contrast medium is tracking along the joint line and into the subacromial space (*1*) indicating a rotator cuff tear (**a, b**). With more contrast medium (**b**) the superior (*2*) and inferior (*3*) surface of the rotator cuff are outlined. The joint cavity has filled poorly with contrast medium and the subcoracoid bursa and the axillary recess not at all. The joint outline is irregular. These findings are diagnostic of adhesive capsulitis

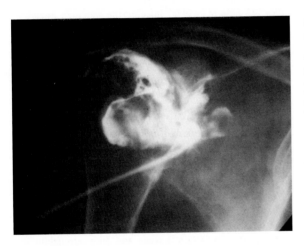

Fig. 2.10. Shoulder arthrogram. Restricted joint capacity with irregularity of the capsular outline and filling defects indicating adhesive capsulitis

matory or degenerative joint disease. MR arthrography of the shoulder joint is particularly well suited to demonstrate such abnormal communications.

2.4
Bursography

Bursography of the subacromial/subdeltoid bursa is achieved by a superior or supero-lateral approach. The patient is placed in a supine position and a 22 G needle is advanced under the anterior margin of the acromion. A „give" is felt as the needle traverses the coracoacromial ligament into the bursa. Alternatively, the needle can be advanced until bony resistance is felt from the back of the acromion. Slight pressure is exerted onto the plunger of a syringe with contrast medium. Loss of resistance indicates intrabursal position. Single or double contrast techniques can be employed and up to 10 ml contrast medium may be injected. Bursography can be combined with therapeutic/diagnostic injections of a local anaesthetic or steroid (RAFII and MINKOFF 1998; RESNICK 1995).

A normal bursogram of the subdeltoid bursa resembles a rotator cuff tear on arthrography but there is no communication with the glenohumeral joint. Contrast medium is seen on the superior surface of the rotator cuff and extending lateral and caudal to the normal outline of the glenohumeral joint capsule (Fig. 2.7a, b).

In the past bursography was used to assess the superior surface of the rotator cuff. Complete and incomplete tears of the superior surface can be demonstrated. It was also used for assessment of impingement where it enables dynamic assessment. In impingement lateral pooling of contrast medium is seen during abduction (RESNICK 1995). Adhesive bursitis can only be diagnosed with bursography but otherwise synovial disease is nowadays assessed by ultrasound or MRI. In adhesive bursitis a distension trial with forceful injection of fluid possibly coupled with a local anaesthetic or corticosteroid can be undertaken (RAFII and MINKOFF 1998; RESNICK 1995).

References

Ahovuo J (1984) Single and double contrast arthrography in lesions of the gleno-humeral joint. Eur J Radiol 4:237–240

Beltran J, Gray LA, Bools JC, Zuelzer W, Weis LD, Unverferth LJ (1986) Rotator cuff lesions of the shoulder: evaluation by direct sagittal CT arthrography. Radiology 160:161–165

Binkert CA, Zanetti M, Gerber C, Hodler J (2001) MR arthrography of the glenohumeral joint: two concentrations of gadoteridol versus ringer solution as the intraarticular contrast material. Radiology 220:219–224

Calvert PT, Packer NP, Stoker DJ, Bayley JI, Kessel L (1986) Arthrography of the shoulder after operative repair of the torn rotator cuff. J Bone Joint Surg Br 68:147–150

El Khoury GY, Kathol MH, Chandler JB, Albright JP (1986) Shoulder instability: impact of gleno-humeral arthrotomography on treatment. Radiology 160:669–673

Farmer KD, Hughes PM (2002) MR arthrography of the shoulder: fluoroscopy guided technique using a posterior approach. AJR 178:433–434

Ferrari FS, Governi S, Burresi F, Vigni F, Stefani P (2002) Supraspinatus tendon tears: comparison of US and MR arthrography with surgical correlation. Eur Radiol 12:1211–1217

Garcia JF (1984) Arthrographic visualization of rotator cuff tears. Optimal application of stress to the shoulder. Radiology 150:595

Goldman AB (1979) Double contrast shoulder arthrography. In: Freiberger RH (ed) Arthrography. Appleton-Century-Crofts, New York, pp 165–188

Hahn Oh C, Schweitzer ME, Spettel CM (1999) Internal derangements of the shoulder: decision tree and cost-effectiveness analysis of conventional arthrography, conventional MRI, and MR arthrography. Skelet Radiol 28:670–678

Hall FM, Goldberg RP, Wyshak G, Kilcoyne RF (1985) Shoulder arthrography: comparison of morbidity after use of various contrast media. Radiology 154:339–341

Hammar M, Wintzell GB, Aström KGO, Larsson S, Elvin A (2001) Role of US in the preoperative evaluation of patients with anterior shoulder instability. Radiology 219:29–34

Kaye JJ, Schneider R (1979) Positive contrast shoulder arthrography. In: Freiberger RH (ed) Arthrography. Appleton-Century-Crofts, New York, pp 137–164

Kilcoyne RF, Matsen FA (1983) Rotator cuff measurement by erect arthropneumotomography. AJR 140:314–319

Lindblom K, Palmer I (1939) Arthrography and roentgenography in ruptures of tendons of the shoulder joint. Acta Radiol 20:548–562

Linkous DM, Gilula LA (1998) Wrist arthrography today. Radiol Clin North Am 36:651–672

Mink JH, Harris E, Rappaport M (1985) Rotator cuff tears: evaluation using double-contrast shoulder arthrography. Radiology 157:621–623

Neviaser RJ (1980) Tears of the rotator cuff. Orthop Clin North Am 11:295–306

Oberholzer J (1933) Arthropneumoradiographie bei habitueller Schulterluxation. Röntgen-Praxis 5:589–590

Peh W, Cassar-Pullicino VN (2001) Magnetic resonance arthrography: current status. Clin Radiol 54:775–778

Rafii M, Minkoff J (1998) Advanced arthrography of the shoulder with CT and MR imaging. Radiol Clin North Am 36:609–633

Resnick D (1981) Shoulder arthrography. Radiol Clin North Am 19:243–253

Resnick D (1995) Diagnosis of bone and joint disorders, vol 1. Saunders, Philadelphia, pp 311–337

Stiles RG, Otte MT (1993) Imaging the shoulder. Radiology 188:603–613

Tallroth K, Vankka E (1985) Iohexol and meglumine iothalamate in shoulder arthrography. A double blind investigation. Acta Radiol 26:757–760

Tirman RM, Nelson CL, Tirman WS (1981) Arthrography of the shoulder joint: State of the art. Crit Rev Diagn Imaging 17:19–76

Totty WG, Murphy WA (1984) Pneumarthrography: re-emphasis of a neglected technique. J Can Assoc Radiolo 35:264–266

Turner PJ, O´Connor PJ, Saifuddin A, Williams J, Coral A, Butt WP (1994) Prone oblique positioning for computed tomographic arthrography of the shoulder. Br J Radiol 67:835–839

Wellings RM, Davies AM, Pynsent PB, Cassar-Pullicino VN (1994) A comparison of a conventional non-ionic contrast medium (iohexol) alone and with adrenaline and an iso-osmolar non-ionic contrast medium (iotrolan) in computed tomographic arthrography of the shoulder. Br J Radiol 67:941–944

3 CT and CT Arthrography

S. Bianchi, A. Keller, J. Fasel, J. Garcia

CONTENTS

3.1 Introduction

In recent years the advent of MR imaging has reduced the utilisation of computed tomography (CT) in the assessment of shoulder diseases. Magnetic resonance imaging (MRI) has multiplanar capability and excellent tissue contrast that are helpful in the assessment of complex anatomic areas such as the shoulder region. CT, however, still remains useful in the evaluation of a variety of shoulder disorders.

In trauma, standard radiography is the first modality to be performed, but often superimposition of different bone structures compromises ability to evaluate the anatomic details. Although specialised projections can be obtained to accurately assess fractures and dislocations, these views can be difficult to achieve in traumatised patients due to movement limitation and pain. CT can be performed on patients in almost every clinical condition and enables an accurate evaluation of fracture fragments, subluxations, dislocations and loose bodies. Moreover, coronal and sagittal reformatted images as well as three-dimensional (3D) reconstructions ease interpretation of the CT images, especially to the referring clinicians. As a general rule, shoulder arthropathies, tumours and infections are best evaluated with MRI. Possible exceptions are osteoid osteoma, in which thin-slice thickness is necessary to demonstrate the nidus, and the assessment of sequestra in osteomyelitis. With the advent of spiral equipment, shoulder CT arthrography has regained popularity as a valuable and accurate modality to investigate rotator cuff tendons, joint capsule, ligaments and glenoid labrum as well as intraarticular loose bodies. Reformatted images can be obtained in any required plane and allow accurate evaluation of size and location of tendon tears as well as dislocation of biceps tendon. The use of thin collimation thickness yields an assessment of the details of capsuloligamentous lesions secondary to shoulder instability.

The aim of this chapter is to present the technical aspects and normal findings of CT and CT arthrography of the shoulder.

3.2 CT

3.2.1 Technique

The patient is examined in the supine position with the shoulder as close to the gantry centre as possible. The upper arm is positioned closely to the body and immobilised in neutral rotation by an elastic bandage. A small pad placed below the elbow and a pillow placed beneath the knees afford a more comfortable position for the patient. To minimise artefacts the opposite arm is abducted and rests above the patient's head. Anteroposterior scanning radiograph is used to plan

S. Bianchi, MD
Department of Radiology, Hopital Cantonal Universitaire, 24 rue Micheli-du-Crest, 1211, Geneva 4, Switzerland
A. Keller, MD
Department of Radiology, Hopital Cantonal Universitaire, 24 rue Micheli-du-Crest, 1211, Geneva 4, Switzerland
J. Garcia, MD
Department of Radiology, Hopital Cantonal Universitaire, 24 rue Micheli-du-Crest, 1211, Geneva 4, Switzerland
J. Fasel, MD
Division of Anatomy, Department of Morphology, University Medical Center, Rue M. Servet 1, 1211 Geneva 4, Switzerland

the level of axial slices. In most patients a traditional acquisition is performed. Depending on the clinical history and on the goal of the examination, slice thickness can vary from 1 to 6 mm. For most patients 2–4 mm thick, contiguous sections reconstructed with bone or soft tissue algorithms are appropriate. If two-dimensional (2D) and 3D reconstructions are needed, a spiral acquisition with small thickness acquisition (1–2 mm), pitch of 1, and reconstruction thickness permitting overlapping is performed. Slices from the acromioclavicular joint to 1 cm below the glenoid are obtained. A 25-cm field of view can usually image the scapula, proximal humerus and the lateral two thirds of the clavicle and permits satisfactory image resolution. Routine comparison images of the contra-lateral shoulder are not obtained.

For the evaluation of the sternoclavicular joint the patient is supine with both arms resting at the side of the trunk. Care must be taken to correctly position the patient inside the gantry to allow symmetrical images of the joints. On an anteroposterior scout view 1 mm axial slices are centred from 1 cm cranial to 1 cm caudal to the medial epiphysis of the clavicle. A 15 cm field of view centred on the midline allows good evaluation of both joints. Coronal reconstructions are obtained to show displacements in the frontal plane.

3.2.2
Results

CT can demonstrate the normal bone anatomy of the shoulder region. Cranially the lateral portion of the clavicle and anterior portion of the scapular spine, the acromion, constitute the AC joint. CT can readily diagnose an os acromiale, that results from a non-union of the distal ossification centre of the acromion with the posterior main centre, and evaluate its size. When present the os acromiale articulates with both the clavicle and the acromion and can be implicated in the pathogenesis of anterior impingement syndrome (GRANIERI and BACARINI 1998). More caudally the spine of the scapula and the coracoid process, respectively anterior and posterior to the glenohumeral joint, are imaged. The round surface of the humeral head and the oval and slightly concave glenoid cavity form the joint surfaces of the glenohumeral joint. The humeral surface is about twice the glenoid surface. The humeral head presents two lateral projections, the anteromedial lesser tuberosity (LT) and the posterolateral greater tuberosity (GT). Humeral torsion can be measured with CT by comparing an image obtained just below the coracoid

process with an image obtained about 2.5 cm proximal to the interepicondylar line. Increased humeral torsion may predispose to recurrent glenohumeral joint dislocation (DIAS et al. 1993). Between the two tuberosities the biceps groove or sulcus is found.

The glenoid cavity is perpendicular to the body of the scapula. Glenoid retroversion can be associated with recurrent posterior glenohumeral instability. CT demonstration of retroversion can be useful in operative treatment (WIRTH et al. 1994). The posterior glenoid rim appears rounded while the anterior one is pointed and thinner. Intraarticular structures can be hardly imaged by CT. The lax and redundant fibrous capsule is reinforced by the glenohumeral ligaments which insert into the humerus and into the fibrocartilaginous glenoid labrum. The labrum, which is attached at the edge of the glenoid fossa, is thought to increase joint stability. The anatomy of muscles and tendons surrounding the shoulder are easily assessed by CT. The rotator cuff is composed of four muscles which surround the glenohumeral joint. Anteriorly the subscapularis muscle is found between the anterior face of the scapula and the chest wall. Its tendon inserts into the internal aspect of the LT. The main function of the subscapularis muscle is adduction and internal rotation of the arm. The supraspinatus muscle, the main abductor of the arm, is located in the homologous bone fossa, delimited posteriorly by the spine of the scapula and anteriorly by the upper third of the body. The muscle continues in a tendon which inserts into the anterior portion of the GT. Posteriorly, inside the infraspinatus fossa, the infraspinatus and teres minor muscles are found. Both allow external rotation of the humerus. Their tendons insert into the middle and posterior facets of the GT respectively. Muscle fatty degeneration can be assessed by CT in the preoperative evaluation of rotator cuff tears. Five degrees of fatty degeneration were described depending on the amount of adipose infiltration of the muscle (GOUTALLIER et al. 1994). A better patient outcome can be expected if surgical treatment of wide tears is made before irreversible muscular damage takes place. Although the degree of fatty degeneration was significantly related to the amount of atrophy of the respective muscles, CT degree of fatty degeneration correlate poorly with MRI findings (FUCHS et al. 1999). The long head of the biceps tendon originates from the muscle in the anterior aspect of the arm, lies inside the biceps groove and enters into the joint between the supraspinatus and subscapularis tendons (interval of the rotator cuff) to insert into the superior edge of the glenoid fossa. The deltoid muscle is separated from the rotator cuff by the subacromial subdeltoid bursa. In normal conditions only the peribursal fat can be imaged at CT while the bursa itself cannot be visualised. Full thickness tears of rotator cuff tendons allow communication between the joint and the bursa. Additional periarticular muscles imaged at CT include the short head of the biceps, which inserts into the tip of the coracoid process together with the coracobrachialis and pectoralis minor muscle, the pectoralis major and triceps muscle.

Normal shoulder axial anatomy and the corresponding CT-anatomy are shown in Fig. 3.1.

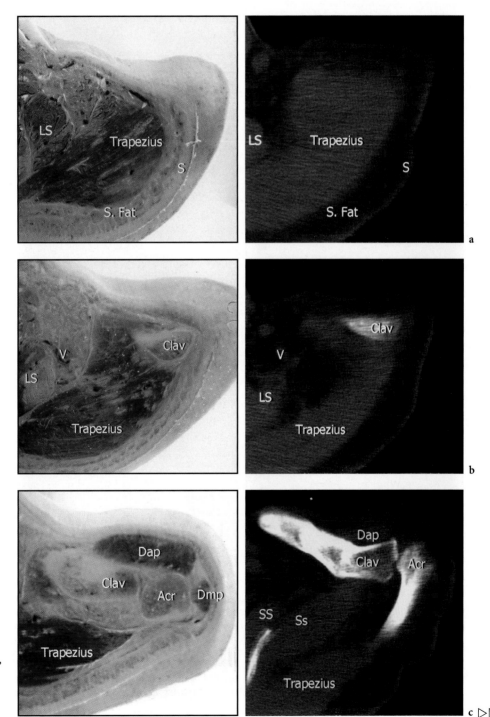

Fig. 3.1a–i. Normal shoulder anatomy revealed by axial sections of a cadaveric preparation and corresponding computed tomography anatomy. **a** *S*, skin; *S. Fat*, subcutaneous fat; *LS*, levator scapulae. **b** *Clav*, clavicle; *V*, vessels; *LS*, levator scapulae. **c** *Clav*, clavicle; *Acr*, acromion; *Dap*, deltoid anterior portion; *Dmp*, deltoid middle portion. ...

c ▷▷

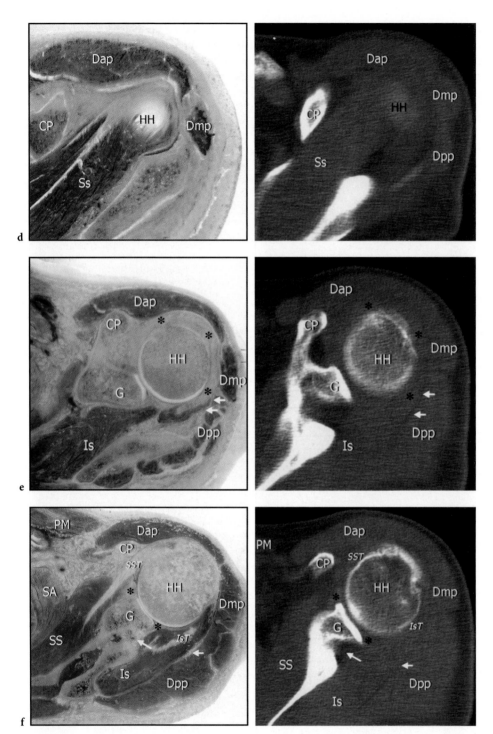

d *CP*, coracoid process; *HH*, humeral head; *Dap*, deltoid muscle anterior portion; *Dmp*, deltoid muscle middle portion; *Dpp*, deltoid muscle posterior portion; *Ss*, supraspinatus muscle. **e** *CP*, coracoid process; *HH*, humeral head; *G*, glenoid; *Dap*, deltoid muscle anterior portion; *Dmp*, deltoid muscle middle portion; *Dpp*, deltoid muscle posterior portion; *Is*, infraspinatus muscle; *asterisks*, rotator cuff tendons; *arrows*, peribursal fat. **f** *CP*, coracoid process; *HH*, humeral head; *G*, glenoid; *Dap*, deltoid muscle anterior portion; *Dmp*, deltoid muscle middle portion; *Dpp*, deltoid muscle posterior portion; *Is*, infraspinatus muscle; *IsT*, infraspinatus tendon; *SS*, subscapularis muscle, *SST*, subscapularis tendon; *asterisks*, glenoid labrum; *arrow*, peribursal fat; *long white arrow*, glenoid notch; *PM*, pectoralis major; *SA*, serratus anterior. **g** *HH*, humeral head; *G*, glenoid; *Dap*, deltoid muscle anterior portion; *Dmp*, deltoid muscle middle portion; *Dpp*, deltoid muscle posterior portion; *Is*, infraspinatus muscle; *Tm*, teres minor; *SS*, subscapularis muscle;

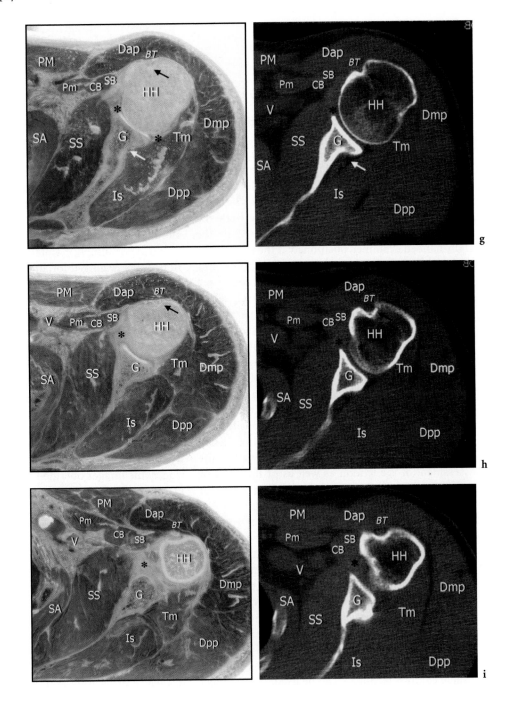

BT, long head biceps tendon; CB, coracobrachialis muscle; SB, short head biceps muscle; Pm, pectorals minor; *asterisks*, glenoid labrum; *white arrow*, glenoid notch; PM, pectoralis mayor; SA, serratus anterior; V, vessels. **h** HH, humeral head; G, glenoid; Dap, deltoid muscle anterior portion; Dmp, deltoid muscle middle portion; Dpp, deltoid muscle posterior portion; Is, infraspinatus muscle; Tm, teres minor; SS, subscapularis muscle; BT, long head biceps tendon; CB, coracobrachialis muscle; SB, short head biceps muscle; Pm, pectorals minor; *asterisks*, glenoid labrum; PM, pectoralis mayor; SA, serratus anterior; V, vessels. **i** HH, humeral head; G, glenoid; Dap, deltoid muscle anterior portion; Dmp, deltoid muscle middle portion; Dpp, deltoid muscle posterior portion; Is, infraspinatus muscle; Tm, teres minor; SS subscapularis muscle; BT, long head biceps tendon; CB, coracobrachialis muscle; SB, short head biceps; Pm, pectorals minor; *asterisks*, glenoid labrum; PM, pectoralis mayor; SA, serratus anterior; V, vessels

3.3
CT Arthrography

3.3.1
Technique

CT arthrography includes two steps: arthrography and CT.

Arthrography is usually performed in a radiological room under fluoroscopic control. The patient is asked to lie supine with the arm in slight external rotation and the elbow close to the trunk. No rotation of the patient is necessary. Usually both the right and the left shoulder can be injected by the right-handed examiner, positioned at the right of the patient. After careful skin asepsis, under fluoroscopic control, a spinal needle (7 cm - 21 gauge), connected with an extension tube to a 20-ml syringe is inserted by an anterior approach into the glenohumeral joint. The extension tube should be used to avoid exposure of the radiologist's hands during contrast injection (OBERMANN 1996) The site of the puncture is at the union between the middle and the lower third of the glenoid cavity. Usually no local anaesthesia is needed. If an accurate evaluation of the anterior structures is desired, attention must be paid to careful positioning of the needle. Inadvertent contrast injection inside the subscapularis tendon can significantly affect the assessment of the tendon as well as of the anterior capsulolabral complex. In this setting a posterior approach to joint puncture can be useful and can be performed under fluoroscopic control (patient prone) or utilising a US-guided technique (patient seated). Confirmation of the correct intraarticular positioning of the needle is obtained by injection of a small quantity of contrast. If the needle position is correct, the injected dye flows quickly away from the needle tip. If the contrast remains around the needle tip the needle is usually located inside the subscapularis tendon. Repositioning of the needle in a deeper position allows intraarticular injection. A single or double contrast technique can be used. We routinely utilise the single contrast technique since we believe that it allows better quality CT arthrography images. Serial plain films are usually obtained during slow injection of 10–15 cc of contrast. The quantity of contrast injected depends on the capacity of the joint that is easily judged at fluoroscopy. In adhesive capsulitis no more then 7 ml can be introduced inside the joint. Adrenaline (0.1–0.3 ml of a 1:1000 solution) is added only if the CT cannot be performed within 30 min. After removal of the needle gentle passive movements of the humerus are performed to obtain homogeneous intraarticular diffusion of the dye. In cases of rotator cuff tears a complete elevation of the arm over the head is suitable, since this can allow the dye to penetrate in small tears. Radiographs are then obtained in the AP view (neutral, internal and external rotation). The patient is then asked to hold the arm close to the trunk in order to avoid shoulder movements and prevent extraarticular contrast leakage.

CT examination is performed with the patient examined in the same position described for the standard CT. Care must be taken to place the glenoid surface perpendicular to the plane of CT sections to allow good evaluation of intraarticular structures. The arm is routinely maintained in a neutral rotation. In patients evaluated for anterior instability, internal rotation of the upper arm can better display tears of the anterior glenoid labrum and filling of the anterior camera. In contrast, if an evaluation of the posterior labrum is needed external rotation of the arm allows optimal imaging since the labrum may be not coated by the contrast in internal rotation. If a double contrast technique is used, a change in the patient posture (prone vs. supine) can induce displacement of the injected air and a more detailed evaluation of the posterior and anterior structures can be obtained. In subjects with a clinical suspicion of medial instability of the biceps tendon, after the standard examination, some images obtained at the level of the biceps groove in forced external rotation can show tendon subluxation or dislocation. Anteroposterior scanning radiograph is used to plan the level of axial slices. Slices from above the acromioclavicular joint to the axillary recess are obtained. A 15 cm field of view can usually image the lateral aspect of the scapula, the humeral head and the rotator cuff muscle. If a traditional acquisition is performed, 3 mm thick, contiguous sections are obtained reconstructed with a bone algorithm. If 2D and 3D reconstructions are required, a spiral acquisition with a collimation of 2 mm, reconstruction at 1 mm, pitch of 1 is performed in order to obtain the maximum amount of information. Comparison images of the contralateral shoulder are obtained if a dysplastic appearance is evident. Because of utilisation of intraarticular contrast, images must be recorded on films by utilising a wide window width (2500–3000) and a window level of 400–600.

Evaluation of the rotator cuff with direct sagittal CT arthrography has been described (BELTRAN et al. 1986). The technique was successful in diagnosing complete and incomplete rotator cuff tears although axial CT scanning was better for diagnosis of Bankart lesions. Direct coronal view of the shoulder, obtained after CT axial sections, has been proposed and was an effective way to improve arthrographic CT (BLUM et al. 1993). The utilisation of a spiral equipment which allows optimal reconstructions in any desired plane has considerably reduced the need for direct coronal and sagittal sections.

3.3.2
Results

Intraarticular injection of contrast greatly enhances the appreciation of internal structures of the glenohumeral joint.

The hyaline cartilages covering the articular surfaces of the glenoid fossa and of the humeral head are demonstrated. The glenoid labrum is imaged in cross section as a triangular structure. The base is attached to the peripheral edge of the glenoid fossa and hyaline cartilage while the apex projects laterally. Usually the anterior labrum is thinner and more pointed than the more rounded posterior labrum. For proper interpretation of CT arthrography images, however, awareness that the normal glenoid labrum presents a wide variety of shapes and sizes is essential. Moreover, considerable variations of labrum attachment can be found in normal subjects (McNIESCH AND CALLAGHAN 1987). At the superior labrum a slight, normal separation between the hyaline cartilage and the labrum (cleaved appearance) is a normal variation and must not be interpreted as a posttraumatic lesion. Occasionally the separation can be complete allowing communication between the joint cavity and the subcoracoid recess (foramen infralabrum).

The joint capsule is loose and redundant to allow wide range of movement of the joint.

The anterior glenohumeral ligaments, superior glenohumeral ligament (SGHL), middle glenohumeral ligament (MGHL) and inferior glenohumeral ligament (IGHL), are fibrous bands which strengthen the lax anterior capsule. A wide range of normal shapes of these structures can be found. The SGHL is the one most commonly identified. The MGHL inserts into the upper portion of the anterior labrum and directs laterally and caudally to reach the anterior region of the anatomic neck of the humerus. The MGHL can be absent or appears as a cordon like structure. In the Buford complex a cord-like MGHL is associated with the absence of the anterosuperior labrum. The IGHL is the ligament that is most frequently torn in anterior dislocation of the shoulder. It is composed of an anterior and a posterior portion.

Variations in the anterior capsule attachment into the neck of the scapula are found. In type 1 the capsule inserts into the glenoid labrum. In type 3 the capsule attaches more medially, into the scapular neck. Type 2 shows an intermediate insertion.

Two synovial recesses are found. The anterior subcoracoid recess and the inferior axillary recess. The subcoracoid recess communicates with the main joint cavity through an opening found between the superior and middle anterior glenohumeral ligaments (the Weitbrecht–Broca foramen) and/or between the middle and inferior ligaments (the Rouvière foramen).

Normal shoulder axial anatomy as visualised by CT arthrography is shown in Fig. 3.2.

In summary, CT arthrography is an accurate and easily performed technique to evaluate intraarticular shoulder structures. An accurate technique for joint puncture and CT examination is required. Awareness of normal variations of glenoid labrum (absence, cleaved appearance, different shape in different locations), as well as of glenohumeral ligaments (absence, Buford complex), is essential for correct interpretation of CT-arthrography images and to avoid false positive results.

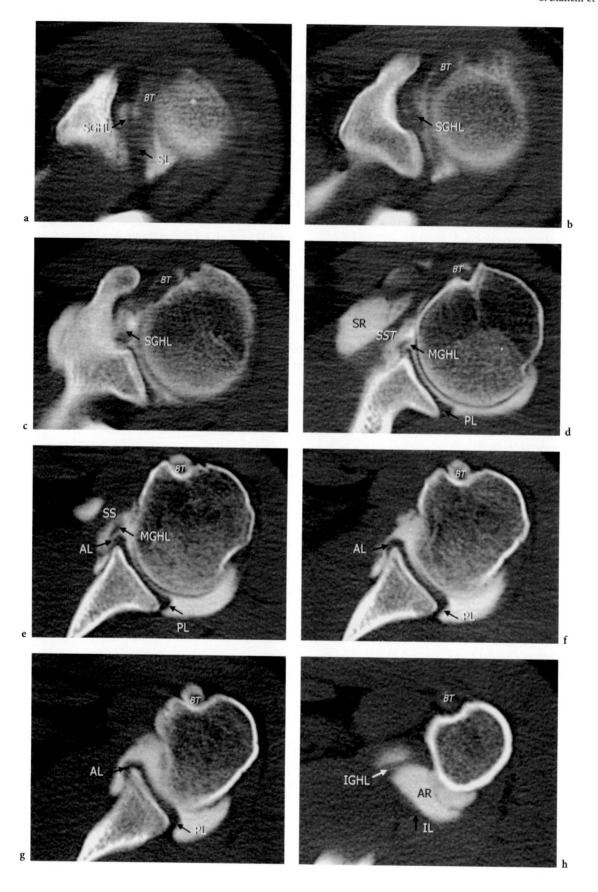

Fig. 3.2a–h. Normal shoulder CT arthrography anatomy revealed by axial images from cranial to caudal. *SL*, superior labrum; *AL*, anterior labrum; *PL*, posterior labrum; *IL*, inferior labrum; *SGHL*, superior glenohumeral ligament; *MGHL*, middle glenohumeral ligament; *IGHL*, inferior glenohumeral ligament; *BT*, long head biceps tendon; *SST*, subscapularis tendon; *SR*, subcoracoid recess; *AR*, axillary recess

References

Beltran J, Gray LA, Bools JC et al (1986) Rotator cuff lesions of the shoulder: evaluation by direct sagittal CT arthrography. Radiology 160:161–165

Blum A, Boyer B, Regent D et al (1993) Direct coronal view of the shoulder with arthrographic CT. Radiology 188: 677–681

Dias JJ, Mody BS, Finlay DB (1993) Recurrent anterior glenohumeral joint dislocation and torsion of the humerus. Injury 24:329–332

Fuchs B, Weishaupt D, Zanetti M et al (1999) Fatty degeneration of the muscles of the rotator cuff: assessment by computed tomography versus magnetic resonance imaging. J Shoulder Elbow Surg 8:599–605

Goutallier D, Postel JM, Bernageau J et al (1994) Fatty muscle degeneration in cuff ruptures. Pre- and postoperative evaluation by CT scan. Clin Orthop 304:78–83

Granieri GF, Bacarini L A (1998) A little-known cause of painful shoulder: os acromiale. Eur Radiol 8:130–133

McNiesch LM, Callaghan JJ (1987) CT arthrography of the shoulder: variations of the glenoid labrum. AJR 149:963–966

Obermann WR (1996) Optimizing joint-imaging: (CT)-arthrography Eur Radiol 6:275–283

Wirth MA, Seltzer DG, Rockwood CA Jr (1994) Recurrent posterior glenohumeral dislocation associated with increased retroversion of the glenoid. A case report. Clin Orthop 308: 98–101

4 MR and MR Arthrography

J. Hodler

CONTENTS

4.1
Introduction

Due to the increasing requirements of modern shoulder surgery MR imaging of the shoulder may be quite demanding. MR imaging should not only confirm obvious clinical or sonographic findings such as major tears of the supraspinatus, but should rather provide additional relevant information such as the detection of rotator cuff abnormalities in unusual positions, fatty degeneration of the muscles of the rotator cuff, abnormalities of the biceps tendon, and others. This chapter should allow the reader to optimally tailor imaging techniques to the indications relevant at his/her institution. The chapter deals with several topics: After a discussion of hardware requirements and patient preparation, various imaging sequences and their role in different indications are discussed. Then, the technique of direct and indirect MR arthrography, as well as their advantages and disadvantages, are described. Finally, some hints for problem solving in difficulties typically encountered during MR imaging of the shoulder are provided.

4.2
Hardware Requirements

4.2.1
Field Strength

Imaging of the shoulder is most commonly performed on mid- to high-field scanners with 0.5–1.5 T field strength. Low-field scanners have certain limitations which may be relevant in shoulder imaging. The choice of available imaging sequences may be limited in low-field scanners. The commonly used T2-weighted images, especially in combination with fat suppression, may not be available on low-field scanners. Moreover, the latter may suffer from the longer imaging times required to compensate for

J. Hodler, MD, MBA
Radiology, Orthopedic University Hospital Balgrist, Forchstrasse 340, 8008 Zurich, Switzerland

their lower signal-to-noise ratio. Longer imaging times may increase the chance of motion artifacts. Low-field scanners, on the other hand, also have certain advantages. The horizontally open designs enable placement of the shoulder in the physically optimal center of the magnetic field, thus avoiding problems relating to off-center imaging. Moreover, patients with claustrophobia may prefer an open-configuration scanner.

Few publications are available regarding the value of low- versus high-field imaging in shoulder abnormalities. Loew et al. (2000) have compared the performance of a 0.2-T and a 1.5-T magnet in patients referred for MR arthrography of the shoulder. They found that images obtained with the low-field scanner were of lower quality and suffered from more motion artifacts when compared to 1.5-T images. However, all rotator cuff tears were correctly diagnosed by both scanners. This unusually good result indicates, however, that the selected patient population had relatively easy-to-diagnose rotator cuff abnormalities. The diagnostic performance of low-field scanners may still be inferior to high field magnets in more discrete but clinically relevant abnormalities.

4.2.2
Coil Selection

Coils are crucial for imaging of the shoulder. For most MR systems dedicated shoulder coils are available either from the MR manufacturer or from a subcontractor. The coil should provide a high signal-to-noise ratio and a homogeneous magnetic field even in the typically eccentric position of the shoulder. The coil should not easily displace during patient positioning. The best available coils are probably phased-array shoulder coils. Other choices include Helmholtz-configuration coils and flexible coils which may be employed as a single coil or in pairs.

4.3
The Patient

Unless MR arthrography is performed, patient preparation is not different from other MR examinations. Preparation includes safety screening, patient information, and, in selected patients, premedication due to claustrophobia or in the case of severe pain.

4.3.1
Patient Screening

The aim of patient screening is to exclude patients from imaging who may suffer inadvertent effects while exposed to the static or variable magnetic fields. The most common contraindications are cardiac pacemakers, neurostimulators, insulin pumps, inner ear implants and other implants which may be dislocated or heated during imaging, or which may temporarily or permanently malfunction. There may be certain situations in which it is possible to image patients in the presence of a cardiac pacemaker under adequate supervision and at intermediate field strengths of 0.5 T (Sommer et al. 2001); however, this does not represent the standard procedure in everyday practice.

Another purpose of screening is detection of ferromagnetic objects introduced into the body by trauma or during surgery. Such objects may damage vital structures due to heat or mechanical forces. The eye, the brain, the myelon, and vessels represent such structures. Orthopedic implants are rarely ferromagnetic and do not usually cause such problems (Augustiny et al. 1987; Shellock and Kanal 1996). Even the occasionally encountered ferromagnetic orthopedic implants rarely cause a problem because they are firmly held in place within bone (Shellock and Kanal 1996). However, they induce susceptibility artifacts.

Another purpose of patient screening is to remove hearing aids, credit cards and other objects potentially damaged by the magnetic field. Moreover, coins, paperclips, keys and other potentially ferromagnetic objects have to be removed because they are attracted by the static magnetic field. although such objects rarely injure the patient or technician they may distort the magnetic field sufficiently to cause visible problems with image quality (Jones and Witte 2000).

4.3.2
Patient Information

Patient information is an important factor in obtaining patient cooperation and to reduce patient anxiety, which has become a relevant factor in medical care. This is confirmed by a number of publications regarding patient questionnaires which relate to this aspect (Cleary et al. 1992). Patients with claustrophobia may be identified early enough to prevent major problems once the patient is in the scanner, for instance by applying a tranquilizer or by special personal attention to the patient.

4.3.3
Patient Premedication

4.3.3.1
Pain

Pain medication may be indicated postoperatively and in the presence of other painful conditions, such as fractures, non-reduced dislocation or infection. If pain medication has not been prescribed by the referring physician, non-steroidal pain medication may be adequate for joint pain. At our institution, 500 mg of mefenamic acid (Ponstan, Parke Davis Europe) are given orally. Maximum plasma levels are reached after 1–3 h. Therefore, medication has to be given some time before the MR examination. More effective pain medication, such as tramadol hydrochloride (Tramal, Grünenthal, Aachen, Germany) may rarely be required in severe pain. It can be applied orally or intravenously. Side effects include vertigo, nausea, vomiting, depressed consciousness, orthostatic problems, tachycardia, and others.

4.3.3.2
Claustrophobia

Claustrophobia does not always require medication. Relatively simple activities may be sufficient to perform the MR examination. This includes reassuring the patient, leaving an accompanying person in the scanner room during the examination and the placing of a wet face flannel over the eyes or the forehead. Patients who believe in alternative types of medication may prefer phytotherapeutic agents such as Valverde (which is marketed in Switzerland by Novartis Consumer Health, Berne, Switzerland). For the remaining patients, the anxiolytic Xanax (Alprazolam, Roche, Basle, Switzerland) is used at our institution. A dose of 0.5 mg is given orally. If required, 7.5 mg of midazolam (Dormicum, Roche, Basle, Switzerland) may be applied orally 20–30 min before the examination. The sedative and anxiolytic effect is reached after 20 min. Midazolam is applied only for inpatients or for outpatients who are aware of the side effects of premedication and thus do not have to drive a car after the examination for 7–8 h. Intravenous injection of midazolam has been employed by many radiologists when more pronounced sedation is required quickly. A dose of 5 mg (1 ml) of midazolam may be diluted in 9 ml of saline and then injected slowly in small portions of 1–2 mg (2–4 ml) intravenously (FRUSH et al. 1996). although midazolam is considered to be a safe sedative and sleeping medication, there are several potential problems. It should not be given intravenously in patients with an addiction to drugs or alcoholism. The normal half life of 1.5–3.5 h may be prolonged in cardiac insufficiency and in renal or hepatic failure. During the effects of midazolam, intravenous access has to remain in place and resuscitation must be possible in case of respiratory depression. After intravenous application, the patients should only be dismissed under supervision and no earlier than 3 h after injection.

Recently, the application of midazolam with an intranasal spray was described by HOLLENHORST et al. (2001). These authors found that none of the 27 patients with midazolam, but 4 of 27 with placebo spray panicked and had to terminate the examination. No problems with patient safety were reported.

4.3.4
Patient Positioning

4.3.4.1
Standard Position

Patients are placed in the supine position with the arm beside the body for most indications. There is no consensus regarding arm rotation. A standardized position of the arm at least within individual institutions is important in order to obtain reproducible images. This can be relevant in structures potentially suffering from the magic angle effect or partial-volume artifacts. At our institution, an approximately neutral position of the arm is obtained by asking the patient to place his hand at the side of the body, with the thumb pointing upwards. We try to avoid both internal and external rotation because in these positions distribution of the contrast medium or joint effusion may no longer be optimal and because anatomy may be distorted. TUITE et al. (1995, 2001), however, describe an examination technique with the arm in external rotation. These authors found a small but statistically significant improvement of sensitivity for anteroinferior labral tears by using external rotation instead of the neutral arm position. KWAK et al. (1998) found an improved detection of the biceps–labrum complex in external rotation. The internal rotation may be less advantageous. DAVIS et al. (1991) found that due to overlap between the supraspinatus and infraspinatus tendon, morphology may become difficult to assess and false diagnoses may result in internal rotation.

4.3.4.2
The ABER Position

The ABER (abduction and external rotation) position has been advocated by several authors (TIRMANN et al. 1994; CVITANIC et al. 1997; KWAK et al. 1998). The ABER position is obtained in the supine position with the patient placing his hand underneath his head, resulting in external rotation and abduction of the humerus. The sections are axial oblique and are planned on a oblique coronal sequence parallel to the axis of the proximal humerus (TIRMANN et al. 1994). In this position, tears of the anteroinferior labrum become more conspicuous because the labrum is pulled from the glenoid by the capsule and glenohumeral ligaments. CVITANIC et al. (1997) found a sensitivity of 89% and a specificity of 95% which compared favorable to standard MR arthrograms (48% and 91%, respectively).

The ABER position may also be useful for the detection of rotator cuff abnormalities (TIRMAN et al. 1994). In a small series of patients, the sensitivity for tears of the undersurface of the rotator cuff and/or of the infraspinatus tendon was improved when the ABER position was employed. However, this sequence requires additional examination time because the patient has to be repositioned and additional localizer sequences have to be obtained in order to obtain ABER images. CVITANIC et al. (1997) describe additional scan times of 10 min only. However, the institutions involved in this investigation were experienced in performing such MR examinations. The ABER position is not comfortable for many patients, including those with shoulder impingement syndrome and anterior instability. The investigation of CVITANIC et al. (1997) had a dropout rate of 20%, or 52 of the included 260 shoulders. The patients were either unwilling, unable, or both, to cooperate in the acquisition of ABER images.

4.3.4.3
ABER Variant

WINTZELL et al. (1999) have described an alternative position similar to that used for clinical apprehension tests. The arm is in 90° of abduction and at maximum tolerable extension. A 0.2 T open-configuration MR scanner was used. Apparently, this position better demonstrates capsulolabral lesions when compared to the classical ABER position (WINTZELL et al. 1998).

4.3.4.4
Traction

Another specialized position has been described by Chan et al. (1999). They have used arm traction by pulling the wrist with 3 kg weights. The authors found that the diagnosis of a SLAP lesion was improved when arm traction and external rotation were combined.

4.3.4.5
Kinematic Imaging

Axial images obtained in various degrees of internal and external rotation have been advocated in order to better depict the labrum and capsule (BONUTTI et al. 1993; SANS et al. 1996; CARDINAL et al. 1996; RHOAD et al. 1998). Some papers regarding imaging in different arm positions refer to CT arthrography (PENNES et al. 1989), but may also be relevant for MR imaging or MR arthrography. PENNES et al. (1989) found a modest (9%) increase in correct diagnoses for anterior and posterior labral lesions when external rotation CT arthrograms were obtained in addition to internally rotated images.

Examinations in internal and external rotation have also been advocated for assessment of subcoracoid impingement. In this type of impingement, soft tissue structures, including the subscapularis tendon, are compressed between the lesser tuberosity and the coracoid. The normal distance between these two structures is 11 mm (mean), with a reduction to 5.5 mm in symptomatic patients (FRIEDMAN et al. 1998).

Beside passive motion studies, MR imaging has also been advocated in combination with physical examinations in instability problems which require an open-design magnet (BEAULIEU et al. 1999).

4.3.4.6
Advanced Image Analysis

Advanced image analysis has occasionally been employed, such as 3D reformations in different body positions, which should allow for a more precise understanding of biomechanically relevant relationships (GRAICHEN et al. 1998).

4.4
Imaging Parameters

The imaging parameters used at the author's institution are presented in Table 4.1 and Figs. 4.1 and 4.2.

4.4.1
General Considerations

Sequence planning depends on the strengths and weaknesses of the available equipment. Fat suppression is an example of a desirable sequence which may not be consistently available on older scanners or on low-field magnets. Heavily T2-weighted or combinations of small slice thickness and field-of-view may be limited due to field strength, gradient strength, slew rates, and other parameters.

The indication for MR imaging in a specific patient, as well as the consequences drawn from the results of imaging are another important aspect in determining imaging parameters. If MR imaging only has to confirm the clinical diagnosis of a full-thickness rotator cuff tear, a simple protocol consisting of a T2-weighted angled coronal spin-echo sequence is adequate. When subtle abnormalities have to be diagnosed or excluded for surgical decision making, such as tendinopathy, partial tears, or unusually located lesions, several imaging planes with different types of sequences, small pixel size and slice thickness, and possibly indirect or direct MR arthrographic sequences have to be considered.

In instability, modern shoulder surgery attempts to restore the abnormal anatomical factors (WARNER 1997). Such anatomical factors should be addressed during MR imaging of the shoulder. They include the capsule, the glenohumeral ligaments, the labrum, the rotator cuff and the biceps tendon. Joint congruity is another relevant aspect. It is determined by the relative sizes and the rotation of the humeral head and glenoid, by the presence of Hill-Sachs and reversed Hill-Sachs lesions associated with anterior and posterior instability, and by the presence of glenoid rim deficiency or fracture (bony Bankart lesion). Therefore, a protocol limited to the axial plane is not sufficient in imaging of instability. The fat-suppressed T1-weighted spin-echo images used in MR arthrography and the gradient-echo images sometimes used for imaging of the labrum may not sufficiently demonstrate small but biomechanically relevant fractures of the glenoid rim. Standard T1-weighted images and — in acute trauma — STIR or frequency-selective fat-suppressed T2-weighted images may assist in this diagnosis.

Most current MR protocols do not specifically take into account another aspect of MR imaging of the shoulder: Osteoarthritis of the glenohumeral joint may be a relevant cause of the patient's symptoms (ELLMAN et al. 1992), which persists after repair of the rotator cuff or other therapy. This diagnosis is probably underreported in the MR literature (HODLER et al. 1995). Little is known, however, about sequences optimized for cartilage imaging. At least theoretically, the sequences used in other joints such as the knee may be employed, such as fat-suppressed gradient-echo techniques or MR arthrography.

Imaging sequences should take into account possible extraarticular findings, such as soft tissue infection or neoplasm. For this reason, the imaging protocol should include T2-weighted images (with or without fat suppression) in at least one imaging plane. Even in MR arthrography with T1-shortening intraarticular contrast the protocol should not be limited to T1-weighted (standard or fat-suppressed) images.

Another important aspect in imaging of extraarticular structures are the muscles of the rotator cuff. The degree of fatty degeneration of the rotator cuff found in rotator cuff tears (GOUTALLIER et al. 1994) influences surgical results. Severe fatty degeneration results in less successful surgery, including reduced function and more severe pain in comparison to patients without such degeneration (GOUTALLIER et al. 1994). The degree of fatty degeneration was originally described on CT images (GOUTALLIER et al. 1989, 1994). Fat can easily be detected on axial or parasagittal standard T1-weighted MR images which should cover part of the supraspinatus fossa (FUCHS et al. 1999).

4.4.1.1
The Value of Standardized Imaging Protocols

Standardized imaging protocols have several advantages over individually tailored imaging techniques: Consistent image quality helps both the radiologist and the clinicians to differentiate subtle findings, avoids time delays caused by the technician waiting for the radiologist and is a prerequisite for quality control and scientific assessment.

4.4.2
Imaging Planes

There are three main imaging planes which are applied in most MR examinations of the glenohumeral joint: the angled coronal, the angled sagittal, and the axial plane. Angled coronal images are

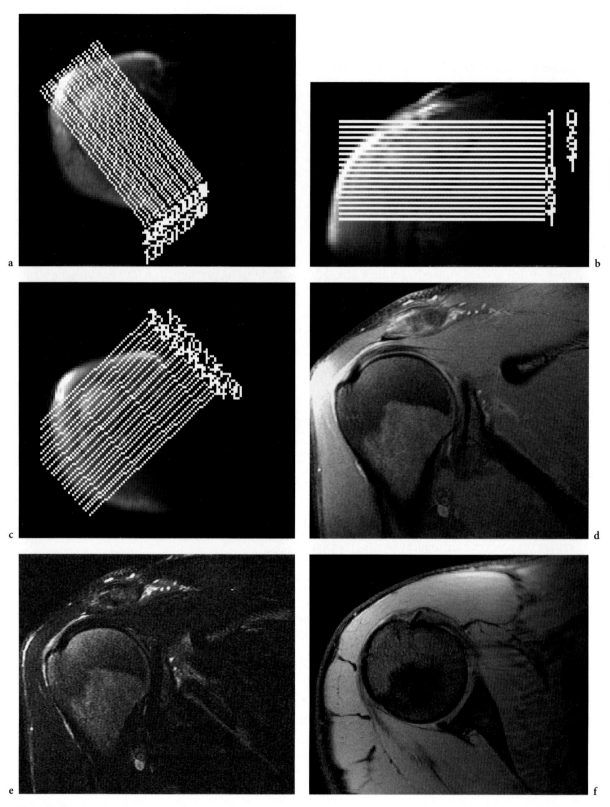

Fig. 4.1a–f

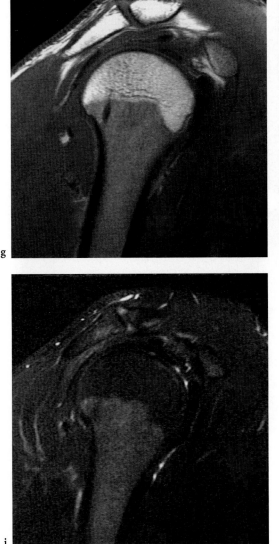
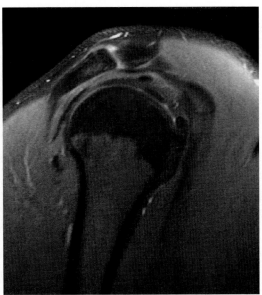

g

h

i

Fig. 4.1a–i. MR sequences as employed at the author's institution. Image parameters are presented in Table 4.1. The second echo of the fat-suppressed long TR sequence is not included in many other imaging protocols. a–c Localizer sequences. d, e Angled coronal fat-suppressed proton-density and T2-weighted sequences. f Axial fat-suppressed proton-density sequence. g–i Angled sagittal T1-weighted and fat-suppressed proton-density and T2-weighted sequences

Table 4.1. Suggested imaging protocol for 1.5-T scanner with phased-array shoulder coil

	Angled coronal			Axial			Angled sagittal		
	Sequence	TR/TE (TI)	FOV, matrix slice thickness, NEX	Sequence	TR/TE	FOV, matrix slice thickness	Sequence	TR/TE	FOV, matrix slice thickness, NEX
Standard MR	PD/T2 TSE FS	3300/14/95	10×16 cm, 256×512 4 mm, 2	PD TSE FS	3300/14	10×16 cm, 256×512 4 mm, 2	T1w SE	621/12	10×16 cm, 256×512 4 mm, 1
							PD/T2 TSE FS	3300/14/95	10×16 cm, 256×512 4 mm, 2
MR arthrography	T1w SE FS	777/12	10×16 cm 256×512 3 mm, 1	T1w SE	600/12	10×16 cm, 256×512 3 mm, 1	T1w SE	621/12	10×16 cm, 256×512 4 mm, 1
	PD/T2 TSE FS	3300/14/95	10×16 cm 256×512 4 mm, 2						

TR, repetition time; TE, echo time; FOV, field of view; SE, spin-echo; TSE, turbo spin-echo; FS, fat suppression; T1w, T1-weighted; T2w, T2-weighted; PD, proton-density; TI, Inversion time

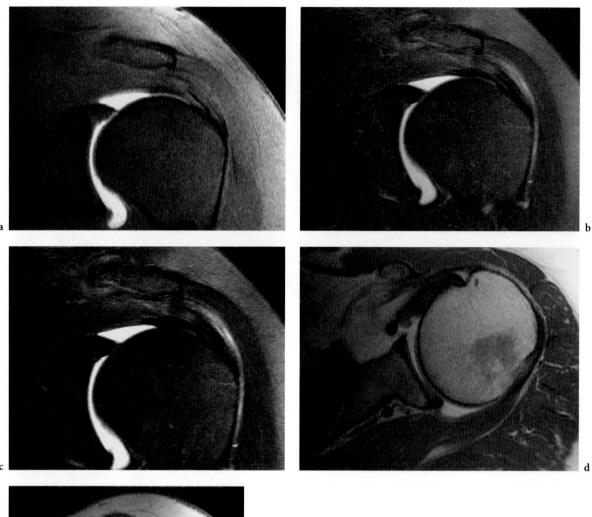

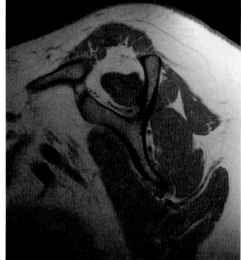

Fig. 4.2a–e. MR arthrographic sequences as employed at the author's institution. Image parameters are presented in Table 4.1. **a–c** Angled coronal T1-weighted and fat-suppressed proton-density and T2-weighted sequences. In the presence of T1-shortening intraarticular contrast the long TR sequences (**b, c**) are not optimal for the assessment of intraarticular structures, but rather for bone and extraarticular soft tissue abnormalities. **d** Axial T1-weighted sequence. Fat suppression would increase lesion conspicuity for intraarticular abnormalities, but may obscure extraarticular abnormalities such as fractures of the glenoid rim. **e** Angled sagittal T1-weighted sequence. Far medial position, demonstrating supraspinatus atrophy

planned on axial localizers parallel to the supraspinatus muscle or perpendicular to the glenoid surface. Slice thickness is 3–4 mm in most published protocols, field-of-view typically between 12 and 16 cm, with an image matrix of 256. Coronal oblique images are most useful for determining abnormalities of the supraspinatus, the superior labrum, the acromioclavicular joint, and the deltoid muscle.

Angled sagittal images are planned perpendicular to the supraspinatus muscle or parallel to the glenoid surface. They should include the entire humeral head and the tuberosities, where the rotator cuff tendons insert. Medially, the sections should cover part of the rotator cuff muscles, at least when the referring physician is interested in the degree of fatty degeneration. In order to provide such coverage, slice thickness may have to be increased to 5 mm which may reduce the diagnostic value of such a sequence in assessing the rotator cuff and the biceps tendon. Other imaging parameters are similar to those used for angled coronal images.

Axial images are best planned on coronal localizers. Typically, slice thickness is 3–4 mm. Slices may be thinner if three-dimensional (3D) gradient-echo sequences are obtained. If the slices should include both the acromioclavicular joint and the axillary recess, slice thickness may have to be increased to 4 mm. Other imaging parameters are similar to those of the angled coronal and axial images.

An additional imaging plane has been introduced by TUITE et al. (2001), who have employed "angled oblique sagittal MR imaging." This sequence is planned on an angled coronal MR image. The sagittal images are then tilted laterally, in order to be perpendicular to the distal supraspinatus tendon. When such images are used in combination with small slice thickness (3 mm instead of 4 mm), the diagnostic performance in rotator cuff abnormalities may be improved compared to standard sequences. In the investigation by TUITE et al. (2001), the involved staff radiologist improved his accuracy to differentiate torn from non-torn rotator cuff abnormalities from 0.76 to 0.88. Similar differences were not found for the fellow included in the investigation, however. The same type of images may also be useful for the assessment of intraarticular biceps tendon abnormalities.

Angled axial images obtained in the ABER position are another additional sequence which have been described previously (see Sect. 4.3.4.2).

4.4.3
Sequence Types

4.4.3.1
Rotator Cuff Lesions

4.4.3.1.1
Spin-Echo Sequences

A combination of angled coronal T1-weighted and T2-weighted spin-echo images is commonly used for assessment of the supraspinatus tendon. T1-weighted images provide anatomical details and information about early degeneration of the supraspinatus tendon. T2-weighted images are superior in detecting partial or full-thickness defects of the rotator cuff. Proton-density images can replace the T1-weighted images in imaging of the rotator cuff. Their sensitivity is inferior, however, to T1-weighted images in bone marrow abnormalities. In the past, dual echo images have commonly been acquired. The repetition time (TR) for standard spin echo sequences was typically close to 2000 ms, the echo times (TE) 20 and 80 ms. There is a tendency to replace such classical sequences by long TR/intermediate TE (40–50 ms) sequences without dual echo.

4.4.3.1.2
Turbo/Fast Spin-Echo Sequences

Turbo or fast spin-echo images have a diagnostic performance which is similar to standard MR images, as demonstrated by SONIN et al. (1996). These authors have used a repetition time of 2000 ms and an echo time of TE of 25 and 75 ms for the standard MR images. The corresponding values for the fast spin-echo images were 3500–5000 ms and 22/90 ms. Imaging times were nearly identical for both types of sequences. They were slightly longer than 6 min. Signal-to-noise ratio was superior for the turbo spin-echo sequence. However, the authors found that there was 100% diagnostic correlation between the two types of sequences regarding full-thickness tears of the rotator cuff. There were no statistically significant differences between the sequences regarding fluid conspicuity, coracoacromial morphology, and bone marrow signal.

4.4.3.1.3
Gradient-Echo Sequences

Gradient-echo images are not commonly used for assessment of the rotator cuff. In a paper published by SAHIN-AKYAR et al. (1998) fat-suppressed fast spin-echo images were compared to gradient-echo images in suspected rotator cuff tears. Imaging parameters were 3633–5300 ms and 40–80 ms (TR/TE) on a GE Signa unit and 1750–1863/50 ms on a Philips Gyroscan unit for the spin-echo images. The corresponding values for the gradient-echo images were 750–850/20/30° (repetition time/echo time/flip angle) and 800/20/30°, respectively. There was relevant diagnostic variability between the four readers but not between the sequences. The gradient-echo images had similar sensitivity (58%–100% versus 71%–96%) for detection of any type of tears. The authors concluded that both sequences could be used instead of classical dual echo spin-echo images because performance was reasonable and imaging times were shorter. Previously, PARSA et al. (1997) had compared T2*-weighted gradient-echo and conventional dual-echo sequences. For differentiation of intact from torn rotator cuffs, the sensitivity was lower for the T2*-weighted images than for the conventional dual-echo T2-weighted images. The specificity decreased for one of the observers for the T2*-weighted images. For differentiation of a partial rotator cuff tear on one hand, intact or full-thickness tears on the other hand, both sensitivity and specificity were lower for the T2*-weighted than the conventional dual-echo T2-weighted images. Image characteristics of gradient-echo images depend on the specific parameters chosen, however, and not all radiologists may make the same experience as these authors (Fig. 4.3).

4.4.3.1.4
Fat Suppressed Sequences

Fat suppression was recognized relatively early on as a means to increase lesion conspicuity and possibly sensitivity, specificity, and accuracy. PALMER et al. (1993) found that by using fat suppression in MR arthrography performed with gadopentetate sensitivity for rotator cuff tears increased from 90%–100%, and specificity from 75%–100%. In an investigation by REINUS et al. (1995) comparing non-enhanced, T2-weighted sequences contrast fat-suppression also proved to be valuable. For the two involved readers sensitivities and specificities in detecting full-thickness rotator cuff tears were 80%/80% and 87%/92%, respectively, for the standard images. The corresponding values for the fat suppressed images were 100%/100% and 77%/87%, respectively. These results indicated that suppression increases lesion conspicuity, but may influence specificity rather negatively.

4.4.3.2
Instability

4.4.3.2.1
Standard MR Imaging

For instability imaging, the axial plane is most important. If non-enhanced MR images are obtained, T2-weighted, proton-density or dual-echo spin-echo images, gradient-echo images (LEGAN et al. 1991; TUITE et al. 1995) or a combination of these two types of sequences (GUSMER et al. 1996) have been recommended. Sensitivities and specificities

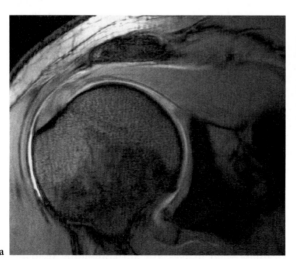 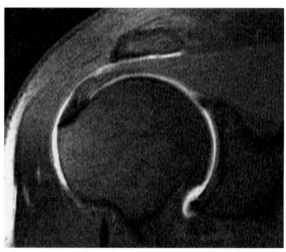

a   b

Fig. 4.3a, b. Gradient-echo sequence. **a** Angled coronal 2D FLASH sequence (TR 600 ms, TE: 12 ms, flip angle 60°). Possible overestimation of supraspinatus tendon signal in comparison to T1-weighted fat-suppressed image (**b**)

reported by GUSMER et al. (1996) were between 74% and 100% for sensitivity, and between 95% and 100%, respectively. LEGAN et al. (1991) found similarly good results for standard MR images. Not all radiologists may agree with these authors, however. Differences in the assessment of labral lesions may relate to patient selection. If sufficient fluid is present, such as immediately after trauma, standard MR performs better than in chronic disease with little or no joint fluid.

Moreover, MR imaging should not be limited to the labrum. Other factors, such as the inferior glenohumeral ligament may be more relevant. For such diagnosis and for the detailed analysis of the labrum (CHANDNANI et al. 1993), MR arthrography may be required.

4.5
MR Arthrography

The role of MR arthrography has been controversial for some time. However, standard MR imaging may not be sufficiently reliable in the assessment of the labrum, the joint capsule and possibly for other structures of the glenohumeral joint. There are two different ways to obtain MR arthrographic images. The first option is to perform indirect MR arthrography by injecting gadolinium-containing contrast media intravenously. The second one is direct MR arthrography which requires intraarticular injection of contrast.

4.5.1
Indirect MR Arthrography

In the shoulder, indirect MR arthrography is probably not as commonly employed as direct MR arthrography (PEH and CASSAR-PULLICINO 1999). It is still worthwhile to consider this alternative MR arthrographic method which has the advantage of avoiding joint injections.

4.5.1.1
Principles

The commonly used gadolinium-containing complexes (0.1 mmol/kg) (WINALSKI et al. 1993; SUH et al. 1996; VAHLENSIECK et al. 1998) appear within the joint space in a concentration sufficient for MR arthrographic effects (VAHLENSIECK et al. 1996, 1998; YAGCI et al. 2001). Intraarticular contrast concentrations may reach 72–170 µmol/l (DRAPÉ et al. 1993). This is less than commonly used concentrations in direct arthrography such as 2 mmol/l or 4 mmol/l but still appear to be adequate for imaging. Contrast concentration may be sufficient after 10 min but may increase up to 45 min after injection (Fig. 4.4).

The pharmacokinetics of contrast enhancement of joint fluid are not completely understood. The signal intensity of vessels and intraarticular space behave in a parallel fashion after intravenous injection (VAHLENSIECK et al. 1998). The contrast media probably pass into joint fluid by diffusion. This is possible because the synovial lining has no basal membrane (VAHLENSIECK et al. 1997). Diffusion alone does not sufficiently explain intraarticular

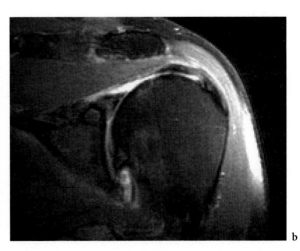

a   b

Fig. 4.4a, b. Indirect MR arthrography. **a** axial T1-weighted image. **b** Angled coronal fat-suppressed proton-density image. In the presence of joint effusion associated with osteoarthritis, intravenous injection of gadopentetate leads to adequate MR arthrographic effect after 15 min

enhancement, however. VAHLENSIECK et al. (1997) have postulated that mechanical factors may be important because arm motion increases intraarticular contrast enhancement.

The importance of arm motion for routine examinations, however, has been debated. ALLMANN et al. (1999) have found diagnostically efficient enhancement of joint fluid (120% 4 min and 145% 8 min after intravenous injection of gadodiamide) without exercising.

Unfortunately, the gadolinium-containing contrast media do not only appear in synovial fluid, but accumulate also in the vascularized connective tissue normally present at the labral base and within granulation tissue found in many abnormalities such as rotator cuff lesions. This can lead to diagnostic difficulties.

4.5.1.2
Advantages of Indirect MR Arthrography

Indirect MR arthrography does not suffer from the side effects potentially associated with direct arthrography such as postarthrographic pain (HALL et al. 1981). Indirect MR arthrography appears to be superior to standard MR imaging: YAGCI et al. (2001) found that agreement between conventional MR imaging and surgery was only moderate (kappa: 0.38–0.57) in detecting rotator cuff tears. It was excellent, however, for indirect MR arthrography (kappa: 0.87–0.94). ALLMANN et al. (1999) found that rotator cuff tears were significantly better delineated by enhanced fat-suppressed T1-weighted gradient-echo sequences when compared to standard MR images.

4.5.1.3
Disadvantages of Indirect MR Arthrography

The diagnostic performance of indirect MR arthrography may suffer when there is not a sufficient amount of joint fluid within the joint space. Another problem is the enhancement of normal and abnormal vascularized structures as described above. Such enhancement may be present at the labral base and may be difficult to differentiate from joint fluid entering a defect associated with labral detachment.

Another disadvantage is the cost of gadolinium-containing contrast media.

Scheduling may be more complicated than for standard MR examinations because the patient has to been seen for an injection some time before the MR examination.

4.5.1.3.1
Side Effects of Indirect MR Arthrography

Clinically diagnosed side effects of intravenously injected gadolinium-containing contrast media appear to be rare. In a database of 21,000 patients, 36 adverse reactions were reported (MURPHY et al. 1996). A total of 15 patients had mild non-allergic reactions such as nausea or vomiting, 12 had mild reactions resembling allergy (hives, diffuse erythema, skin irritation), seven had moderate reactions (respiratory symptoms) and two had life threatening reactions with respiratory distress. A fatal reaction was reported by JORDAN and MINTZ (1995). Known hypersensitivity to gadolinium-containing contrast media is a contraindication for intravenous injections. Indications should be limited in children, patients with known allergic tendencies, severe renal insufficiency, and pregnancy. Theoretically, intraarticular gadolinium could damage cartilage or the synovial membrane. No such effects have been proved to date, however. Additional information about this aspect is provided in the section about direct MR arthrography.

4.6
Non-arthrographic Indications for Intravenous Injections of Contrast Media

Intravenous contrast injections may not only be used for indirect MR arthrography but are also indicated in infection, synovitis associated with systemic inflammatory disease, and neoplasm. Enhanced MR images may differentiate between vascularized inflammatory or neoplastic tissue from necrotic tissue, abscess fluid, or bleeding. Spin-echo sequences may be combined with fat-suppression for this purpose.

4.7
Direct MR Arthrography

4.7.1
Patient Preparation

In addition to the standard information and screening procedures performed for non-enhanced MR examinations, written information should be provided to the patients regarding the specific procedures associated with MR arthrography. This information should include potential side effects, as described below.

4.7.2
Imaging Guidance of Intraarticular Injections

Most radiologists employ imaging guidance for joint injections and do not perform them blindly. Fluoroscopy is the most commonly employed guiding method, although ultrasonography or even CT and MR imaging may be considered as an alternative.

4.7.2.1
Fluoroscopy

The injection of intraarticular contrast required for MR arthrography has most commonly been performed under fluoroscopic guidance (BELTRAN et al. 1997; SHANKMAN et al. 1999) (Fig. 4.5). Fluoroscopy is a fast, easily available guiding method. Sterile handling of needles is much easier on a fluoroscopy unit when compared to CT or even MR. Moreover, many radiologists are well trained to perform the injection with fluoroscopy. Disadvantages of fluoroscopy include radiation and the requirement to transfer the patient from the fluoroscopic unit to the MR suite between injection and image acquisition. Radiation dose, however, if applied by a trained radiologist, is negligible when compared to standard radiographs.

At our institution, fluoroscopy times were between 6 and 18 s in a series of 50 consecutive shoulder injections performed by either a musculoskeletal fellow or staff person.

4.7.2.2
Ultrasonography

The advantages of ultrasonography for guiding intraarticular injections include: No radiation, real time guidance, speed, and few requirements regarding room (size and radiation protection). Disadvantages include potential problems with sterility and, as with fluoroscopy, patient transfers.

4.7.2.3
CT

CT has also been used as a guiding method for joint injections (Fig. 4.6). CT is a very precise method. The examination may be as fast as fluoroscopy. In a series of patients injected at our institution by either fluoroscopy, CT, or intermittent CT fluoroscopy, the times spent in the room by the radiologist were as follows: fluoroscopy, 8.7 min (7–11 min) (mean and range); CT, 10.5 min (7–15 min); and CT fluoroscopy, 9.5 min (7–14 min). Disadvantages of CT include scheduling problems, cost and local irradiation. In addition, sterility problems may occur and there is a patient transfer between injection and MR imaging.

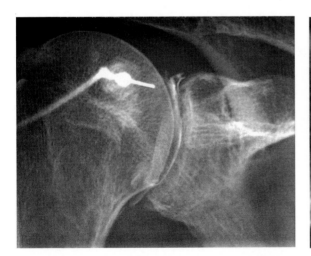

Fig. 4.5. Fluoroscopic guidance for joint injection. Cranial injection site. Small amounts of contrast material in glenohumeral joint space and subscapular recess demonstrate intraarticular position of needle tip. Many radiologists prefer a more caudal needle position

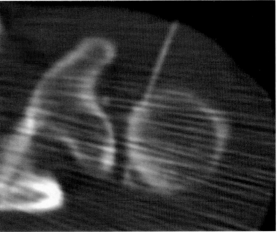

Fig. 4.6. CT guidance for joint injection. This CT fluoroscopic image was acquired with reduced matrix and tube current. It demonstrates needle position within the cranial joint space and a small amount of iodinated contrast medium within dorsal joint recess

4.7.2.4
MR Imaging

MR imaging may also be used for guiding intraarticular injections (PETERSILGE et al. 1997). MR imaging has advantages such as the lack of irradiation and the fact that patient transfers between rooms are not required. However, sterile handling may represent a problem, especially in the classically designed, closed magnets. Moreover, the time required for the injection has a relatively high opportunity cost because during arthrography another exam cannot be performed and therefore not be billed.

4.7.3
Patient Positioning for Fluoroscopic Injections

Patient position is supine. We prefer slight external rotation of the arm and elevation of the patient's contralateral side. In this position, the scapula becomes more or less parallel to the table top and the glenohumeral joint space parallel to the radiographic beam.

4.7.4
Needles

We usually employ 20 G (0.9 mm) 7-cm long needles for injection of the shoulder joint. This needle is relatively stiff and can easily be maneuvered even in obese or uncooperative patients. alternatively, thinner needles such as a 23 G (0.6 mm) 6 cm long needles may be used. Longer needles are rarely required, at least not when a cranial injection site is chosen, as described below. Needles which are shorter than 6 cm may not be sufficiently long in obese or athletic patients.

4.7.5
Puncture Site

Injection is commonly recommended at or below the equator of the humeral head (RESNICK 1995). An anterosuperior approach (PETERSILGE et al. 1997) has also been employed. This latter option has certain advantages: It avoids painful conflicts with a downward pointing coracoid. Injections appear to be more consistently intraarticular, even for beginners. This probably relates to the fact that the anterior joint recess is wide cranially. The distance between skin and humeral head may be shorter in the anterosupe-

rior approach. A potential disadvantage of the cranial needle position is the leaking of contrast material into the superior subscapularis. This may mimic abnormalities of the subscapularis tendon such as those associated with lesions of the reflection pulley of the biceps tendon (WEISHAUPT et al. 1999).

It is possible, but not necessary, to place the needle tip within the glenohumeral joint space between the humeral head and the glenoid. Advancing the needle between these two bones may be painful due to needle contact with bone or the labrum.

The dorsal approach may be used in order to avoid contrast leakage into diagnostically important anterior structures but may not be as easily performed as the anterior or anterosuperior approach.

4.7.6
Local Anesthetics

The skin, the joint capsule and the surface of the humeral head most commonly cause pain. We inject a total of 2–3 ml of mepivacaine (Scandicain, AstraZeneca, Södertälje, Sweden) preferentially close to these anatomical structures. with approximately 1 ml injected intraarticularly.

4.7.7
Contrast Media

4.7.7.1
Gadolinium-Containing Complexes

Gadolinium-containing complexes are most commonly employed for direct MR arthrography. Gadopentetate (Magnevist, Schering, Berlin, Germany), gadoterate (Gd-DOTA) (Dotarem, Guerbet, Aulnaysous-bois, France) (DRAPÉ et al. 1993) and gadoteridol (ProHance, Bracco, Milan, Italy) (BINKERT et al. 2001) have been employed for this purpose. Concentrations of 2 mmol/l (1:250 of the intravenous concentration of 0.5 mol/l) are commonly employed. BINKERT et al. (2001) found that 4 mmol/l gadoteridol produced significantly higher CNR when compared to 2 mmol/l concentrations. However, the differences in diagnostic accuracy for suspected rotator cuff disease were not significant.

Gadolinium-containing contrast may significantly contribute to the cost of the MR examination, depending on the available vial size. KAMISHIMA et al. (2000) have tested the safety of reusing vials with gadolinium-containing contrast. The authors found no culture growth and no side effects when reusing contrast during a period of up to 3 days. According to the authors and for the price setting valid in the US the cost of intraarticular contrast could be reduced significantly by reusing vials.

The local medicolegal situation has to be taken into account when gadolinium-containing contrast is injected intraarticularly. In the US, MR arthrography with gadolinium-containing complexes can be performed during routine imaging, based on a rule permitting off-label use of FDA-approved drugs. In a study context, however, Institutional Review Board approval is required. In European countries there is no uniform policy at present. Many countries at least require a special permit for the intraarticular use of gadolinium-containing contrast media.

4.7.7.1.1
Combination of Gadolinium-Containing and Iodinated Contrast

In order to avoid extraarticular injections, many radiologists use iodinated contrast media prior to the application of MR contrast. Iodinated contrast may be injected before the gadolinium-containing complex or as a mixture. Mixtures appear to be safe. A mixture of gadopentetate, lidocaine and epinephrine has been analyzed using spectrophotometry by BROWN et al. (2000). No significant dissociation of the gadolinium ion from its complex was found. Such dissociation would be highly undesirable because the free gadolinium ion is toxic.

In the presence of iodinated contrast, however, signal intensity of gadolinium-containing contrast appears to decrease on T1-weighted spin-echo and gradient-echo images when compared to dilution in saline (MONTGOMERY et al. 2001). Moreover, the optimal gadolinium concentration may be different from arthrograms performed with MR contrast diluted in saline. The peak signal intensity, which was lower in the presence of iodinated contrast in the investigation by MONTGOMERY et al. (2001), was reached at lower gadolinium concentrations (0.625 mmol/l for a gadopentetate/iodinated contrast mixture versus 2.5 mmol/l for a gadopentetate/saline mixture, for a field strength of 1.5 T).

4.7.7.2
Saline

Saline does not require Institutional Review Board approval. Moreover, saline is an inexpensive, physi-

ological and well-tolerated type of contrast medium (TIRMAN et al. 1993; ZANETTI and HODLER al. 1997). alternatively, Ringer solution can be used (sodium chloride 0.9%, potassium chloride 0.03%, calcium chloride 0.015%, sodium hydrocarbonate 0.017%; Braun Medical, Melsungen, Germany) (BINKERT et al. 2001). Apparently, Ringer solution is less irritant to joint cartilage than saline (BULSTRA et al. 1994). For both Ringer solution and saline, the types of sequences have to be adapted. In the presence of a gadolinium-containing contrast, T1-weighted spin-echo with or without fat suppression or adapted gradient-echo sequences may be employed. In saline arthrograms, T2- or T2*-weighted (WILLEMSEN et al. 1998) sequences have to be employed (Fig. 4.7). Depending on the parameters chosen, this may result in longer imaging times, motion artifacts and lower signal-to-noise ratios in comparison to the gadolinium arthrograms based on T1-weighted sequences.

In the previously mentioned study by BINKERT et al. (2001) regarding different types of intraarticular contrast media, Ringer solution (in combination with a T2-weighted sequence) was compared to 2-mmol/l and 4-mmol/l types of gadoteridol (with a T1-weighted sequence). The contrast-to-noise ratios were slightly superior to 2-mmol/l gadoteridol arthrograms, but not statistically different to 4-mmol/l gadoteridol arthrograms. However, regarding qualitative criteria (overall quality, motion artifacts, image contrast, and joint distention), Ringer arthrograms were inferior to

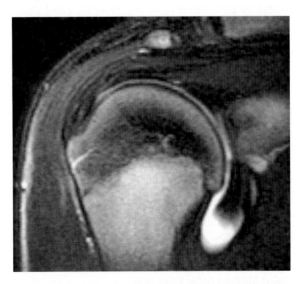

Fig. 4.7. Saline/Ringer MR arthrogram: Angled coronal fat-suppressed T2-weighted MR image demonstrates adequate contrast between intraarticular fluid and articular surface of supraspinatus tendon, cranial labrum and humeral head cartilage

their gadoteridol counterparts. Moreover, sensitivity and specificity may be different between the different types of arthrograms. In BINKERT et al. (2001), Ringer arthrograms were more sensitive but less specific than gadoteridol arthrograms in the detection of supraspinatus abnormalities.

4.7.7.3
Iodinated Contrast Media

Iodinated contrast media have also been considered to be potential agents in MR arthrography (HAJEK et al. 1987). Such contrast has the advantage that it is widely accepted for standard arthrography and does not cause medicolegal problems. Iodinated contrast media may have visible effects on T1 and/or T2 relaxation times (JINKINS et al. 1992). However, such effects do not appear to be sufficient for clinical imaging (HAJEK et al. 1987). In this investigation, Renografin provided inadequate contrast on T1-weighted images. T2-weighted sequences were required for sufficient image contrast. Therefore, iodinated contrast does not have diagnostic advantages compared to saline or Ringer solution.

4.7.7.4
Joint Effusion

Joint effusions are found after trauma, in diseases of the synovial membrane such as rheumatoid arthritis, in chronic rotator cuff tears, in osteoarthritis of the glenohumeral joint, and in other conditions. Joint effusions may be used as naturally occurring contrast medium. Relaxation times may differ from saline. HAJEK et al. (1987) simulated joint fluid by placing various albumin concentrations into cadaveric joints. They found that an albumin concentration of 12%, similar to that found in arthritis, produced adequate contrast to articular cartilage on T1-weighted images. In this same investigation, intraarticular blood had insufficient contrast differences with articular cartilage on T1-weighted images.

In general, however, T2-weighted images are most useful in the presence of effusions.

4.7.8
Joint Motion After Injection

Joint motion after intraarticular injection is recommended by many radiologists because it may improve delineation of rotator cuff tears or labral lesions. On the other hand, joint motion may lead to contrast leakage into surrounding soft tissue. Such effects were not proved in a formal study by BRENNER et al. (2000). They found that arm swinging 1 min both before and after injection were neither beneficial nor detrimental for image quality. On one hand there was no difference in the delineation of the labrum and rotator cuff; on the other hand no increased prevalence of extraarticular contrast leakage was found.

4.7.9
Advantages of Direct MR Arthrography

Direct MR arthrography, in trained hands, is performed quickly and with little discomfort for the patient. It provides consistent joint distention and quite consistent contrast. In selected cases the possibility to obtain joint fluid may be of interest.

In comparison to standard MR examinations, there is evidence that additional information can be obtained for subtle lesions of the rotator cuff (HODLER et al. 1992). However, MR arthrography has more consistently been employed in patients with instability (PALMER and CASLOWITZ 1995; BACHMANN et al. 1998; SHANKMAN et al. 1999; SANDERS et al. 1999). T1-weighted spin-echo sequences with fat suppression are probably most commonly used for this purpose. Standard T1-weighted images (PALMER and CASLOWITZ 1995) and gradient-echo images have also been employed (ZANETTI and HODLER al. 1997). Such sequences are less dependent on a homogeneous magnetic field than fat-suppressed spin-echo images.

4.7.9.1
Test Injection with Local Anesthetics

There is also the possibility to inject local anesthetics during arthrography which provides additional diagnostic information. If the usual pain is gone after arthrography, there is additional evidence that intraarticular abnormalities detected during MR arthrography are related to the patient's symptoms. If there is no pain reduction, the message is not as clear. The intraarticular abnormalities seen on MR images may not be relevant for the patient's symptoms. However, any pain reduction produced by intraarticular local anesthetic may simply be offset by the negative effects of joint distention or direct effects of contrast on the synovial membrane. If both MR arthrography and diagnostic injections have to be performed in one session, the gadolinium concentration should be increased from 2 mmol/l to 4 mmol/l, and the volume of intraarticular local anesthetic from 1 ml to 5 ml.

Pain response to diagnostic injections should be measured in a consistent fashion. For this purpose visual analogue scales (VAS) are commonly employed. They may take the form of a 10 cm long line with anchors at each end. The anchor on the left may be called "unchanged pain," the one of the right "pain completely gone." The patient is then asked to place a mark between the two anchors. The distance between the anchor on the left and the patient's mark is measured and commonly communicated as a percentage of pain reduction (the entire 10 cm representing 100%, a mark in the middle of the two marks representing 50%).

4.7.10
Disadvantages of Direct MR Arthrography

MR arthrography has several disadvantages. Beside medicolegal problems, side effects and patient anxiety are probably the most relevant.

4.7.10.1
Side Effects of Direct MR Arthrography

4.7.10.1.1
Possible Effects on Synovial Membrane or Articular Cartilage

Although there is no evidence that intraarticular gadolinium-containing contrast media damage the synovial membrane or articular cartilage, there may be non-specific reactions to the injection itself (HAJEK et al. 1990). In this investigation, 26 knee joints of New Zealand white rabbits were injected with either 500 μmol of gadopentetate with the rest of the knees serving as controls. In one injected knee, minimal joint effusion was found and in one, mild hyperemia. During microscopic examinations, four knees had mild focal synovial hyperplasia and three, minimal focal mononuclear infiltration. Gadopentetate was not found with X-ray fluorescent spectroscopy either in the synovial membrane or within articular cartilage.

BASHIR et al. (1997), however, found increased concentrations of gadolinium-containing complexes within articular cartilage. The concentrations depended on the extent of cartilage degeneration. The concentrations of contrast within cartilage were sufficient to provide diagnostic signal differences. In spite of this fact, long-term side effects have not been reported to date.

4.7.10.1.2
Non-specific Side Effects

MR arthrography is associated with the side effects found in all types of joint injections or arthrograms, regardless of the choice of injected contrast.

The patient may suffer from allergic reactions which may not be related to the contrast medium but rather to the local anesthetic used during the intraarticular injection. Such allergies may be caused by the local anesthetic itself, such as mepivacaine (Scandicain, AstraZeneca, Södertälje, Sweden) or additional constituents of local anesthetics such as the methyl parahydroxybenzoate found in Scandicain. In general, allergic reactions in arthrography are rare. Severe cases with anaphylactic shock are the exception. Treatment follows the usual guidelines for allergic reactions.

Vasovagal reactions or nausea are not uncommon in intraarticular injections (NEWBERG et al. 1985). They are an unpleasant experience for the patient, but are not dangerous and have no sequelae. Care should be taken, however, that the patients do not fall on the floor during vasovagal episodes. Such incidents may occur during patient transfer to the MR unit.

Infection is an extremely rare complication of joint injections. Its incidence appears to be below $1/10^4$ injections. NEWBERG et al. (1985) reported three infections in 126,000 arthrograms, and HUGO et al. (1998) 45 infections in 262,000 arthrograms. In patients with infection, predisposing factors are commonly present such as diabetes mellitus or orthopedic implants.

Bleeding is not a common problem with MR arthrography or arthrography in general. Hematomas may be found, but usually appear to be minor. HUGO et al. (1998) have reported five "vascular" complications in 262,000 arthrograms.

Patients may complain about pain after the injection. Such pain commonly starts a few hours after the procedure, presumably when the effects of local anesthetics are no longer present. In an investigation with iodinated contrast (alone or mixed with either local anesthetics or air), HALL et al. (1981) described such side effects. A total of 74% of their 72 patients complained about moderate or severe increase in their shoulder pain in the 24–48 h after arthrography. The pain usually began 4–6 h after the procedure. Pain may persist for 2–3 days. Because no relationship with age, gender, baseline discomfort or arthrographic diagnosis was found, the authors attributed pain to direct effects of the injected contrast or to the increased joint volume. Patients should be informed about the possibility of such pain. Standard non-steroidal pain medication such as mefenamic acid (Ponstan, Parke Davis Europe, Zaventem, Belgium) are effective in treating arthrography-related pain. If pain persists after 72 h or if it still increases after 24 h, however, the possibility of infection should be considered. The patient should immediately call the radiologist in such cases and arrangements for adequate diagnosis and treatment have to be made.

4.7.10.2
Patient Anxiety

Arthrography performed by a trained radiologists is not experienced as a major problem by the patients, although many of them are anxious before the examination. In a study performed at our institution with 193 consecutive patients referred for MR arthrography of the shoulder, we found that 34% considered the arthrographic procedure to produce discomfort identical to the MR examination itself; 40% found that the MR examination caused more discomfort, mainly due to claustrophobia or the obligation to lie still. The remaining 26% (the smallest group) indicated that arthrography caused more discomfort than the MR examination.

4.8
Problem Solving in MR Imaging of the Shoulder

4.8.1
Rotator Cuff

4.8.1.1
Magic Angle Effects

Normal tendons are supposed to be hypointense on standard MR sequences. However, normal supraspinatus tendons are usually slightly hyperintense on T1-weighted and proton-density images. Such signal is not always easy to differentiate from tendinopathy. It may be caused by the magic angle effect (ERICKSON et al. 1991). Because this effect is reduced on T2-weighted sequences, such sequences may be added to the protocol if they are not part of the standard protocol. Another possibility is to reexamine the patient with the arm in a different position, such as in abduction if the magnet bore allows this.

4.8.1.2
Tendinopathy Versus Partial Tear

Tendinopathy is associated with increased signal best seen on T1-weighted or proton-density spin-echo images or on gradient-echo sequences. It is more circumscribed than the signal associated with the magic angle. It may be difficult to differentiate from a partial tear or small full-thickness tear. Again, T2-weighted images may represent the solution. On T2-weighted images, true defects associated with partial tears are hyperintense, contrary to tendon degeneration.

Another possibility to differentiate tendinopathy from articular surface partial tears is the use of MR arthrography.

4.8.2
Biceps Tendon Abnormalities

4.8.2.1
Biceps Tendon Subluxation

Biceps tendon subluxation may not be apparent on images obtained in the neutral position of the humerus. It may become apparent, however, when the arm is examined in external rotation.

4.8.2.2
SLAP Lesion

Lesions of the biceps anchor (SLAP lesions) may be difficult to differentiate from a recess commonly present at the labral base. Increased signal may be found at the labral base due to articular cartilage undercutting the labral base or fibrovascular tissue present in this location. MR arthrography may help to differentiate an SLAP lesion or a recess from such anatomical structures. SLAP lesions may even more reliably be differentiated from a normal recess in the ABER position, or when images obtained with arm traction are applied. Admittedly, some of these procedures are not routinely used.

4.8.3
Instability

Increased signal at the labral base is also a problem at the anterior labrum. The possible solutions are similar to suspected SLAP lesions and include MR arthrography and examinations in the ABER position.

4.8.4
Synovitis

MR imaging probably underestimates early synovitis. The synovial membrane may not be sufficiently thickened for detection with standard protocols, or synovial fluid may not be present in amounts sufficient to delineate synovial irregularities. In such a situation, intravenous contrast increases lesion conspicuity.

4.8.5
Orthopedic Implants

Susceptibility artifacts associated with orthopedic implants may cause relevant problems in postoperative shoulders. There are various possibilities to improve imaging in this situation. Spin-echo sequences are less susceptible to such artifacts than gradient-echo images which should be avoided in the postoperative situation. Turbo or fast spin-echo images are less susceptible than standard spin-echo images. In a study involving gradient-echo imaging, PORT and POMPER (2000) found several additional factors reducing artifact size, including a short TE, increasing the frequency matrix, and decreasing the slice thickness. When feasible, implanted prostheses should be aligned with the main magnetic field to minimize artifact size. Parameters with negligible effect on artifact size in this study included bandwidth, phase encode matrix, and field of view.

If fat-suppressed images have to be acquired, STIR sequences should be employed instead of frequency-selective fat-suppressed images. Image quality may not be as good. However, STIR sequences are far less susceptible to field inhomogeneities than frequency-selective fat-suppressed images (HILFIKER et al. 1995).

4.8.6
Motion Artifacts

Motion artifacts are common in imaging of the shoulder. They may be caused by lack of patient cooperation which commonly relates to pain or claustrophobia. They may also occur due to breathing. Breathing artifacts may be most pronounced in patients who are overdoing cooperation with regard to breathing. Another source of motion artifacts encountered during MR imaging of the shoulder are pulsation artifacts originating from the heart or from major vessels.

In patients suffering from pain or claustrophobia, adequate medication is the obvious choice. Patient information prior to and feedback during the examination are possible solutions in patients lacking cooperation, although repeat examinations commonly do not improve image quality significantly.

Respiration artifacts can occasionally be reduced by instructing the patient to breath normally. Moreover, presaturation pulses over the thoracic cage may help to reduce breathing-related and pulsation artifacts.

Motion artifact reduction with (McGEE et al. 1997) and without (MANDUCA et al. 2000) navigator echoes have been described for shoulder imaging. Such techniques require advanced MR scanner hard- and software, however, which are not universally available.

4.9
Synopsis of MR and MR Arthrographic Examination Technique

Standardization of imaging techniques has several advantages such as faster throughput, consistent diagnostic quality, reliable image quality which remains stable over time, and facilitation of quality control. With the exception of minimized protocols such as a single coronal sequence in order to prove or rule out a full-thickness rotator cuff tear, three imaging planes should be obtained in imaging of the glenohumeral joint. Many institutions typically apply a slice thickness of 3–4 mm. Slightly thicker slices may be adequate when there is a need to increase coverage. Pixel size should also be as small as possible. With a matrix of 256×256, a typical field of view is between 12 and 16 cm. Fat suppression plays an important role in MR imaging of the shoulder. Not all scanners are able to consistently produce homogeneous fat suppression in eccentric positions as typically present in shoulder imaging, however. The role of MR arthrography versus standard MR sequences has been debated because it increases cost, time, patient anxiety, and because in many countries medicolegal issues have to be addressed. It appears, however, that MR arthrography increases diagnostic performance of MR imaging in instability and other indications. Indirect MR arthrography as a possible alternative to direct arthrographic techniques, although it has weaknesses such as the differentiation of vascularized tissue at the base of the labrum and joint fluid entering a true defect. A number of problems occurring during MR imaging of the glenohumeral joint can be addressed by adapting imaging protocols and better patient guidance. There are no perfect tools for avoiding all problems, pitfalls and artifacts. However, many of them can at least be reduced by using different tools including patient guidance, premedication, and appropriate MR imaging protocols.

References

Allmann KH, Schafer O, Hauer M et al. (1999) Indirect MR arthrography of the unexercised glenohumeral joint in patients with rotator cuff tears. Invest Radiol 34:435–440

Augustiny N, von Schulthess GK, Meier D et al. (1987) MR imaging of large nonferromagnetic metallic implants at 1.5 T. J Comput Assist Tomogr 11:678–683

Bachmann G, Bauer T, Jürgensen I et al. (1998) Diagnostische Sicherheit und therapeutische Relevanz von CT-Arthrographie und MR-Arthrographie der Schulter. Fortschr Roentgenstr 168:149–156

Bashir A, Gray ML, Boutin RD et al. (1997) Glycosaminoglycan in articular cartilage: in vivo assessment with delayed Gd(DTPA)(2-)-enhanced MR imaging. Radiology 205: 551–558

Beaulieu CF, Hodge DK, Bergman AG et al. (1999) Glenohumeral relationships during physiologic shoulder motion and stress testing: Initial experience with open MR imaging and active imaging-plane registration. Radiology 212: 699–705

Beltran J, Rosenberg ZS, Chandnani VP et al. (1997) Glenohumeral instability: evaluation with MR arthrography. RadioGraphics 17:657–673

Binkert CA, Zanetti M, Gerber C et al. (2001) MR arthrography of the glenohumeral joint: Two concentrations of gadoteridol versus Ringer solution as the intraarticular contrast material. Radiology 220:219–224

Bonutti PM, Norfray JF, Friedman RJ et al. (1993) Kinematic MRI of the shoulder. J Comput Assist Tomogr 17:666–669

Brenner ML, Morrison WB, Carrino JA et al. (2000) Direct MR arthrography: Is exercise prior to imaging beneficial or detrimental? Radiology 215:491–496

Brown RR, Clarke DW, Daffner RH (2000) Is a mixture of gadolinium and iodinated contrast material safe during MR arthrography? AJR Am J Roentgenol 175:1087–1090

Bulstra SK, Kuijer R, Eerdmans P et al. (1994) The effect in vitro of irrigating solutions on intact rat articular cartilage. J Bone Joint Surg Br 76:468–470

Cardinal E, Buckwalter KA, Braunstein EM (1996) Kinematic magnetic resonance imaging of the normal shoulder: assessment of the labrum and capsule. Can Assoc Radiol J 47:44–50

Chan KK, Muldoon KA, Yeh L et al. (1999) Superior labral anteroposterior lesions: MR arthrography with arm traction. AJR 173:1117–1122

Chandnani VP, Yeager TD, DeBerardino T et al. (1993) Glenoid labral tears: Prospective evaluation with MR imaging, MR arthrography, and CT arthrography. AJR 161:1229–1235

Cleary PD, Edgman-Levitan S, McMullen W et al. (1992) A national survey of hospital patients: the relationship between reported problems with care and patient evaluations. Qual Rev Bull 18:53–59

Cvitanic O, Tirman PF, Feller JF et al. (1997) Using abduction and external rotation of the shoulder to increase the sensitivity of MR arthrography in revealing tears of the anterior glenoid labrum. AJR 169:837–844

Davis SJ, Teresi LM, Bradley WG et al. (1991) Effect of arm rotation on MR imaging of the rotator cuff. Radiology 181: 265–268

Drapé J-L, Thelen P, Gay-Depassier P et al. (1993) Intraarticular diffusion of Gd-DOTA after intravenous injection in the knee: MR imaging evaluation. Radiology 188:227–234

Ellman H, Harris E, Kay SP (1992) Early degenerative joint disease simulating impingement syndrome: arthroscopic findings. Arthroscopy 8:482–487

Erickson SJ, Cox IH, Hyde JS et al. (1991) Effect of tendon orientation on MR imaging signal intensity: a manifestation of the "magic angle" phenomenon. Radiology 181: 389–392

Friedman RJ, Bonutti PM, Genez B (1998) Cine magnetic resonance imaging of the subcoracoid region. Orthopedics 21: 545–548

Frush DP, Bisset GS, Hall S (1996) Pediatric sedation in radiology: the practice of safe sleep. AJR 167:1381–1387

Fuchs B, Weishaupt D, Zanetti M et al. (1999) Fatty degeneration of the muscles of the rotator cuff: Assessment by computed tomography versus magnetic resonance imaging. J Shoulder Elbow Surg 8:599–605

Goutallier D, Bernageau J, Patte D (1989) L'évaluation par le scanner de la trophicité des muscles des coiffes des rotateurs ayant une ruptur tendineuse. Rev Chir Orthop 75: 126–127

Goutallier D, Postel JM, Laveau L et al. (1994) Fatty muscle degeneration in cuff ruptures. Pre- and postoperative evaluation by CT scan. Clin Orthop 304:78–83

Graichen H, Bonel H, Stammberger T et al. (1998) A technique for determining the spatial relationship between the rotator cuff and the subacromial space in arm abduction using MR and 3D image processing. Magn Reson Med 40:640–643

Gusmer PB, Potter HG, Schatz JA et al. (1996) Labral injuries: accuracy of detection with unenhanced MR imaging of the shoulder. Radiology 200:519–524

Hall FM, Rosenthal DI, Goldberg RP et al. (1981) Morbidity from shoulder arthrography: etiology, incidence, and prevention. AJR 136:59–62

Hajek PC, Sartoris DJ, Neumann CH et al. (1987) Potential contrast agents for MR arthrography: in vitro evaluation and practical observations. AJR 49:97–10

Hajek PC, Sartoris DJ, Gylys-Morin V et al. (1990) The effect of intra-articular gadolinium-DTPA on synovial membrane and cartilage. Invest Radiol 25:179–183

Hilfiker P, Zanetti M, Debatin J et al. (1995) Fast spin-echo inversion-recovery imaging versus fast T2-weighted spin-echo imaging in bone marrow abnormalities. Invest Radiol 30:110–114

Hodler J, Brahme SK, Snyder SJ et al. (1992) Rotator cuff disease: Assessment with MR arthrography versus standard MR imaging in 36 patients with arthroscopic confirmation. Radiology 182:431–436

Hodler J, Loredo RA, Longo C et al. (1995) Assessment of articular cartilage of the humeral head: MR-anatomic correlation in cadavers. AJR 165:615–620

Hollenhorst J, Munte S, Friedrich L et al. (2001) Using intranasal midazolam spray to prevent claustrophobia induced by MR imaging. AJR 176:865–868

Hugo PC, Newberg AH, Newman JS et al. (1998) Complications of arthrography. Semin Musculoskelet Radiol 2:345–348

Jinkins JR, Robinson JW, Sisk L et al. (1992) Proton relaxation enhancement associated with iodinated contrast agents in MR imaging of the CNS. AJNR 13:19–27

Jones RW, Witte RJ (2000) Signal intensity artifacts in clinical MR imaging. RadioGraphics 20:89–901

Jordan RM, Mintz RD (1995) Fatal reaction to gadopentetate dimeglumine. AJR 164:743–744

Kamishima T, Schweitzer ME, Awaya H et al. (2000) Utilization of "used" vials: cost-effective technique for MR arthrography. JMRI 12:953–955

Kwak SM, Brown RR, Trudell D et al. (1998) Glenohumeral joint: comparison of shoulder positions at MR arthrography. Radiology 208:375–380

Legan JM, Burkhard TK, Goff WB et al. (1991) Tears of the glenoid labrum: MR imaging of 88 arthroscopically confirmed cases. Radiology 179:241–246

Loew R, Kreitner K-F, Runkel M et al. (2000) MR arthrography of the shoulder: Comparison of low-field (0.2T) vs high-field (1.5T) imaging. Eur Radiol 10:989–996

Manduca A, McGee KP, Welch EB et al. (2000) Autocorrection in MR imaging: Adaptive motion correction without navigator echoes. Radiology 215:904–909

McGee KP, Grimm RC, Felmlee JP et al. (1997) The shoulder: adaptive motion correction of MR images. Radiology 205: 541–545

Montgomery DD, Morrison WB, Schweitzer M et al. (2001) Effects of iodinated contrast and field strength on gadolinium enhancement: implications for direct MR arthrography. Proc Int Soc Mag Reson Med 9:2140

Murphy KJ, Brunberg JA, Cohan RH (1996) Adverse reactions to gadolinium contrast media: a review of 36 cases. AJR 167:847–849

Newberg AH, Munn CS, Robbins AH (1985) Complications of arthrography. Radiology 155:605–606

Palmer WE, Caslowitz PL (1995) Anterior shoulder instability: diagnostic criteria determined from prospective analysis of 121 MR arthrograms. Radiology 197:819–825

Palmer WE, Brown JH, Rosenthal DI (1993) Rotator cuff: evaluation with fat-suppressed MR arthrography Radiology 188: 683–687

Parsa M, Tuite M, Norris M et al. (1997) MR imaging of rotator cuff tendon tears: comparison of T2*-weighted gradient-echo and conventional dual-echo sequences. AJR 168: 1519–1524

Peh WC, Cassar-Pullicino VN (1999) Magnetic resonance arthrography: current status. Clin Radiol 54:575–587

Pennes DR, Jonsson K, Buckwalter K et al. (1989) Computed arthrotomography of the shoulder: comparison of examinations made with internal and external rotation of the humerus. AJR 153:1017–1019

Petersilge CA, Lewin JS, Duerk JL et al. (1997) MR arthrography of the shoulder: Rethinking traditional imaging procedures to meet the technical requirements of MR imaging guidance. AJR 169:1453–1457

Port JD, Pomper MG (2000) Quantification and minimization of magnetic susceptibility artifacts on GRE images. J Comput Assist Tomogr 24:958–964

Reinus WR, Shady KL, Mirowitz SA et al. (1995) MR diagnosis of rotator cuff tears of the shoulder: Value of using T2-weighted fat-saturated images. AJR 164:1451–1456

Resnick D (1995) Shoulder - Arthrography of the glenohumeral joint. In: Resnick D (ed) Diagnosis of bone and joint disorders. Saunders, Philadelphia, pp 311–333

Rhoad RC, Klimkiewicz JJ, Williams GR et al. (1998) A new in vivo technique for three-dimensional shoulder kinematics analysis. Skeletal Radiol 27:92–97

Sahin-Akyar G, Miller TT, Staron RB, McCarthy DM, Feldman F. (1998) Gradient-echo versus fast-suppressed fast spin-echo MR imaging of the rotator cuff tears. AJR 171: 223–227

Sanders TG, Tirman PFJ, Linares R et al. (1999) The glenohumeral articular disruption lesion: MR arthrography with arthroscopic correlation. AJR 172:171–175

Sans N, Richardi G, Railhac JJ et al. (1996) Kinematic MR imaging of the shoulder: Normal patterns. AJR 167: 1517–1522

Shankman S, Bencardino J, Beltran J (1999) Glenohumeral instability: evaluation using MR arthrography of the shoulder. Skeletal Radiol 28:365–382

Shellock FG, Kanal E (1996) Magnetic resonance. Bioeffects, safety, and patient management. Lippincott Williams and Wilkins, Philadelphia, pp 127–155

Sommer T, Vahlhaus C, Lauck G et al. (2001) MR imaging and cardiac pacemakers: in vitro evaluation and in vivo studies in 51 patients at 0.5 T. Radiology 215:869–879

Sonin AH, Peduto AJ, Fitzgerald SW et al. (1996) MR imaging of the rotator cuff mechanism: comparison of spin-echo and turbo spin-echo sequences. AJR 167:333–338

Suh JS, Cho JH, Shin KH et al. (1996) Chondromalacia of the knee: evaluation with a fat-suppression three-dimensional SPGR imaging after intravenous contrast injection. J Magn Reson Imaging 6:884–888

Tirman PF, Stauffer AE, Crues JV (1993) Saline magnetic resonance arthrography in the evaluation of glenohumeral instability. Arthroscopy 9:550–559

Tirman PF, Bost FW, Steinbach LS et al. (1994) MR arthrographic depiction of tears of the rotator cuff: benefit of abduction and external rotation of the arm. Radiology 192:851–856

Tuite MJ, De Smet AA, Norris MA et al. (1995) MR diagnosis of labral tears of the shoulder: value of T2*-weighted gradient-recalled echo images made in external rotation. AJR 164:941–944

Tuite MJ, Asinger D, Orwin JF (2001) Angled oblique sagittal MR imaging of the rotator cuff tears: comparison with standard obilque sagittal images. Skeletal Radiol 30:262–269

Vahlensieck M, Peterfy CG, Wischer T et al. (1996) Indirect MR arthrography: optimization and clinical applications. Radiology 200:249–254

Vahlensieck M, Lang P, Sommer T et al. (1997) Indirect MR arthrography: techniques and applications. Semin Ultrasound CT MR 18:302–306

Vahlensieck M, Sommer T, Textor J et al. (1998) Indirect MR arthrography: Techniques and applications. Eur Radiol 8: 232–235

Warner JJP (1997) Overview: avoiding pitfalls and managing complications and failures of instability surgery. In: Warner JJP, Iannotti JP, Gerber C (eds) Complex and revision problems in shoulder surgery. Lippincott-Raven, Philadelphia, pp 3–8

Weishaupt D, Zanetti M, Tanner A et al. (1999) Lesions of the reflection pulley of the long biceps tendon. MR arthrographic findings. Invest Radiol 34:463–469

Willemsen UF, Wiedemann E, Brunner U et al. (1998) Prospective evaluation of MR arthrography performed with high-volume intraarticular saline enhancement in patients with recurrent anterior dislocations of the shoulder. AJR 170:79–84

Winalski CS, al.iabadi P, Wright RJ et al. (1993) Enhancement of joint fluid with intravenously administered gadopentetate dimeglumine: technique, rationale, and implications. Radiology. 187:179–185

Wintzell G, Larsson H, Larsson S (1998) Indirect MR arthrography of anterior shoulder instability in the ABER and the apprehension test positions: a prospective comparative study of two different shoulder positions during MRI using intravenous gadodiamide contrast for enhancement of the joint fluid. Skeletal Radiol 27: 488–494

Wintzell G, Haglund-Akerlind Y et al. (1999) Open MR imaging of the unstable shoulder in the apprehension test position: description of an alternative MR examination position. Eur Radiol 9:1789–1795

Yagci B, Manisali M, Yilmaz E et al. (2001) Indirect MR arthrography of the shoulder in detection of rotator cuff ruptures. Eur Radiol 11:258–262

Zanetti M, Hodler J (1997) Contrast media in MR arthrography of the glenohumeral joint: intra-articular gadopentetate vs saline: preliminary results. Eur Radiol 7: 498–502

5 Ultrasound

M. Zanetti

CONTENTS

examiner performing the investigation. In addition, evidence regarding the diagnostic value of ultrasound for certain abnormalities such as labral or capsular lesions, determination of muscle atrophy and fatty degeneration and articular cartilage damage is very limited (HAMMAR et al. 2001). Ultrasound is not useful for the assessment of intraosseous abnormalities unless they cause abnormalities of bone surfaces, such as fractures with cortical disruption. Finally, although a single ultrasound examination is inexpensive in most fee schedules from the point of view of national health care systems, ultrasound may be a relevant cost factor due to the large number of examinations performed. In Germany in 1993, the total fees paid for ultrasound was higher than for CT and MR imaging (DELORME and VAN KAICK 1996). For such reasons, adequate equipment, examination technique and documentation of imaging findings is crucial if ultrasound not only has to act as a confirmatory imaging test, but rather as an accepted determinant in an imaging algorithm.

This chapter reviews imaging technique and sonographic anatomy, followed by a review of sonographic abnormalities. Finally, the diagnostic efficacy and clinical impact of ultrasonography for various abnormalities is discussed and compared to other imaging methods, mainly MR imaging.

5.1
Introduction

Ultrasound of the shoulder has several advantages compared to competing imaging methods such as computed tomography (CT), CT arthrography, magnetic resonance (MR) imaging, and MR arthrography. It is non-invasive, provides good spatial and excellent contrast resolution, allows for routine dynamic investigations, is widely available and relatively inexpensive on a per-examination basis. On the other hand, ultrasound appears to depend on the experience of the

M. ZANETTI, MD
Radiology, Orthopedic University Hospital Balgrist,
Forchstrasse 340, 8008 Zurich, Switzerland

5.2
Imaging Technique

5.2.1
Transducers

Currently, linear transducers with frequencies in the range of 5–13 MHz are used for ultrasound of the musculoskeletal system. Frequencies in the range of 9–13 MHz allow an in-plane spatial resolution of 0.2 to 0.4 mm (SEIBOLD et al. 1999), which is higher than the spatial resolution of currently used MR protocols.

However, such high ultrasound frequencies can be used for superficially located structures only. For deep-lying structures and in patients with hypertrophic muscles or obesity, lower frequencies (typically 5–7.5 MHz) are most commonly employed.

5.2.2
Patient Positioning, Transducer Positions

Proper positioning of the patient is important for the performance of shoulder ultrasound. We examine the patients in the upright (seated) position, facing the ultrasound screen, with the radiologist standing behind the patient (Figs. 5.1–5.5). In this position, the

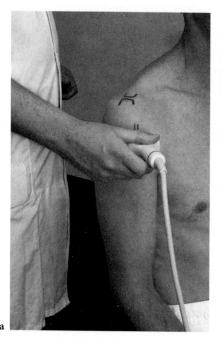

Fig. 5.1. Examination technique: Acromioclavicular (AC) joint. This image demonstrates the transducer position for assessing the AC joint. The contours of the AC joint are marked on the skin. Note that the investigator stands behind the patient

patient's arm can be externally rotated and placed behind his back, two important positions for complete examination of the shoulder. Moreover, the patient can follow the examination on the screen, which enhances patient collaboration. We use a standardized examination protocol starting with an examination of the acromioclavicular joint (Fig 5.1) (capsular hypertrophy, osteophytes, subchondral cysts, ganglia) and continue with transverse and longitudinal scans of each of the following structures: the long biceps tendon (Fig. 5.2) (tendon tears, tendon subluxation or dislocation, tendinitis, tendon sheath effusion, synovial proliferation), subscapularis (Fig. 5.3) (tears, calcifications), supraspinatus (Fig. 5.4) and infraspinatus tendons (tears, calcification, abnormalities of the subacromial/subdeltoid bursa). The acromioclavicular joint and the biceps tendon are examined with the patient placing his hand on his knee. The subscapularis is best seen in external rotation of the arm (Fig. 5.3c). We commonly perform this examination in a dynamic fashion because subscapularis tears may not easily been seen otherwise. The supraspinatus tendon is best demonstrated with the arm placed behind the back (Fig. 5.4), thereby distending any tears and by moving hidden (more medial parts) of the supraspinatus from underneath the acromial arch. The more anteriorly located lesions can be missed with the arm placed behind the back. Anteriorly located lesions are better seen with the arm in a neutral position with the patient's hand on the knee (Fig. 5.4c). In suspected bursitis and impingement syndrome we also perform a dynamic

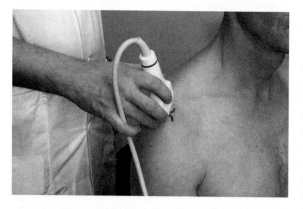

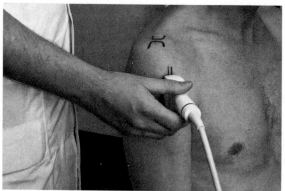

Fig. 5.2a, b. Examination technique: Long biceps tendon. **a** The transducer position for assessing the long biceps tendon with a transverse scan is demonstrated. **b** The transducer position for assessing the long biceps tendon with a longitudinal scan is demonstrated

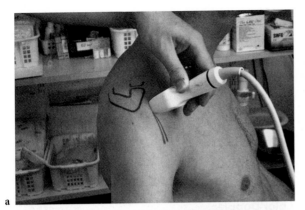

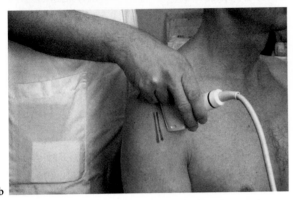

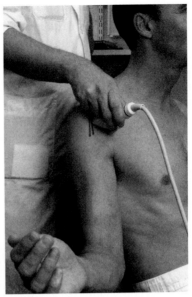

a

b

c

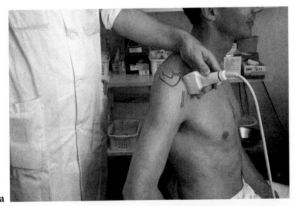

Fig. 5.3a–c. Examination technique: Subscapularis (SSC) tendon. **a** The transducer position for assessing the SSC tendon with a longitudinal scan is demonstrated. **b** The transducer position for assessing the SSC tendon with a transverse scan is demonstrated. **c** The arm can be rotated externally for better demonstration of the SSC tendon lesions. This position enables diagnosis of dislocation of the long biceps tendon

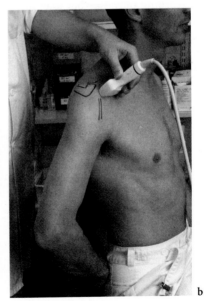

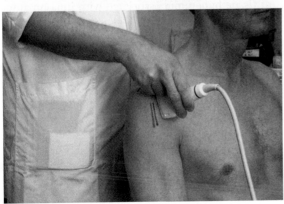

a

b

c

Fig. 5.4a–c. Examination technique: Supraspinatus (SSP) tendon. **a** The transducer position for assessing the SSP tendon with a longitudinal scan is demonstrated. The arm is placed behind the back. **b** The transducer position for assessing the SSC tendon with a transverse scan is demonstrated. The arm is placed behind the back. **c** The arm has to be moved into a neutral position for the detection of the most anteriorly located

type of examination with the transducer placed on the subacromial bursa during forward and/or lateral flexion of the arm (Fig. 5.3c). Any bursal effusions may become better visible and movements between tissue layers may no longer by continuous and harmonic in chronic bursitis. Glenohumeral effusion is especially sought with a dorsally placed transducer and an increased field of view.

The posterior transverse scan is also recommended for the assessment of the dorsal glenoid labrum (HAMMAR et al. 2001). The labrum is best seen on anterior or posterior transverse scans with or without dynamic examination. Some authors place the patient in the supine position, with the arm abducted and externally rotated. The transducer is oriented parallel to the inferior border of the major pectoral muscle resulting in ventrocaudal tilting of the transducer (WITTNER and HOLZ 1996).

5.2.3
Dynamic Examination Technique

Descriptions of imaging techniques such as those provided in this chapter may give the impression that ultrasound examinations of the shoulder can be performed with a few standardized images. This approach may be useful for teaching purposes but may result in inadequate imaging results. Certain abnormalities tend not to be seen on a few standardized sections. A typical example is the small anterior tear of the supraspinatus insertion which may be missed on a single standard image of the supraspinatus with the arm in internal rotation. Moreover, certain abnormalities are more conspicuous when a dynamic type of examination is performed. A typical example is biceps tendon subluxation in the presence of lesions of the superior border of the subscapularis tendon and the reflection pulley of the biceps tendon (WEISHAUPT et al. 1999). A dynamic examination technique may involve both arm motion (for instance for the detection of biceps tendon subluxation) as well as continuous, systematic motion of the transducer in order to cover the entire diameter of structures such as the rotator cuff.

5.2.4
Documentation

Documentation of ultrasonographic images has occasionally been a debated subject. However, we believe that documentation of both normal and abnormal findings are crucial for ultrasonography to gain or

maintain acceptance, as well as for quality control purposes. Admittedly, standardized documentation is not as easily performed as for CT or ultrasonography. We have the following minimal protocol for documentation: acromioclavicular joint, transverse and longitudinal scans of the long biceps tendon, subscapularis, supraspinatus and infraspinatus tendons. This documentation also includes also any bony abnormalities in the humeral head.

5.2.5
Color Doppler

Color Doppler is well suited for evaluating the flow in the vessels, particularly in large vessels. Most commonly, an anterior approach is used. The transducer is put parallel or transverse to the vessels. As in any other region of the body, arterial as well as the venous systems can be evaluated.

The theoretical advantages of color Doppler sonography in the assessment of inflammatory or reparative tissue have not been thoroughly evaluated, although a few papers relate to the diagnosis of hypervascular tissue in the musculoskeletal system (see Sect. 5.2.6).

5.2.6
Power Doppler

Power Doppler ultrasound has been available for several years but has only rarely been used for musculoskeletal indications (NEWMAN et al. 1994). In contrast to the conventional color Doppler examination brightness of the color signal in power Doppler does not depend on the orientation of the vessels in relation to the transducer. With the power Doppler technique small blood vessels may be detected. As such, it may prove a sensitive means of assessing soft tissue hyperemia associated with inflammatory conditions of the musculoskeletal system.

Color gain has to be adjusted below a level at which all color noise disappears. First, when the transducer is placed on the patient surface and any movement of the hand has stopped, the gain will be increased until color is visible. Second, the gain is reduced until the color has disappeared from all regions where capillary flow is not present. The cortical bone echo in the corresponding image can be used as internal control structure where capillary flow should be absent. Criteria for pathologic flow include subjective increase in vessel number within tendon structures or other surrounding soft-tissue parts (BREIDAHL et al. 1996). This can be used to differentiate hypoechoic rims as fluid rim or vascularized synovium (BREIDAHL et al. 1998).

5.2.7
Tissue Harmonic Imaging

The recent introduction of tissue harmonic imaging could resolve the problems related to ultrasound in technically difficult areas by providing a marked improvement in image quality (TRANQUART et al. 1999). Tissue harmonic images are formed by utilizing the harmonic signals that are generated by tissue and by filtering out the fundamental echo signals that are generated by the transmitted acoustic energy. This imaging mode could be used in different organs with a heightening of low-contrast lesions through artifact reduction, as well as by the induced greater intrinsic contrast sensitivity of the harmonic imaging mode. So far, this imaging technique has been most commonly used in cardiac and abdominal ultrasound – especially in the evaluation of pancreas (SHAPIRO et al. 1998) and focal liver lesions (TANAKA et al. 2000).

To our knowledge, published experiences with tissue harmonic imaging in the musculoskeletal system are lacking. Presumably, tissue harmonic imaging may provide better contrast in rotator cuff tears than standard ultrasound resulting in higher conspicuity of the lesions.

5.2.8
Intravenous Contrast Agents

The recent introduction of ultrasound contrast medium to clinical practice has enabled the detec-tion of otherwise invisible vessels in tumors and tumor-like abnormalities. For musculoskeletal purposes only few experiences have been published (MAGARELLI et al. 2001). MAGARELLI et al. reported a qualitative increase of vessels in patients with early signs of inflammatory synovitis. The clinical importance of such findings is not yet assessed.

5.3
Normal and Abnormal Ultrasound Findings

5.3.1
Acromioclavicular Joint

The superior and anterior surface of the acromiocla-vicular joint can be examined with ultrasound, but the potentially more important inferior surface of the acromioclavicular can not be inspected. The normal acromioclavicular joint has smoothly rounded borders at the acromioclavicular joint (Fig. 5.5). The joint space itself is characterized by a hypoechoic small band. Capsular hypertrophy can be diagnosed when the capsule is thickened in the cranial portion of the joint. Osteophytes are visible when directed cranially (Fig. 5.6). Subchondral cysts as signs of osteoarthritis can also be detected. However, cyst or an erosion should not be diagnosed merely in the presence of an osteophyte where insonation is not perpendicular to the surface. Non-perpendicular insonation may produce a dramatic reduction of echogenicity that may be mistaken for an erosion. Ganglia originating from the acromioclavicular joint can easily be demonstrated as a hypoechoic, well demarcated structure originating from the joint.

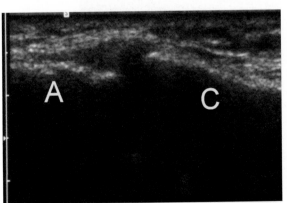
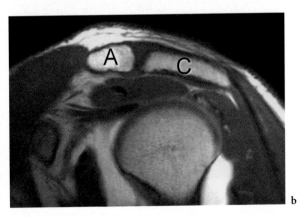

a   b

Fig. 5.5. Normal acromioclavicular (AC) joint (A, C). **a** Ultrasound image demonstrates the normal AC joint. **b** The corresponding parasagittal T1 MR arthrogram demonstrates the normal AC joint

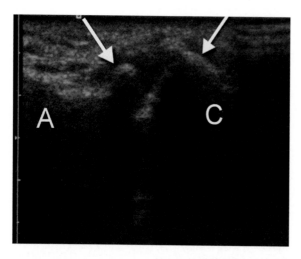

Fig. 5.6. Degenerated AC joint: Osteophytes (*arrows*) are demonstrated on ultrasound

5.3.2
Long Biceps Tendon

The demonstration of fluid collections within the tendon sheath of the long biceps (Figs. 5.7, 5.8) is one of the most straightforward but also one of the most unspecific abnormalities which can be identified with ultrasound. Small amounts of fluid within the biceps tendon sheath represent a normal finding. Larger quantities may be seen in a number of abnormalities, such as rotator cuff tears, biceps tendinitis, and any abnormality involving the glenohumeral joint space (Fig. 5.8). In spite of this non-specificity, many authors believe that biceps tendon fluid is a sign of rotator cuff tears and therefore increase

their index of suspicion. Rotator cuff tears have been found to be related with fluid collections within the biceps tendon sheath in more than half of the cases (HOLLISTER et al. 1995; MIDDLETON et al. 1986b). The ultrasound criteria for a biceps tendinopathy are the same as in tendinopathy of other tendons. This diagnosis can be suspected with increased amounts of fluid in the tendon sheath, when the tendon is focally thickened or thinned, or when the border becomes irregular (FARIN 1996). The normal tendon has a fibrillar appearance. Absence of the fibrillar pattern is abnormal. It indicates severe degeneration, rupture, or dislocation of the tendon with replacement by fibrous and granulation tissues (PTASZNIK and HENNESSY 1995). This granulation or scar tissue may fill the bicipital groove, mimicking the appearance of an at least partially intact tendon. Non-visualization of the tendon is evidence of a complete tear (Fig. 5.9). However, a false positive diagnosis of tear may be made when the transducer is not perpendicular to the biceps tendon. This is due to the fact that the biceps tendon is highly ordered and anisotropic, leading to an artifact similar to the one described for the rotator cuff. Subluxation (the tendon overlies the medial prominence of the bicipital groove) and dislocation (tendon completely displaced from the bicipital groove) of the biceps tendon can be diagnosed in transversal scans during external rotation of the arm. Displacements always occur in the medial direction. The dynamic demonstration of a subluxation or dislocation of the biceps tendon represents a relevant advantage of ultrasound over more or less static imaging methods (CT and MR imaging).

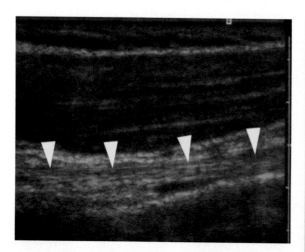

Fig. 5.7. Normal long biceps tendon (*arrowheads*) is demonstrated on a longitudinal ultrasound scan. A small amount of fluid between the tendon humerus is normal. Note the clearly visible fibrillar appearance of the normal long biceps tendon

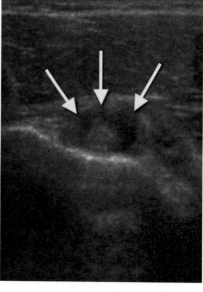

Fig. 5.8. Effusion in the tendon sheath of the long biceps tendon is demonstrated

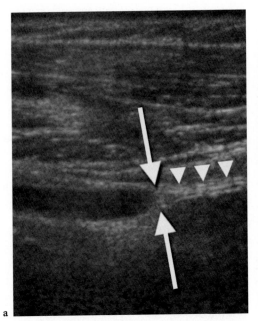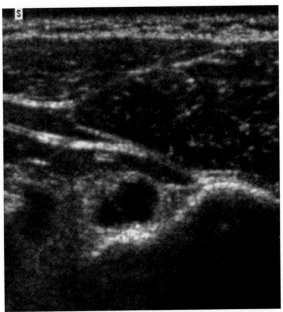

Fig. 5.9a, b. Complete rupture of the longs biceps tendon. **a** The longitudinal ultrasound (US) image demonstrates a discontinuity of the long biceps tendon. **b** The corresponding US scan above the rupture of the long biceps tendons shows an empty intertubercular groove

5.3.3
Rotator Cuff

In comparison to the overlying deltoid muscle the normal rotator cuff is slightly hyperechoic. The echogenicity is, however, significantly influenced by the angle of insonation and the age of the patient. The transducer should be perpendicular to the tendon. Even minor deviations from this orientation lead to a relevant loss of echogenicity which may be mistaken for a tendon tear. This pitfall is caused by the tendon's anisotropy. The well-ordered tendon fibers reflect the energy in a direction slightly different from the incoming sound waves which leads to the signal loss described above. Hypoechogenicity caused by tendon anisotropy can easily be differentiated from a true abnormality by slightly rotating the transducer. An artifact will move depending on the transducer position, but not a true abnormality.

Abnormality of echogenicity as criteria for lesions is much more critical than abnormality of the form. Beneath the problems with tendon anisotropy the echogenicity is also age related. This age dependency means that the usually greater echogenicity of the rotator cuff than the deltoid muscle is absent. Occasionally, the echogenicity of the rotator cuff may be equal or less than that of the deltoid muscle. This occurs most often in older patients (>50 years), but it is still relative

uncommon (50–60, 24%; 60+, 28%; MIDDLETON et al. 1986). The age related decreased echogenicity should not be interpreted as rotator cuff lesion. It can, however, be confused with non-visualization of the cuff by those less experienced with the technique.

5.3.3.1
Supraspinatus

The supraspinatus tendon assumes a convex curvilinear course when it passes over the humeral head (Fig. 5.10). Ultrasound findings for a full-thickness tear include non-visualization of tendon tissue, localized hypoechoic zones throughout the entire cuff thickness and loss of convexity of the outer contour (Figs. 5.11, 5.12). The lesion may become more conspicuous when the transducer compresses the deltoid muscle against the humeral head. Proposed criteria for partial-thickness tear include a hypoechoic defect that involves the articular or bursal surface but not the entire cuff thickness (Fig. 5.13). Other published criteria for partial-thickness tears overlap with those for full-thickness tears: thinning of the cuff and straight outer cuff border with loss of convexity. Criteria such as echogenic foci (MIDDLETON et al. 1986b) are not reliable and may be caused by tendon degeneration or calcification. A further potential pitfall exists from a lack of familiarity with the anatomy of the anterior

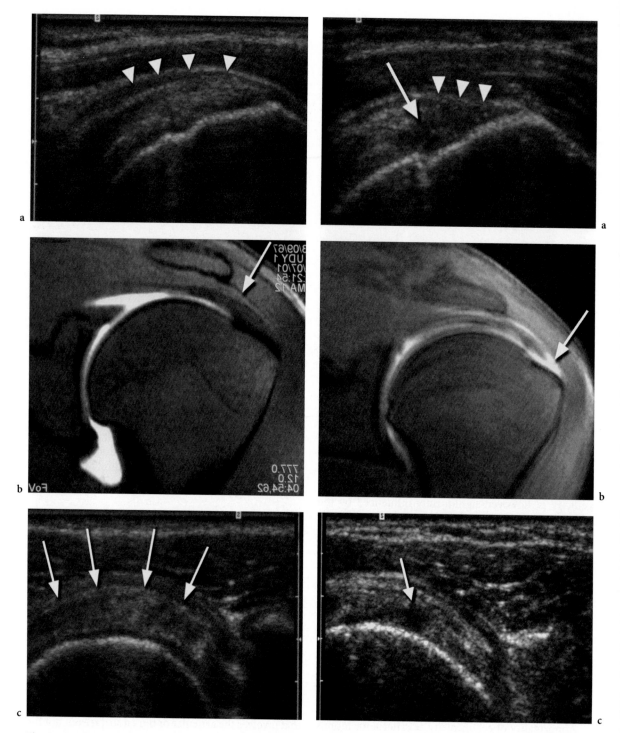

Fig. 5.10a–c. Normal supraspinatus (SSP) tendon. **a** Normal SSP tendon on a longitudinal ultrasound (US) scan. Note the normal convex curvilinear course when it passes over the humeral head. **b** Corresponding coronal T1-weighted fat-suppressed MR arthrogram demonstrates the normal longitudinal course of the SSP tendon. **c** Normal SSP tendon on transverse US scan

Fig. 5.11a–c. Small full-thickness tear of the supraspinatus (SSP) tendon. **a** Small, full-thickness SSP tendon tear on longitudinal US scan. Hypoechogenicity (*arrow*) demonstrates the tear, note also the concavity of the outer contour (*arrowheads*) of the SSP tendon. **b** Small full-thickness tear (*arrow*) on a corresponding coronal T1-weighted MR arthrogram. **c** Small full-thickness SSP tendon tear on a transverse ultrasound scan is visible (*arrow*); however, differentiation from a partial-thickness tear is barely possible

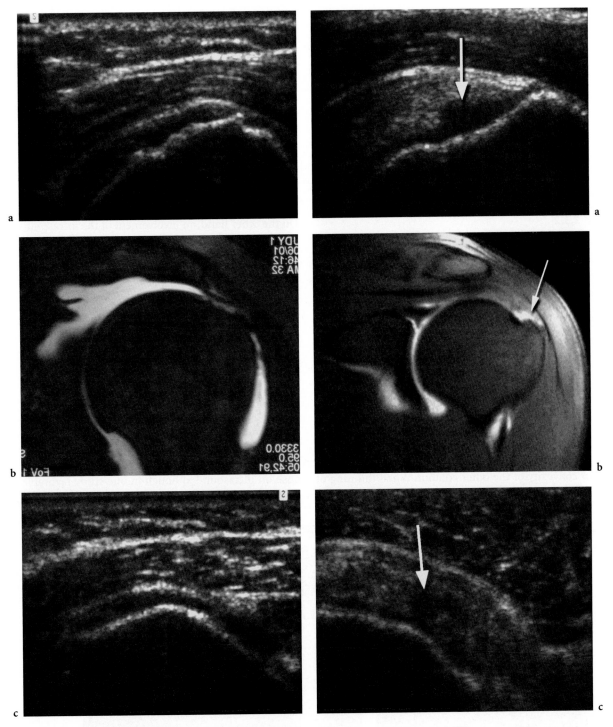

Fig. 5.12a–c. Large full-thickness tear of the supraspinatus (SSP) tendon. **a** Large full-thickness SSP tendon tear on longitudinal ultrasound (US) scan. **b** Large full-thickness tear on a corresponding coronal T2-weighted fat suppressed MR arthrogram. **c** Large full-thickness SSP tendon tear on a transverse US scan

Fig. 5.13a–c. Articular partial thickness tear of the supraspinatus tendon. **a** Articular partial-thickness SSP tendon tear on longitudinal ultrasound (US) scan with internal rotation of the arm. **b** Articular partial-thickness SSP tear and corresponding coronal T1-weighted fat suppressed MR arthrogram. **c** Articular partial-thickness SSP tendon tear on a transverse US scan

part of the rotator cuff. On transverse view of the anterior cuff, the intraarticular biceps tendon itself appears as an echogenic focus opposed to the humeral head located between the supraspinatus and subscapularis part of the rotator cuff. Failure to recognize this echogenic focus as the biceps tendon could result in diagnostic error. In addition, a focal area of decreased echogenicity is often observed immediately posterior to the intraarticular biceps tendon. This appearance most likely results from a void of tissue between the biceps tendon and the anterior aspect of the supraspinatus (MIDDLETON et al. 1986a).

5.3.3.2
Infraspinatus

The tendon of the infraspinatus (Fig. 14) can not easily be differentiated from the supraspinatus tendon. Such differentiation is difficult even during arthroscopy. Therefore, TEEFEY et al. (1999) have suggested that on transverse views the first 1.5 cm of the rotator cuff located posterolateral to the intraarticular portion of the biceps tendon represent the supraspinatus and the next 1.5 cm the infraspinatus tendon. Sonographic findings for a full-thickness tear of the infraspinatus tendon include the same criteria as noted for the supraspinatus tendon: non-visualization of tendon tissue, localized hypoechoic zones throughout the entire cuff thickness and loss of convexity of the outer contour. When thinning of the infraspinatus is described the normal anatomy

should not be misinterpreted. The thickness of the anterior and posterior parts of the normal rotator cuff are different. The normal rotator cuff is thinned posteriorly. BRETZKE et al. (1985) measured the thickness of the normal rotator cuff in the anterior and posterior part. In their study, the anterior part averaged 6 mm in thickness, while the posterior cuff averaged 3.6 mm. Normal posterior thinning of the cuff should not be evidence for infraspinatus tear.

Moreover, an isolated full thickness tear of the infraspinatus tendon should be cautiously diagnosed because this occurs rarely. Infraspinatus tears are most commonly associated with supraspinatus tears. On the other hand, an involvement of the infraspinatus tendon should be considered when the size of the supraspinatus tendon exceeds 3 cm.

5.3.3.3
Subscapularis

The ultrasound literature generally focuses on lesions of the supraspinatus lesions but rarely on the subscapularis tendon. In contrast to the problems of differentiation between infraspinatus and supraspinatus, the subscapularis tendon can be differentiated easily from the supraspinatus. The subscapularis tendon (Fig. 15) is separated from the supraspinatus tendon by the long biceps tendon and also based on their course.

Subscapularis lesions may be more difficult to diagnose on ultrasound although in one study favorable results (sensitivity of 82%) have been demonstrated

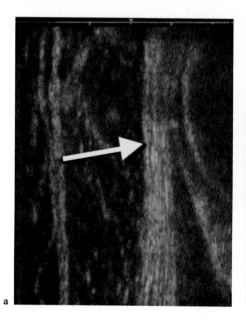
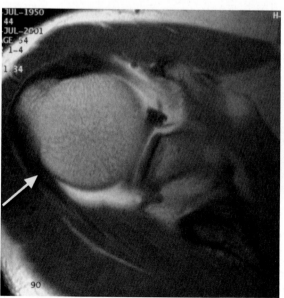

Fig. 5.14a, b. Normal infraspinatus (ISP) tendon. **a** Normal ISP tendon (*arrow*) on a longitudinal scan. **b** Corresponding axial T1-weighted MR arthrogram demonstrates the normal longitudinal course of the ISP tendon (*arrow*)

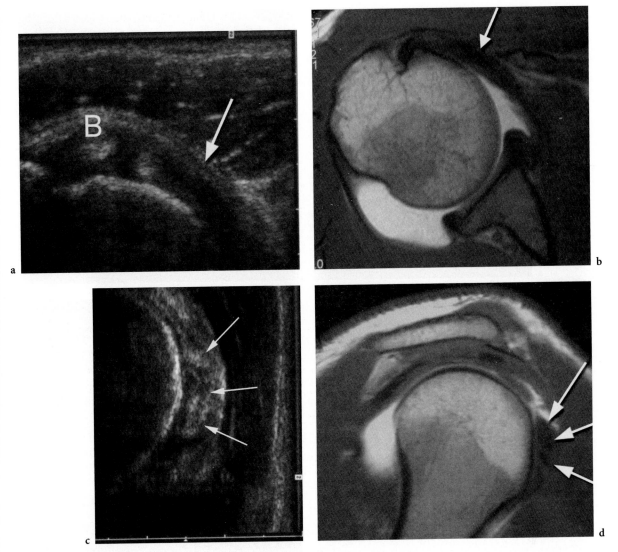

Fig. 5.15a–d. Normal subscapularis (SSC) tendon. **a** Normal SSC tendon beneath the long biceps (B) tendon on a longitudinal ultrasound (US) scan. **b** Corresponding axial T1-weighted MR arthrogram demonstrates the normal longitudinal course of the SSC tendon. **c** Normal SSC tendon on transverse US scan. The various tendon fibers (*arrows*) of the SSC are visible. **d** Corresponding parasagittal T1-weighted MR arthrogram also demonstrates the various normal tendon fibers of the distal SSC tendon (*arrows*)

(FARIN and JAROMA 1996). The diagnostic difficulties with subscapularis lesions may relate to the fact that tendon degeneration and tears are commonly limited to the cranial border of the tendon. Complete detachment is rarer. The resulting ultrasound signs may be subtle and may be missed when a single standardized transverse to the humeral shaft ultrasound image is obtained where the supscapularis tendon is seen longitudinally. The cranial part of the subscapularis tendon should probably be scrutinized with the same care as it has recently been published with regard to MR imaging (WEISHAUPT et al. 1999; ZANETTI et al. 1999b). This means that parasagittal and transverse ultrasound images perpendicular and parallel to the long fibers of the subscapularis tendon, with emphasis on the cranial border of the tendon should be performed (Figs. 5.15, 5.16), and that an examination limited to a few standardized sonographic images may not be sufficient. Transverse images perpendicular to the long fibers of the subscapularis tendon are preferred in our clinic for the assessment of partial tears on the cranial border. Apart from the location being different to supraspinatus tears, the ultrasound findings of subscapularis tendon tears are similar to those seen with tears of the supraspinatus. Focal thinning and non-visualization are reliable signs for full thickness tears. More than half of the patients have secondary abnormalities associated with subscapu-

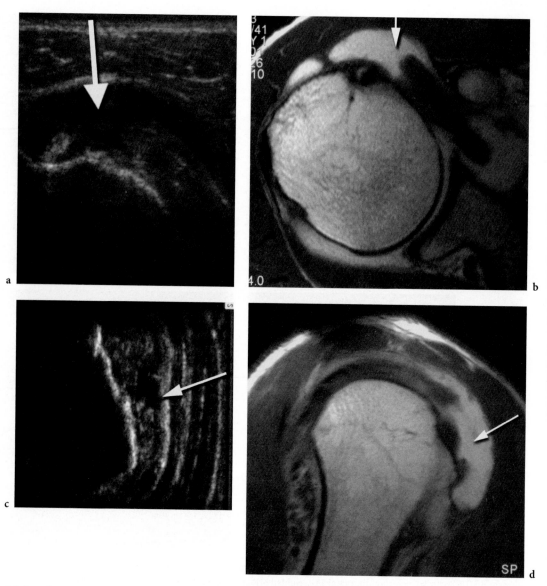

Fig. 5.16a–d. Subtotal tear of the subscapularis (SSC) tendon. **a** The transverse ultrasound scan along the fibers of the SSC demonstrates a large defect at the insertion of the SSC tendon. **b** Corresponding axial T1-weighted MR arthrogram demonstrates a beautiful correlation of the SSC tear visible on the ultrasound image. **c** A parasagittal ultrasound scan perpendicular to the fibers of the SSC tendon also demonstrate the defect in the SSC tendon. **d** Corresponding parasagittal T1-weighted MR arthrogram shows again a beautiful correlation of the SSC tear visible on the ultrasound image

laris tears. These secondary abnormalities include: fluid collections in the subacromial subdeltoid bursa or in the glenohumeral joint, or biceps tendon medial displacement. However, only medial displacement of the biceps tendon is a specific sign for subscapularis abnormality.

A subscapularis tendon should more likely be considered when the patient has reported an injury since anteriorly located rotator cuff lesions (subscapularis) are more commonly associated with trauma than posteriorly located ones (infraspinatus) (NOVÉ-JOSSERAND et al. 1997; ZANETTI et al. 1999b).

5.3.4
Subacromial/Subdeltoid Bursa

Depending on the resolution of the transducer even very small amounts of fluid or synovial proliferation are visible as a hypoechoic line between two hyperechoic stripes formed by peribursal fat and other peribursal structures. Fluid collections may become more conspicuous during provocation maneuvers such as forward or lateral flexion of the arm because fluid will not easily enter the compressed subacromial space and is collected close to the acromion. In fibrinous bursitis motion between the superficial and deep layer of the peribursal tissue planes is no longer harmonic but may be intermittently interrupted. Occasionally, the deltoid may present with internal hyperechoic septations. When such septa are close to the bursa the hypoechoic part of the deltoid muscle between the septum and the bursa may mimic a thickened bursa. This pitfall can be avoided by following the structures laterally (the deltoid septum will be lost within the deltoid muscle, the true bursa will follow a course underneath the deltoid and finally end at the proximal humerus).

Power Doppler ultrasound may help to distinguish between inflammatory and infectious fluid collections in the subacromial bursa from those that are non-inflammatory. In general, hyperemia detected by power Doppler ultrasound around fluid collections in the musculoskeletal system is associated with inflammatory or infectious disease (BREIDAHL et al. 1996, 1998). Effusions associated with degenerative lesions do not usually demonstrate hyperemia. Unfortunately, in shoulder abnormalities exceptions from this rule have also been reported. Increased perfusion has been shown, in relation to rotator cuff arthropathy, that the clinical importance of hyperemia detected with power Doppler ultrasound in the shoulder remains unclear (BREIDAHL et al. 1996, 1998).

5.3.5
Differentiation Between Chronic (Degenerative) and Acute (Posttraumatic) Lesions

Most rotator cuff lesions are thought to relate to chronic tendon degeneration. Impingement underneath the acromial arch, attrition and ischemia are considered to be possible causes of tendon failures (COFIELD 1985). In a minority of patients acute tears may be caused by trauma. The differentiation between patients with acute traumatic lesions and those with chronic lesions is of major importance in the case of insurance queries. Imaging findings in patients with acute traumatic lesions are occasionally characteristic. FARIN et al. found a so-called "defect tear pattern" with separated ends of the ruptured tendon (FARIN and JAROMA 1995) in acute injury. Focal thinning of

the rotator cuff indicating a full-thickness tear was less commonly found by this author in acute tears. In some cases the convexity of the cuff is preserved in full-thickness tears because the gap is filled by hematoma (FARIN and JAROMA 1995). IANNOTTI (1991) found different configurations in acute and chronic tendon tears. Transverse or L-shaped defects were detected in acute tears, and oval or triangular defects in chronic tears, respectively.

TEEFEY et al. (2000b) also identified differences between acute and chronic rotator cuff lesions. A mid-substance location and the presence of joint or bursal fluid were more commonly associated with an acute tear. On the other hand, a non-visualized cuff due to a massive tear and the absence of joint and bursal fluid were more commonly observed with a chronic tear.

The assessment of the rotator cuff muscle quality can also be used for differentiating between acute and chronic lesions. Clinical and experimental studies have demonstrated that rotator cuff tears result in muscle atrophy (BJORKENHEIM 1989; GOUTALLIER et al. 1994). In an experimental study with rabbits, fatty infiltration and atrophy of the supraspinatus muscle have been shown as early as 4 weeks after detachment of the tendon from the osseous insertion (BJORKENHEIM 1989). However, the assessment of the muscle quality with ultrasound is critical. Fatty tissue and muscle tissue have similar appearances on ultrasound images (Figs. 5.17, 5.18). Possibly, a dedicated ultrasound examination for the assessment of the rotator cuff would enable differentiation between normal and fatty degenerated muscle. REIMERS et al. (1993) (REIMERS and FINKENSTAEDT 1997) have shown that ultrasound is useful in the assessment of various muscle diseases. However, contrary to CT and MRI there are no reports of assessment of the rotator cuff muscles with ultrasound (GOUTALLIER et al. 1994; ZANETTI et al. 1998). Moreover, CT and MRI allow a quantitative assessment of the rotator cuff muscles. The classification of GOUTALIER et al. (1994) is frequently used among orthopedic shoulder surgeons. Grade 1 is characterized by some fatty streaks, grade 2 by substantial fatty streaks but still more muscle tissue than fatty tissue, grade 3 by an equal amount of fat and muscle, and grade 4 by fatty degeneration with more fat than muscle. A recent study has demonstrated that the CT classification suggested by GOUTALIER et al. (1994) can be also administered on MR images (FUCHS et al. 1999). So far, it is unknown if ultrasound is also capable of assessing muscle atrophy.

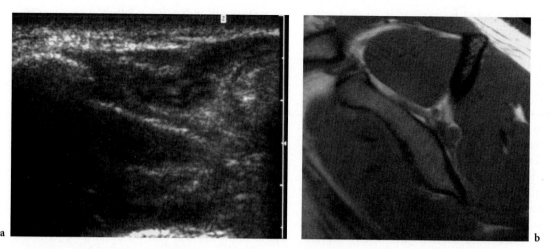

Fig. 5.17a, b. Normal supraspinatus (SSP) muscle. **a** Transverse ultrasound scan through the SSP muscle between spina scapulae and the cranial border of the scapulae is demonstrated. **b** Corresponding parasagittal MR image demonstrates much better the normal SSP muscle

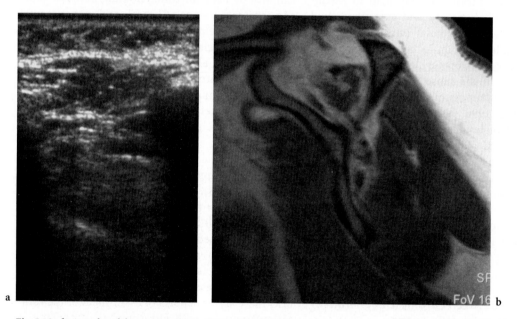

Fig. 5.18a, b. Atrophy of the supraspinatus (SSP) muscle. **a** On transverse ultrasound scan the atrophy of the SSP muscle is hardly visible. **b** On the corresponding parasagittal T1-weighted MR scan the atrophy of the SSP is conspicuous

In our experience, non-displaced fractures of the greater tuberosity and subscapularis tendon tears are not uncommonly encountered in patients where an acute rupture of the rotator cuff is suspected. Greater tuberosity fractures are especially commonly seen in younger patients aged under 40 years. In these patients, non-displaced fractures should be looked for specifically when ultrasound is performed for suspected acute rupture of the rotator cuff (ZANETTI et al. 1999b). Ultrasound is capable of revealing non-displaced fractures of the greater tuberosity (Fig. 5.19) (PATTEN et al. 1992). However, the ultrasound findings of cortical irregularity and discontinuity of the humeral head are not 100% specific. Cortical irregularity of the greater tuberosity is not uncommon in degenerative disease.

5.3.6
Instability

Posterocranial impression fractures of the humeral head (Hill-Sachs lesions) can be easily demonstrated

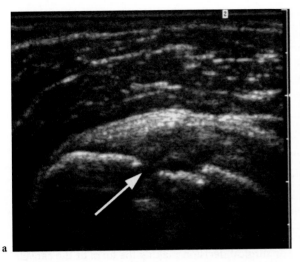
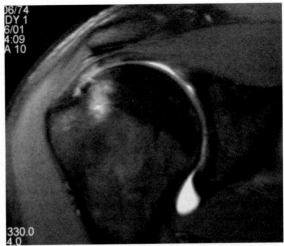

a

b

Fig. 5.19a, b. Greater tuberosity fracture. a Longitudinal ultrasound scan of the supraspinatus tendon demonstrates contour irregularity compatible with fracture. b Corresponding T2-weighted MR arthrogram confirms the greater tuberosity fracture

with ultrasound (CICAK et al. 1998; HAMMAR et al. 2001). The depiction of labral tears is more difficult. In the literature specific criteria have been suggested. HAMMAR et al. (2001) used the following criteria for a labral tear: Hypoechoic zone, larger than 2 mm at the base of the labrum, vacuum phenomenon between the glenoid and labrum, absence of the labrum, or movement of the labrum when dynamic examination is performed. The criterion for a degenerated labrum was a small anterior labrum, with an altered configuration, that was smaller than the ipsilateral posterior labrum and smaller than the anterior labrum on the normal side.

5.4
Accuracies and Clinical Role in Abnormalities of the Rotator Cuff and Biceps Tendon Abnormalities

The accuracy of ultrasound in rotator cuff abnormalities is operator-dependent. The learning curve is steep. However, accepting these limitations, an adequate accuracy can be achieved with dedicated ultrasound technique as outlined above. Recent reports on the accuracy of ultrasound in rotator cuff abnormality note constantly high values for full thickness-tears (Table 5.1). There is no consensus on the accuracy of partial-thickness tears. Although ultrasound has several potential advantages compared to MRI it has not gained universal acceptance by radiologists and ortho-

pedic surgeons in preoperative evaluation of rotator cuff abnormalities. Contrary to MRI (BLANCHARD et al. 1997; ZANETTI et al. 1999a), ultrasound has not yet demonstrated that it influences the clinician's diagnostic certainty and treatment concept. It is intriguing to note that the clinical examination is very reliable in the diagnosis of full-thickness tears of the supraspinatus. A sensitivity of up to 91% and a specificity of between 75% and 89% have been recorded for clinical examinations (HERMANN and ROSE 1996; LYONS and TOMLINSON 1992). In this situation it is difficult for every imaging test to compete with the clinical examination. Further studies should demonstrate that ultrasound can still influence the clinician concerning diagnostic thinking and therapeutic procedures as it has been performed for standard MRI and MR arthrography (BLANCHARD et al. 1997; ZANETTI et al. 1999a). MRI led to a change in management in 44 (62%) of the 71 patients in one study (BLANCHARD et al. 1997). Changes of therapeutic decision after MR arthrography were noted in 36 of the 73 patients (49%) in another study (ZANETTI et al. 1999a). In our institution orthopedic surgeons prefer MRI to ultrasound because it enables a reliable assessment of muscle atrophy and fatty degeneration which is associated with rotator cuff lesions (ZANETTI et al. 1998). Based on orthopedic publications, atrophy and fatty infiltration are important for the outcome after rotator cuff repair (GOUTALLIER et al. 1994). This may be explained by the fact that repair of the ruptured tendon has no effect when sufficient muscle function is lacking. The lack of reliable muscle information is probably the larg-

Table 5.1. Diagnostic accuracy of ultrasound in rotator cuff lesions

		Sensitivity	Specificity	Literature
Rotator cuff	Full-thickness	100	97	READ and PERKO (1998)
		90	100	FARIN et al. (1996)
		81	94	SWEN et al. (1999)
		100	85	TEEFEY et al. (2000a)
	Partial- or full-thickness	86	91	VAN MOPPES et al. (1995)
	Partial-thickness	46	97	READ and PERKO (1998)
		93	94	VAN HOLSBEECK et al. (1995)
		67	85	TEEFEY et al. (2000a)
		80	98	FARIN et al. (1996)
	Subscapularis	82	100	FARIN and JAROMA (1996)
Biceps tendon	Tendinitis	80	95	READ and PERKO (1998)
	Rupture	75	95	READ and PERKO (1998)
		64	88	Teefey et al. (2000a)

est drawback of ultrasound compared to MRI in the assessment of the rotator cuff.

5.5
Role in Instability

In our experience, the quality of labral images obtained with ultrasound is limited, presumably due to the location of this structure deep beneath the body surface. Moreover, the coracoid process may obscure parts of the labrum. Nevertheless, extremely high accuracy for labral tears has been reported in the ultrasound literature with a sensitivity of up to 98% and a specificity of up to 92% (WITTNER and HOLZ 1996; HAMMAR et al. 2001). However, we prefer not to use ultrasound for the assessment of soft tissue lesions associated with instability. Even if reasonable images of the labrum are obtained the clinical value of any findings remains questionable. The normal labrum is highly variable, a fact which has been demonstrated in several studies using CT or MRI in asymptomatic volunteers (CHANDNANI et al. 1992; McNIESH and CALLAGHAN 1987) or in arthroscopically normal labrum parts (ZANETTI et al. 2001). On MR arthrograms, only 121 of 241 (50%) arthroscopically normal labral parts demonstrated normal (low) signal intensity and normal form. Increased linear or globular signal intensity was present in 74 of 241 (31%) normal labral parts, deformed or fragmented labra in 28 (12%), complete separation of the labrum from the glenoid in four (2%), a cleft in five (2%), attenuation in four (2%), and complete absence in five (2%), respectively. These data underline the general problems in assessing the glenoid labrum. Many described abnormalities detected by imaging may represent possibly not the same importance to the orthopedic surgeon.

For surgical decision making the form of the capsule and the glenohumeral ligaments, most importantly the inferior glenohumeral ligament, and glenoid rim fractures may be far more relevant than labral lesions (PALMER et al. 1994).

5.6
Role in Various Abnormalities

5.6.1
Infection

Ultrasound is a useful tool in the management of septic arthritis (MNIF et al. 1997). The early detection of joint effusion is crucial. A negative result concerning joint effusion is a strong indicator for absence of septic arthritis. Joint effusion is easily visible within the tendon sheath of the long biceps tendon. Joint effusion should be looked for also in the anterior or posterior recess of the glenohumeral joint. Joint effusion is a sensitive sign but not specific for infection. The thickness of synovial and joint capsule is also not specific of septic arthritis. More specific for septic arthritis is the presence of a hyperechoic or mixed aspect of the fluid joint. The ultrasound examination allows a one-step investigation in the management of septic arthritis. When a localized fluid collection is seen aspiration for microbacterial analysis can be performed under ultrasound guidance. When the ultrasound result is negative but the clinical suspicion is nevertheless high a glenohumeral joint puncture can be performed under ultrasound guidance. However, in such situations we prefer to perform aspiration from the glenohumeral joint under fluoroscopy due to the more sterile conditions.

Table 5.2. Ultrasound indications at the shoulder

Abnormality	Established indications	Some experiences reported	Not recommended or no reported experiences in the literature
Tendon lesion rotator cuff	×		
Muscle degeneration rotator cuff			×
Biceps tendon lesion	×		
Subdeltoid bursitis	×		
Fracture		×	
Labrum lesion		×	×
Ligament lesion			×
Rheumatoid arthritis		×	
Ganglion		×	
Soft tissue tumor		×	
Infection		×	

5.6.2
Soft Tissue Swelling

Ultrasound can be used initially to assess soft tissue swelling. Differentiation between localized or diffuse soft tissue lesions narrows the differential diagnosis. Moreover, ultrasound is able to differentiate between cystic and solid lesion. However, the characteristic of echogenicity of a cystic lesion with absence of any echoes may be atypical. Occasionally, a fluid-containing cyst may be relatively bright on ultrasound images. This is typically found in acute hematoma, e.g. after surgery or in septic abscess. Aspiration should be performed when fluid is suspected within a lesion.

When a solid soft tissue lesion is detected during ultrasound, a subsequent MR examination is usually required to plan surgical resection. However, there are notable exceptions where ultrasound may obviate further imaging (SINTZOFF et al. 1992). Usually, no further imaging is required when a benign subcutaneous lipoma is detected. A subcutaneous lipoma may present as a smoothly delineated mass with iso- or hyperechogenic striated structures. Typically, lipomas are elongated, with their greatest diameter parallel to the skin (FORNAGE and TASSIN 1991). Foreign bodies may also demonstrate a characteristic ultrasound image.

5.6.3
Ganglion Cyst

Ganglion cysts are most commonly found in association with labrum lesions, especially with superior labrum anterior posterior (SLAP) lesions (LEITSCHUH et al. 1999). Ganglion cysts originating from the posterocranial labrum may compress the suprascapular nerve (LEVY et al. 1997). These patients may have non-specific pain, weakness, and atrophy of the spinatus musculature.

Decompression of the suprascapular nerve can be performed by ultrasound guided aspiration (LEITSCHUH et al. 1999).

References

Bjorkenheim JM (1989) Structure and function of the rabbit's supraspinatus muscle after resection of its tendon. Acta Orthop Scand 60:461–463

Blanchard TK, Mackenzie R, Bearcroft PW, Sinnatamby R, Gray A, Lomas DJ, Constant CR, Dixon AK. (1997) Magnetic resonance imaging of the shoulder: assessment of effectiveness. Clin Radiol 52:363–368

Breidahl WH, Newman JS, Taljanovic MS, Adler RS (1996) Power Doppler sonography in the assessment of musculoskeletal fluid collections. AJR 166:1443–1446

Breidahl WH, Stafford Johnson DB, Newman JS, Adler RS (1998) Power Doppler sonography in tenosynovitis: significance of the peritendinous hypoechoic rim. J Ultrasound Med 17:103–107

Bretzke CA, Crass JR, Craig EV, Feinberg SB (1985) Ultrasonography of the rotator cuff. Normal and pathologic anatomy. Invest Radiol 20:311–315

Chandnani V, Ho C, Gerharter J, Neumann C, Kursunoglu-Brahme S, Sartoris DJ, Resnick D (1992) MR findings in asymptomatic shoulders: a blind analysis using symptomatic shoulders as controls. Clin Imaging 16:25–30

Cicak N, Bilic R, Delimar D (1998) Hill-Sachs lesion in recurrent shoulder dislocation: sonographic detection. J Ultrasound Med 17:557–560

Cofield RH (1985) Rotator cuff disease of the shoulder. J Bone Joint Surg Am 67-A:974–979

Delorme S, van Kaick G (1996) Cui bono? Comments on cost-benefit analysis in ultrasound diagnosis. Radiologe 36:285–291

Farin PU (1996) Sonography of the biceps tendon of the shoulder: normal and pathologic findings. J Clin Ultrasound 24:309–316

Farin PU, Jaroma H (1995) Acute traumatic tears of the rotator cuff: value of sonography. Radiology 197:269–273

Farin PU, Jaroma H (1996) Sonographic detection of tears of the anterior portion of the rotator cuff (subscapularis tendon tears). J Ultrasound Med 15:221–225

Farin PU, Kaukanen E, Jaroma H, Vaatainen U, Miettinen H, Soimakallio S (1996) Site and size of rotator-cuff tear. Findings at ultrasound, double-contrast arthrography, and computed tomography arthrography with surgical correlation. Invest Radiol 31:387–394

Fornage BD, Tassin GB (1991) Sonographic appearances of superficial soft tissue lipomas. J Clin Ultrasound 19:215–220

Fuchs B, Weishaupt D, Zanetti M, Hodler J, Gerber C (1999) Fatty degeneration of the muscles of the rotator cuff: assessment by computed tomography versus magnetic resonance imaging. J Shoulder Elbow Surg 8:599–605

Goutallier D, Postel JM, Bernageau J, Lavau L, Voisin MC (1994) Fatty muscle degeneration in cuff ruptures. Pre- and postoperative evaluation by CT scan. Clin Orthop Relat Res 304:78–83

Hammar MV, Wintzell GB, Astrom KG, Larsson S, Elvin A (2001) Role of US in the preoperative evaluation of patients with anterior shoulder instability. Radiology 219:29–34

Hermann B, Rose DW (1996) Value of anamnesis and clinical examination in degenerative impingement syndrome in comparison with surgical findings – a prospective study. Z Orthop 134:166–170

Hollister MS, Mack LA, Patten RM, Winter TC III, Matsen FA III, Veith RR (1995) Association of sonographically detected subacromial/subdeltoid bursal effusion and intraarticular fluid with rotator cuff tear. AJR 165:605–608

Iannotti JP (1991) Rotator cuff disorders: evaluation and treatment. American Academy of Orthopedic Surgeons, Rosemount, IL

Leitschuh PH, Bone CM, Bouska WM (1999) Magnetic resonance imaging diagnosis, sonographically directed percutaneous aspiration, and arthroscopic treatment of a painful shoulder ganglion cyst associated with a SLAP lesion. Arthroscopy 15:85–87

Levy P, Roger B, Tardieu M, Ghebontni L, Thelen P, Richard O, Grenier P (1997) Cystic compression of the suprascapular nerve. Value of imaging. Apropos of 6 cases and review of the literature. J Radiol 78:123–130

Lyons AR, Tomlinson JE (1992) Clinical diagnosis of tears of the rotator cuff. J Bone Joint Surg 74-B:414–415

Magarelli N, Guglielmi G, Di Matteo L, Tartaro A, Mattei PA, Bonomo L (2001) Diagnostic utility of an echo-contrast agent in patients with synovitis using power Doppler ultrasound: a preliminary study with comparison to contrast-enhanced MRI. Eur Radiol 11:1039–1046

McNiesh LM, Callaghan JJ (1987) CT arthrography of the shoulder: variations of the glenoid labrum. AJR 149:963–966

Middleton WD, Reinus WR, Melson GL, Totty WG, Murphy WA (1986a) Pitfalls of rotator cuff sonography. AJR Am J Roentgenol 146:555–560

Middleton WD, Reinus WR, Totty WG, Melson CL, Murphy WA (1986b) Ultrasonographic evaluation of the rotator cuff and biceps tendon. J Bone Joint Surg Am 68:440–450

Mnif J, Khannous M, Keskes H, Louati N, Damak J, Kechaou MS (1997) Ultrasonography in the diagnostic approach of

septic arthritis. Rev Chir Orthop Reparatrice Appar Mot 83:148–155

Newman JS, Adler RS, Bude RO, Rubin JM (1994) Detection of soft-tissue hyperemia: value of power Doppler sonography. AJR 163:385–389

Nové-Josserand L, Gerber C, Walch G (1997) Lesions of the antero-superior rotator cuff. Lippincott-Raven, Philadelphia

Palmer WE, Brown JH, Rosenthal DI (1994) Labral-ligamentous complex of the shoulder: evaluation with MR arthrography. Radiology 190:645–651

Patten RM, Mack LA, Wang KY, Lingel J (1992) Nondisplaced fractures of the greater tuberosity of the humerus: sonographic detection. Radiology 182:201–204

Ptasznik R, Hennessy O (1995) Abnormalities of the biceps tendon of the shoulder: sonographic findings. AJR 164:409–414

Read JW, Perko M (1998) Shoulder ultrasound: diagnostic accuracy for impingement syndrome, rotator cuff tear, and biceps tendon pathology. J Shoulder Elbow Surg 7:264–271

Reimers CD, Finkenstaedt M (1997) Muscle imaging in inflammatory myopathies. Curr Opin Rheumatol 9:475–485

Reimers CD, Fleckenstein JL, Witt TN, Muller-Felber W, Pongratz DE (1993) Muscular ultrasound in idiopathic inflammatory myopathies of adults. J Neurol Sci 116:82–92

Seibold CJ, Mallisee TA, Erickson SJ, Boynton MD, Raasch WG, Timins ME (1999) Rotator cuff: evaluation with US and MR imaging. Radiographics 19:685–705

Shapiro RS, Wagreich J, Parsons RB, Stancato-Pasik A, Yeh HC, Lao R (1998) Tissue harmonic imaging sonography: evaluation of image quality compared with conventional sonography. AJR 171:1203–1206

Sintzoff SA Jr, Gillard I, van Gansbeke D, Gevenois PA, Salmon I, Struyven J (1992) Ultrasound evaluation of soft tissue tumors. J Belge Radiol 75:276–280

Swen WA, Jacobs JW, Algra PR, Manoliu RA, Rijkmans J, Willems WJ, Bijlsma JW (1999) Sonography and magnetic resonance imaging equivalent for the assessment of full-thickness rotator cuff tears. Arthritis Rheum 42:2231–2238

Tanaka S, Oshikawa O, Sasaki T, Ioka T, Tsukuma H (2000) Evaluation of tissue harmonic imaging for the diagnosis of focal liver lesions (in process citation). Ultrasound Med Biol 26:183–187

Teefey SA, Middleton WD, Yamaguchi K (1999) Shoulder sonography. State of the art. Radiol Clin North Am 37:767–785, ix

Teefey SA, Hasan SA, Middleton WD, Patel M, Wright RW, Yamaguchi K (2000a) Ultrasonography of the rotator cuff. A comparison of ultrasonographic and arthroscopic findings in one hundred consecutive cases. J Bone Joint Surg Am 82:498–504

Teefey SA, Middleton WD, Bauer GS, Hildebolt CF, Yamaguchi K (2000b) Sonographic differences in the appearance of acute and chronic full-thickness rotator cuff tears. J Ultrasound Med 19:377–378; quiz 383

Tranquart F, Grenier N, Eder V, Pourcelot L (1999) Clinical use of ultrasound tissue harmonic imaging. Ultrasound Med Biol 25:889–894

van Holsbeeck MT, Kolowich PA, Eyler WR, Craig JG, Shirazi KK, Habra GK, Vanderschueren GM, Bouffard JA (1995) US depiction of partial-thickness tear of the rotator cuff. Radiology 197:443–446

van Moppes FI, Veldkamp O, Roorda J (1995) Role of shoulder ultrasonography in the evaluation of the painful shoulder. Eur J Radiol 19:142–146

Weishaupt D, Zanetti M, Tanner A, Gerber C, Hodler J (1999) Lesions of the reflection pulley of the long biceps tendon. MR arthrographic findings. Invest Radiol 34:463–469

Wittner B, Holz U (1996) Ultrasound imaging of the ventrocaudal labrum in ventral instability of the shoulder. Unfallchirurg 99:38–42

Zanetti M, Gerber C, Hodler J (1998) Quantitative assessment of the muscles of the rotator cuff with MR imaging. Invest Radiol 33:163–170

Zanetti M, Jost B, Lustenberger A, Hodler J (1999a) Clinical impact of MR arthrography of the shoulder. Acta Radiol 40:296–302

Zanetti M, Weishaupt D, Jost B, Gerber C, Hodler J (1999b) MR imaging for traumatic tears of the rotator cuff: high prevalence of greater tuberosity fractures and subscapularis tendon tears. AJR 172:463–467

Zanetti M, Carstensen T, Weishaupt D, Jost B, Hodler J (2001) MR arthrographic variability of the arthroscopically normal glenoid labrum: qualitative and quantitative assessment. Eur Radiol 11:559–566

6 Interventional Procedures

H. Yoshioka, B. Wollman, P. Lang

CONTENTS

6.1
Introduction

Many interventional techniques of the shoulder require imaging guidance by X-ray fluoroscopy, computed tomography (CT), and ultrasound. In more recent studies, magnetic resonance imaging (MRI) has been proposed as a promising method. This chapter will consider those imaging techniques, in particular MRI, and clinical applications including distention arthrography for frozen shoulder, aspiration for calcific tendinitis, and aspiration of cystic lesions. The technique of bone and soft tissue tumor biopsy and abscess drainage is not specific to the shoulder, and not discussed here.

6.2
Hardware, Needles

The needle approach to the shoulder using conventional X-ray fluoroscopy has been widely published. The needle tip is easily controlled with fluoroscopic guidance. The X-ray beam can be tilted to confirm the needle tip location (Normandin et al. 1988). Biplane

H. Yoshioka, MD; P. Lang, MD, MBA
Department of Radiology, Brigham and Women's Hospital, 75 Francis Street, ASB I, Floor L1, Room 003E, Boston, MA 02115, USA
B. Wollman, MD
Department of Radiology, Stanford University, California, USA

fluoroscopy may be more comfortable for checking the needle position. A CT-guided procedure may be another option. The patient lies on the CT table and the point of skin puncture is decided in conjunction with metallic indicators on the skin and positioning lights of the gantry. CT fluoroscopy may be available using spiral CT. The principal advantage of CT is better soft tissue contrast than fluoroscopy. However, a vertical approach to the shoulder with a long needle may be difficult because of the limited size of the gantry opening. The combination of fluoroscopy and CT guidance has also been introduced. The common disadvantage of X-ray fluoroscopy and CT is patient exposure to ionizing radiation during the intervention procedure.

With ultrasound there is no ionizing irradiation and it has the advantage of real-time imaging capabilities. Ultrasound is also cost-effective. A high-resolution transducer (7.5 MHz) is preferable to provide a high resolution image of the shoulder lesions. However, determining the site of skin puncture using ultrasound is limited, and the contrast of ultrasound is inferior to that of CT and MRI. Technical difficulties may also be encountered in obese patients.

MRI has been introduced as a promising tool for shoulder interventions (Schenck et al. 1995; Beaulieu et al. 1999; Penner 1998). The open magnet technology and real-time imaging sequences are mandatory for interventional MRI. There are two types of open magnet MRI: vertically and horizontally open magnets. The vertically open MRI system (Signa SP; GE Medical Systems, Milwaukee, Wisconsin) allows radiologists and surgeons direct vertical access to the patient through an opening, with near real-time imaging. The Signa SP system is a whole-body scanner operating with a 0.5 T superconducting magnet with a 58-cm vertical gap and 60-cm patient bore actively shielded gradients. The flexible RF coil with sterile covers is placed on the patient shoulder when an intervention is performed (Fig. 6.1). MR compatible needles, catheters, and surgical supplies (drapes, disposable procedure

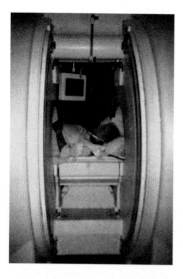

Fig. 6.1. The vertically open MRI system. The flexible radio-frequency coil is placed on the patient's shoulder when the intervention is performed. The liquid crystal display monitor inside the gap provides MR images during procedures

trays, etc.) should be prepared prior to the intervention. Stainless steel or titanium alloy needles are acceptable, due to their limited artifact. The liquid crystal display monitor inside the gap displays MR images during procedures. Fast imaging sequences like steady-state gradient-echo sequences are chosen to provide higher signal-to-noise ratio images, and better discrimination of lesions from adjacent structures. The near real-time reconstruction also allows arthrographic injection during MR fluoroscopy (Fig. 6.2).

The ideal skin entry point can be determined with a "finger pointing technique." With this approach, the radiologist pushes the skin with his fingertip to mimic needle insertion, and MR images are scanned with a couple of contiguous sections using fast sequences. The point of skin puncture is easily identified from MR images of the fingertip and the skin dimpling. The low field horizontally open MRI (0.2–0.35 T) is used for a variety of interventional procedures, because of its wide openness and patient comfort, but it limits intervention capabilities for the shoulder, as the horizontal opening generally extends only 35–45 cm. Thus, vertical access from above the patient is not possible in this configuration.

MRI has several advantages over other equipment for interventional guidance: MRI does not expose patients, radiologists, or surgeons to ionizing radiation; it provides excellent soft tissue contrast; has multiplanar imaging capability; and provides real-time or near real-time imaging capability.

6.3
Clinical Applications

Three clinical entities are currently treatable via interventional radiologic techniques: frozen shoulder syndrome (adhesive capsulitis), calcific tendinitis, and cystic lesions about the shoulder. The following is a brief discussion of the disease processes, followed by a description of the techniques, as well as a review of therapeutic outcomes.

6.3.1
Frozen Shoulder Syndrome

Frozen shoulder syndrome, also known as adhesive capsulitis, was first described in 1872 by DUPLAY. This disease progresses in three stages: a painful period of weeks to months, followed by several months of stiffness, after which spontaneous gradual resolution occurs with variable degrees of residual functional restriction. A multitude of therapies have been studied, but the self-limiting nature of the disease makes evaluation difficult. For example, BULGEN et al. (1984) reported no long-term differences in outcomes between intraarticular steroids, physical therapy, ice therapy, or no treatment at all. However, for this clinical entity the focus of a particular therapeutic modality should be to palliate the months of potentially disabling stiffness.

As the period of decreased range of motion is associated with a dramatic decrease in glenohumeral joint capacity – usually only a few cc (PARLIER-CUAU et al. 1998) – it is not surprising that distention of the joint during arthrography has emerged as a therapeutic modality, first described in 1965 by ANDRÉN and LUNDBERG. In the supine position on the fluoroscopy table, the patient holds the palm up in order to keep the shoulder in external rotation. The skin is then prepared, draped and anesthetized in the usual fashion and, under fluoroscopic guidance, a 20-gauge needle is advanced into the anterior glenohumeral joint. Injection of contrast confirms appropriate positioning within the joint space. The joint is subsequently distended with 20–40 cc of fluid, during which the patient is expected to have increased pain. Composition of the fluid depends on physician preference and a variety of protocols have been proposed. Generally, 15–30 cc of normal saline or water soluble contrast, either mixed with or injected after 5–10 cc of corticosteroids and local anesthetic, would be reasonable (PARLIER-CUAU et al. 1998; RIZK et al. 1994; ELKUND and RYDELL 1992). Even air has been used as a distending agent instead of saline or contrast

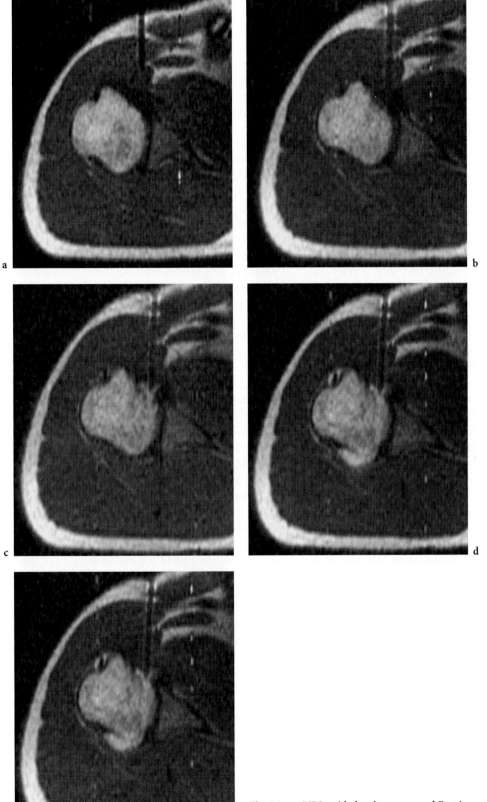

Fig. 6.2a–e. MRI-guided arthroscopy. **a–d** Fast image sequence allows radiologists to confirm the needle tip location in real time. **e** Three-point Dixon spin-echo image shows successful MR arthroscopy

(Jacobs et al. 1991; Mulcahy et al. 1994). The desired result is also variable; while some consider capsular rupture to be essential to the procedure (Andrén and Lundberg 1965; Rizk et al. 1994; Mulcahy et al. 1994), others view this as counter-productive and attempt to cause maximal distention without extravasation (Parlier-Cuau et al. 1998). Regardless, after the procedure the patient is encouraged to continue physical therapy and the appropriate exercises.

Most of the studies regarding outcomes of distention arthrography for frozen shoulder have been noncontrolled trials. A review of those papers describing similar procedures (fluid distention) with comparable endpoints, i.e., pain at varying follow-up intervals, is presented in Table 6.1. In general, the percentage of patients reporting complete or near-complete resolution of pain was 78% after 2 weeks, 88% after 4–6 weeks, 94% at 6 months and 95% 1 year after the procedure (Parlier-Cuau et al. 1998; Rizk et al. 1994; Elkund and Rydell 1992; Sharma et al. 1993). Laroche et al. (1998) quantified 40 patients' pain and range of motion and found statistically significant improvements in both parameters when comparing measurements from pre-procedure and 5 days afterwards. Further improvement was also noted in pain and range of motion comparing day five to day 30. Mulcahy et al. (1994) noted that while 73% of patients without rotator cuff tears had decreased pain after intra-articular steroids and air distention, this was the case in only 56% of those with cuff tears and 19% of these individuals actually had increased pain.

Two studies have compared distention arthrography with intra-articular corticosteroid injection only. The first, by Jacobs et al. (1991) evaluated quantitative range of motion 16 weeks after therapy. Both steroid injection and steroids with distention had statistically significantly greater improvements when compared to distention alone. Distention with steroids also resulted in an increased range of motion in all movements measured, compared to steroids alone. While these differences were not statistically significant, to dismiss

the value of the better results with distention would be incorrect due to the small number of patients (33 between the two treatment arms) and the relatively low distention volume of only 10 cc (1 cc triamcinolone, 6 cc bupivacaine and 3 cc air). Similarly, a second study (Corbeil et al. 1992) reporting no significant difference between intra-articular steroids only and steroids with distention (20 cc lidocaine) is also highly limited by the small patient population of 45 cases. Statistically speaking, in order to suggest the presence (or lack) of benefit of distention arthrography, a much larger series would be required. Regardless, the likely utility of articular distention is not lost on our clinical colleagues, some of whom have proposed performing the procedure in an office-based setting without image guidance (Fareed and Gallivan 1989).

In terms of complications, the theoretical risks of bleeding or infection certainly exist, but have not been reported. One paper did describe two cases of transient facial flushing after injection of intra-articular steroids (Jacobs et al. 1991), but no adverse effects from joint distention have been described.

6.3.2
Calcific Tendinitis

Calcific tendinitis is a sequela of hydroxyapatite deposition disease and most commonly present in the shoulder. Although the crystals are often asymptomatic, inflammation caused by the presence of calcium may result in this chronically painful syndrome (Fig. 6.3). Surgical excision of the calcific deposits, mostly via arthroscopy today, can be highly effective for symptomatic relief. However, percutaneous treatments via image-guided aspiration have been proposed in order to provide a less invasive alternative.

Clinical selection criteria for percutaneous aspiration of calcific deposits include worsening of pain at night and exacerbation of symptoms with all shoulder movements (Parlier-Cuau et al. 1998). This is to dif-

Table 1. Follow-up outcomes of distention arthrography for frozen shoulder

Reference	Cases (n)	2 Weeks	4–6 Weeks	6 Months	Years
Parlier-Cuau et al. (1998)	30	53% very good; 27% good		80% very good; 10% good	
Rizk et al. (1994)	16	75% better	87% better	87% no pain; 7% tolerable	
Elkund and Rydell (1992)	23		48% no pain; 43% slight pain		71% no pain; 19% slight pain
Sharma et al. (1993)	20				75% no pain; 25% slight pain
Overall lessened symptoms		78%	88%	94%	95%

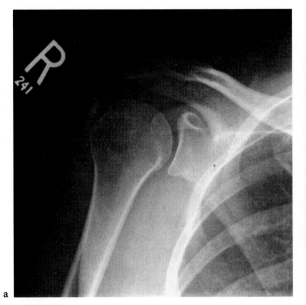

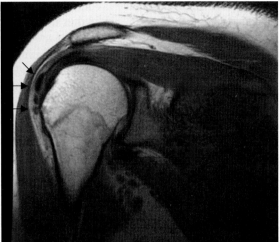

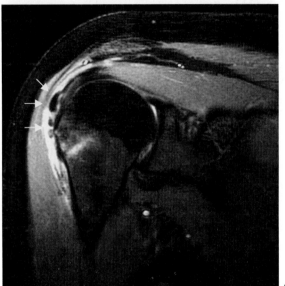

Fig. 6.3. a–c Calcific tendinitis as seen on plain radiograph (**a**), T1-weighted image (**b**), and short tau inversion recovery (STIR) image (**c**). Calcifications show low signal intensity on T1-weighted and STIR images (*arrows*)

ferentiate this disease from pain due to an impingement syndrome (i.e., not the calcific lesions), where absence of night discomfort and a painful arc are more characteristic. Radiographic evaluation of the deposits is also important. Irregular striate radiodensities are usually sequelae of degenerative tendinitis and aspiration is not indicated (PARLIER-CUAU et al. 1998). Recent changes in appearance of the calcific bodies may also warrant deferral of the procedure, as spontaneous resolution may occur, although this is controversial (PARLIER-CUAU et al. 1998; PFISTER and GERBER 1997). While dense, well-defined deposits may be more difficult to aspirate than those with a faint, fuzzy contour, fragmentation with the needle itself may provide similar outcomes.

Two modalities have been utilized for image-guided percutaneous needle aspiration of calcific tendinitis: fluoroscopy and ultrasound.

6.3.2.1
Fluoroscopy

Fluoroscopically-guided needle aspiration in the shoulder was first described in 1978 by COMFORT and ARAFILES. The patient is placed on the fluoroscopy table in the supine position and the skin prepared, draped and anesthetized in the usual fashion. An 18- to 19-gauge needle is then advanced into the anterior aspect of the subacromial space in the direction of the X-ray beam. As desired, the image intensifier can be tilted cranially and caudally to confirm the appropriate position of the needle tip within the calcific deposits. Repeated passes into and out of the lesion can be made in an attempt to cause fragmentation of a harder mass. Using a syringe, normal saline and/or lidocaine is injected into the deposit and then aspirated, with calcific fragments or a milky white fluid being recovered. After a maximal amount is aspirated, many authors inject a few cubic centimeters of corticosteroids, although others disagree with this practice (Parlier-Cuau et al. 1998; Pfister and Gerber 1997; Comfort and Arafiles 1978). One-quarter to one-third of patients may experience actual exacerbation of the pain after the procedure lasting up to a few days, likely due to inflammation induced by the crystals being deposited in adjacent tissues. Patients should be warned accordingly and instructed to use ice packs, non-steroidal anti-inflammatory medications, and analgesics to provide relief.

The seminal paper describing this technique (Comfort and Arafiles 1978) presented a series of nine patients. Post-procedure calcifications had essentially resolved and good to excellent subjective and objective clinical results were observed with about a 9-year mean follow-up in all cases. Pfister and Gerber (1997) reported a prospective series of 62 cases. After the procedure, the area of crystal deposits on radiography was approximately halved on average, with complete resolution in 26%. At a 6-month follow-up, quantified pain was reduced an average of 50%, with 35% of patients having complete relief and an equal number with only mild residual symptoms. Interestingly, clinical outcomes were independent of the pre-procedural appearance of the calcific deposits. The same authors have also published a retrospective questionnaire of 212 patients, which also suggests that long-term prognosis is favorable (Pfister and Gerber 1994). After a median interval of 5 years post-procedure, 60% of individuals were pain-free, another 34% had marked relief, and only 6% had no improvement.

Only one complication was reported in these series: a crystal-induced tenosynovitis of the long head of the biceps muscle (Pfister and Gerber 1997).

6.3.2.2
Ultrasound

Another method of treating symptomatic rotator cuff calcific deposits percutaneously is via ultrasound-guided aspiration, first described in 1995 by Farin et al. (1995) and Bradley et al. (1995). The main advantages of this over the fluoroscopic technique are the lack of radiation dose to patient and physician, as well as being able to examine the rotator cuff tendons.

The patient is placed in the oblique decubitus position and the shoulder prepared, draped and anesthetized in the usual fashion. Depending on the location of the calcifications, optimal positioning may vary. Supraspinatus tendinous deposits are often best identified with the arm in internal rotation. For the subscapularis tendon, slight external rotation may be useful, and positioning the hand on the opposite shoulder with backward extension allows for infraspinatus tendon visualization (Farin et al. 1996).

The calcific deposits are localized using a 7.5 MHz linear transducer; they appear as hyperechoic foci with variable degrees of posterior acoustic shadowing. Under ultrasound guidance, the deposits are punctured with an 18- to 19-gauge needle (often repeatedly to promote disruption). One technique (Bradley et al. 1995) merely entails simple aspiration with a 20-cc syringe to obtain the gritty calcified fragments or milky fluid. A more involved method (Farin et al. 1995) includes placement of a second needle into the area of concern. Through one needle a small amount of normal saline is lavaged into the lesion and subsequently aspirated out of the second. This is repeated until the aspirated fluid is clear.

Bradley et al. (1995) reported the results of the more basic procedure in 11 patients. Complete resolution of calcification was noted in six patients immediately after the procedure, and in all cases by 2 weeks. In terms of pain relief, 55% had complete resolution by 1 week, 91% by 2 weeks and no recurrence occurred on 6-month follow-up. The one case with persistent pain was noted to have had a rotator cuff tear during ultrasound scanning.

Results of the more involved technique have been described for 61 procedures by Farin et al. (1996). A total of 74% of calcifications were noted to decrease in size with complete resolution in 28%. After the initial treatment, 84% had complete or significant improvement in symptoms. Repeat treatments in a few patients increased the percentage with clinical improvement to 90% (74% being totally asymptomatic). The relief was sustained at 1-year follow-up.

No complications were reported with either technique.

6.3.3
Cystic Lesions

Cystic lesions in the shoulder can be symptomatic for reasons such as local mass effect or compressive neuropathy. Since they are generally not visible on radiography, fluoroscopy cannot be utilized for percutaneous drainage, and thus surgical treatment was the standard until relatively recently. With the advent of newer technologies (i.e., CT, ultrasound, and MRI) has come the means for minimally invasive therapies and all of these modalities have been used for cyst treatment.

6.3.3.1
CT

Ironically, although CT-guided procedures are extremely common elsewhere in the body, its use for therapy in the shoulder has been rarely discussed. FRITZ et al. (1992) commented briefly about three patients with spinoglenoid notch cysts in whom CT-guided aspiration was performed. No description of technique was provided and the outcomes presented were limited to the patients being asymptomatic after therapy for at least 2 months, with an average of 6 months follow-up.

6.3.3.2
Ultrasound

Ultrasound provides a therapeutic modality that spares patients the radiation doses associated with CT. As described by CHIOU et al. (1999), the patient is placed in the sitting position and the skin prepared, draped, and anesthetized in the standard fashion. Using a 5- to 7-MHz linear (CHIOU et al. 1999) or 3-MHz sector (HASHIMOTO et al. 1994) transducer, an 18-gauge needle is advanced into the cyst and the contents aspirated. At this point the needle may be removed, although some authors have described performing a cystogram using iodinated contrast or injecting corticosteroids (TUNG et al. 2000).

HASHIMOTO et al. (1994) authored one of the first reports of this procedure, describing three patients with spinoglenoid notch cysts who reported decreased pain lasting for at least 2 months after aspiration. In a larger series of 15 individuals with cystic lesions in a variety of locations about the shoulder (CHIOU et al. 1999), all patients had improved symptoms immediately after the procedure. By 2 months the pain was noted to return in two patients, but overall 86% had marked decrease or complete resolution with mean 6-month follow-up. Four cases of paraglenoid cysts in a separate report (TUNG et al. 2000) did not respond as well, however, as the cysts recurred in 75% of subjects within 4 months. No complications have been reported with this procedure.

6.3.3.3
MRI

Although not commonly utilized currently, MRI is another means for performing image-guided aspiration of cystic lesions. Advantages include better depiction of bony anatomy than ultrasound and superior delineation of soft tissue compared to CT. The following relates the methods and results for the authors' series of five patients with shoulder cysts – four in the spinoglenoid notch and one in the supraspinatus muscle belly.

After providing informed consent, the patients are placed in a 0.5 T vertically open MRI unit. Initial axial supine images of the shoulder are obtained, as well as prone or other planes as needed, primarily using T2-weighted fast spin-echo pulse sequences. Once the optimal needle path is determined, the shoulder is prepared, draped and anesthetized in the usual fashion. Under MR guidance, an 18 or 20-gauge MR-compatible needle is inserted into the lesion (Fig. 6.4). The cyst fluid is then aspirated and 1–2 cc of corticosteroids is injected into the remnant before removal of the needle.

The procedure was technically successful in all five patients, each reporting immediate symptomatic improvement. Follow-up was obtainable in all but one of the patients (mean 6 months, range 2–10 months). Two patients demonstrated suprascapular neuropathy on initial electromyography (EMG), and while one patient had improved findings after therapy, the other did not have significant change and cyst recurrence was later noted in this patient. A follow-up MRI on another patient revealed no evidence of cyst recurrence. No complications were noted.

6.4
Conclusion

In this chapter, interventional procedures for the shoulder were presented, including a description of the techniques and a review of therapeutic outcomes from previous literature. For all of the percutaneous therapeutic procedures described above, there are generally few patients reported, and further data, ideally obtained in a prospective controlled fashion, would be needed to determine if the outcomes are improved over the surgical techniques in the future. Similar data is lacking to allow comparison between the various imaging modalities available to perform these procedures. New equipment, such as real-time CT fluoroscopy and the ability for percutaneous techniques on open magnet MRI, gives the radiologist even more therapeutic options.

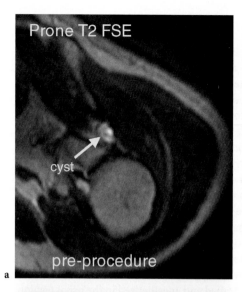
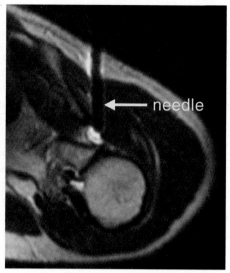
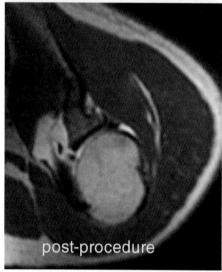

Fig. 6.4a–c. Spinoglenoid notch cyst aspiration under MR guidance. Pre-procedure MR image (**a**), mid-procedure MR image (**b**), and post-procedure MR image (**c**)

References

Andrén L, Lundberg BJ (1965) Treatment of rigid shoulders by joint distention during arthrography. Acta Orthop Scand 36:45–53

Beaulieu CF, Hodge DK, Bergman AG et al. (1999) Glenohumeral relationships during physiologic shoulder motion and stress testing: initial experience with open MR imaging and active imaging-plane registration. Radiology 212: 699–705

Bradley M, Bhamra MS, Robson MJ (1995) Ultrasound guided aspiration of symptomatic supraspinatus calcific deposits. Br J Radiol 68:716–719

Bulgen DY, Binder AI, Hazleman BL, Dutton J, Roberts S (1984) Frozen shoulder: prospective clinical study with an evaluation of three treatment regimens. Ann Rheum Dis 43:353–360

Chiou HJ, Chou YH, Wu JJ et al. (1999) Alternative and effective treatment of shoulder ganglion cyst: ultrasonographically guided aspiration. J Ultrasound Med 18:531–535

Comfort TH, Arafiles RP (1978) Barbotage of the shoulder with image-intensified fluoroscopic control of needle placement for calcific tendinitis. Clin Orthop 135:171–178

Corbeil V, Dussault RG, Leduc BE, Fleury F (1992) Capsulite rétractile de l'épaule: étude comparative de l'arthrographie avec corticothérapie intra-articulaire avec ou sans distension capsulaire. Can Assoc Radiol J 43:127–130

Duplay ES (1872) De la périarthrite scapulo-humérale et des raideurs de l'epaule qui en sont la consequences. Archiv Gen Med 20:513–542

Elkund AL, Rydell N (1992) Combination treatment for adhesive capsulitis of the shoulder. Clin Orthop 282:105–109

Fareed DO, Gallivan WR (1989) Office management of frozen shoulder syndrome: treatment with hydraulic distention under local anesthesia. Clin Orthop 242:177–183

Farin PU, Jaroma H, Soimakallio S (1995) Rotator cuff calcifications: treatment with US-guided technique. Radiology 195:841–843

Farin PU, Räsänen H, Jaroma H, Harju A (1996) Rotator cuff calcifications: treatment with ultrasound-guided percutaneous needle aspiration and lavage. Skeletal Radiol 25: 551–554

Fritz RC, Helms CA, Steinbach LS, Genant HK (1992) Suprascapular nerve entrapment: evaluation with MR imaging. Radiology 182:437–444

Hashimoto BE, Hayes AS, Ager JD (1994) Sonographic diagnosis and treatment of ganglion cysts causing suprascapular nerve entrapment. J Ultrasound Med 13:671–674

Jacobs LGH, Barton MAJ, Wallace WA, Ferrousis J, Dunn NA, Bossingham DH (1991) Intra-articular distention and steroids in the management of capsulitis of the shoulder. BMJ 302:1498–1501

Laroche M, Ighilahriz O, Moulinier L, Constantin A, Cantagrel A, Mazieres B (1998) Adhesive capsulitis of the shoulder: an open study of 40 cases treated by joint distention during arthrography followed by an intraarticular corticosteroid injection and immediate physical therapy. Rev Rhum Engl Ed 65:313–319

Mulcahy KA, Baxter AD, Oni OOA, Finlay D (1994) The value of shoulder distention arthrography with intraarticular injection of steroid and local anaesthetic: a follow-up study. Br J Radiol 67:263–266

Normandin C, Seban E, Laredo JD (1988) Aspiration of tendinous calcific deposits. In: Bard M, Laredo JD (eds) Interventional radiology in bone and joint. Springer, Berlin Heidelberg New York, pp 258–270

Parlier-Cuau C, Champsaur P, Nizard R, Wybier M, Bacque MC, Laredo JD (1998) Percutaneous treatments of painful shoulder. Radiol Clin N Am 36:589–596

Penner EA (1998) Interventional MR with a mid-field open system. In: Debatin JF, Adam G (eds) Interventional magnetic resonance imaging. Springer, Berlin Heidelberg New York, pp 11–18

Pfister J, Gerber H (1994) Behandlung der periarthropathia humero-scapularis calcarea mittels schulterkalkspülung: retrospektive fragebogenanalyse. Z Orthop 132:300–305

Pfister J, Gerber H (1997) Chronic calcifying tendinitis of the shoulder – therapy by percutaneous needle aspiration and lavage: a prospective open study of 62 shoulders. Clin Rheum 16:269–274

Rizk TE, Gavant ML, Pinals RS (1994) Treatment of adhesive capsulitis (frozen shoulder) with arthrographic distention and rupture. Arch Phys Med Rehabil 75:803–807

Schenck JF, Jolesz FA, Roemer PB et al. (1995) Superconducting open-configuration MR imaging system for image-guided therapy. Radiology 195:805–814

Sharma RK, Bajekal RA, Bhan S (1993) Frozen shoulder syndrome: a comparison of hydraulic distention and manipulation. Int Orthop 17:275–278

Tung GA, Entzian D, Stern JB, Green A (2000) MR imaging and MR arthrography of paraglenoid labral cysts. AJR 174: 1707–1715

Clinical Problems

7 Congenital and Developmental Disorders

K. Johnson and A. M. Davies

CONTENTS

7.1
Introduction

The development of the upper limb and shoulder depends not only upon normal skeletal maturation but also neural, vascular, muscular and cartilaginous

K. Johnson, MD
Radiology Department, Birmingham Children's Hospital,
Steelhouse Lane, Birmingham, B4 6NH, UK
A. M. Davies, MD
MRI Centre, Royal Orthopaedic Hospital, Birmingham,
B31 2AP, UK

maturation. As a result abnormalities in any one of these structures can significantly affect surrounding tissue. In addition disorders of the shoulder may be more than just localised anomalies but form part of a wider spectrum of disease such as in skeletal dysplasias and metabolic bone disease. Shoulder development can also be affected by upper arm traction and nerve damage at birth.

In view of this complex intra-relationship of structures, classification of congenital and developmental disorders of the shoulder is difficult. For instance disorders of the scapula may affect the humerus through its articulation at the glenoid and also the musculature of the posterior abdominal wall. In this chapter we have dealt with the disorders primarily on an anatomical basis dealing with each structure in turn. As a result there is an element of repetition. This chapter has concentrated on those shoulder abnormalities that primarily affect upper limb appearance and function. Only those systemic disorders that primarily affect the shoulder or shoulder as the major site have been covered in any detail. The humeral head, clavicle and upper ribs are very common sites for a very large number of congenital disorders but covering these in any detail is beyond the scope of this chapter.

7.2
Birth Injuries

7.2.1
Brachial Plexus Injury in the Newborn

Brachial plexus injury in the newborn is caused by traction on the nerve roots by forced abduction of the arm during delivery and is more common in high birth weight infants and breech deliveries. It results in paralysis of the arm; the muscles involved depend on the nerve roots injured (Greenwald et al. 1984). There are three types of nerve root injury: (1) Erb's palsy where there is damage to the C5/6 nerve roots.

This causes denervation of the deltoid, anterior serratus, biceps and brachioradialis muscles, the classical clinical finding is with the arm held loosely at the side and internally rotated at the shoulder and extended at the elbow, pronation of the forearm and flexion of wrist (headwaiters tip position); (2) Klumpke palsy which is a C8/T1 lesion with denervation of the intrinsic hand and wrist muscles; (3) Erb–Duchenne–Klumpke is caused by denervation of C5–8, T1 and causes paralysis involving the upper limb (HENSINGER 1986). The newborn child who has a brachial plexus paralysis will not move their arm. The differential diagnosis in the neonatal period includes a fractured clavicle, proximal humeral fracture, humeral growth plate injury, humeral dislocation or septic arthritis of the shoulder joint. With a brachial plexus injury the child will allow passive movement of the arm, as it is a painless condition. Radiographs of the upper limb in the acute situation show no evidence of trauma or infection but will demonstrate internal rotation of the humerus. Ultrasound has been used to diagnose separation of the proximal humeral epiphysis in the newborn when there is diagnostic confusion. Ultrasound demonstrates the relationship of the unossified humeral epiphysis with respect to the metaphysis. The fracture in all cases has been classified as a Salter Harris types I or II (BROKER and BURBACH 1990).

The prognosis for uncomplicated brachial plexus injuries is good with over 95% making a full recovery (GREENWALD et al. 1984).

Magnetic resonance imaging (MRI) of the cervical spine is of prognostic value for the clinical outcome in brachial plexus injury. The presence of a pseudomeningocele extending lateral to the spinal cord into the neural foramina, suggests a persisting neurological deficit. Those children expected to have a good clinical recovery will have a normal cervical MRI (Fig. 7.1) (MILLER et al. 1993).

If the paralysis persists there is significant residual shoulder deformity. Radiologically there is hypoplasia of the humeral head, elevation of the scapula with a shallow glenoid fossa and an abnormally developed coracoid and acromion with deformity of the clavicle (Fig. 7.2) (POLLOCK and REED 1989). Abnormalities around the elbow joint have also been described.

Posterior subluxation or dislocation of the shoulder can occur with a brachial plexus injury and may be the result of muscle imbalance or may occur at the same time as the nerve root damage occurs. Posterior dislocation may be difficult to detect clinically and standard radiographs may be unhelpful, as the humeral head will be poorly ossified. Both CT and ultrasound

have been used to diagnose the posterior dislocation (HUNTER et al. 1998).

CT and MRI of the shoulder in children with Erb's palsy demonstrate deformity of the posterior lip with thinning of the posterior cartilage of the glenoid fossa and posterior subluxation of the humeral head (HERNANDEZ and DIAS 1988; GUDINCHET et al. 1995).

7.2.2
Birth Fractures

The clavicle is the most commonly fractured bone during delivery occurring in up to 3.5% of deliveries.

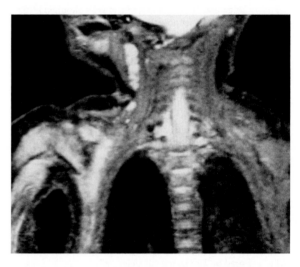

Fig. 7.1. Coronal T2-weighted image of a 2-week-old girl. There is a pseudomeningocele of the cervical 5th and 6th nerve roots on the right. This is demonstrated by the high signal fluid adjacent to the spinal cord. This finding was confirmed at surgery

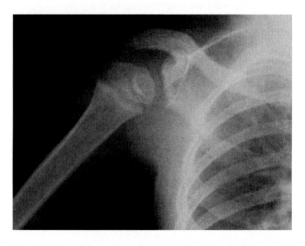

Fig. 7.2. AP radiograph of the right shoulder of a 7-year-old boy who had a brachial plexus injury at birth. The glenoid is shallow and there is an abnormally shaped acromion

The majority of fractures are through the mid-clavicle and are asymptomatic in up to 80% of cases presenting as a painless lump under the skin. Alternatively the child may be irritable or have reduced arm movement. The clinical differential diagnosis will include humeral fracture, brachial plexus injury or septic arthritis. Radiographically the fracture shows a significant periosteal reaction and callus formation. In the majority of cases there is no long-term residual deformity.

Other sites for birth related fractures are the humerus, femur and ribs. These often occur through the diaphysis or at the metaphyseal junction. As the epiphysis is unossified radiological detection of these fractures can be difficult and ultrasound and MRI have been shown to be of value.

Dislocations can occur but are uncommon. Widening of the joint space may be related to dislocation of the shoulder joint, epiphyseal separation or a brachial plexus injury (BANAGLE and KUHNS 1983; BARRETT et al. 1984; DIAZ and HEDLUND 1991; JOSEPH and ROSENFELD 1990).

7.3
Congenital High Scapula
(Sprengel's Shoulder)

The congenitally high scapula was first described by EULENBIG in 1863, 18 years before SPRENGEL in 1891. The high scapula is the result of inadequate caudal movement during the 9th and 12th weeks of foetal life (JEANNOPOULOS 1952.) The condition is usually noted at birth but will progress with growth, with the arm position being altered and shoulder movement restricted. It is up to three times more common in girls, more commonly affects the left side and may be bilateral in up to 14% of cases (CAVENDISH 1972). It can cause significant cosmetic and functional impairment with the scapula being elevated between 2 and 10 cm.

The scapula is hypoplastic and is tilted up by an angle of 25° to the horizontal, with the glenoid being inferiorly positioned and the superior angle forming a lump in the web of the neck. The acromion may be elongated and the scapular musculature deficient or hypoplastic (CARSON et al. 1981; CONFORTY 1979). Compensatory hypermobility may develop at the scapulohumeral joint to improve functional ability (HAMNER and HALL 1995; CARSON et al. 1981).

Up to 98% of cases are associated with other congenital abnormalities, the commonest being an omovertebral body, which is found in approximately one third of cases and, when present, is diagnostic of a Sprengel's deformity (CAVENDISH 1972). The omovertebral body is an osseous or cartilaginous bar that connects one or more of the lower cervical vertebrae with the superior medial aspect of the scapula. This bar occasionally occurs in combination with hypoplasia or fibrosis of the levator scapulae and scalenus muscles that limit motion of the scapula (Fig. 7.3).

Kyphosis of the cervicothoracic spine is very common. Scoliosis is present in 39% of cases being more common on the side of the deformity. Other vertebral anomalies include hemivertebrae, vertebral fusion, Klippel-Feil syndrome, meningomyeloceles

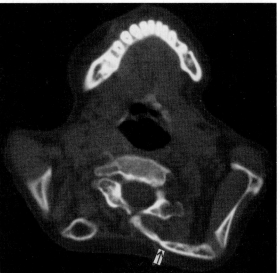

a

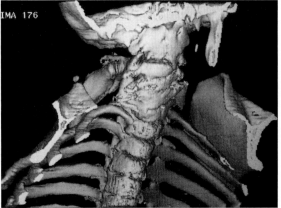

b

Fig. 7.3. a Axial computed tomography through the neck at the C2 level of a 15-year-old boy who has a Sprengel's deformity of both shoulders. There is an ossified omovertebral body on the left that goes from the spinal process of the vertebral body to the scapula (arrow). b Three-dimensional reconstruction demonstrating the relationship of the omovertebral body to the elevated scapula. The reconstruction is viewed from an anterior position

and diastematomyelia (BANNIZA VON BAZAN 1979). Bifid, fused or absent ribs are seen in 25% of cases (CAVENDISH 1972).

Antero-posterior radiographs of the shoulders with the arms by the side in maximum abduction give the best assessment of scapula elevation. Lateral and oblique radiographs of the cervical spine improve detection of an omovertebral body and any vertebral anomalies.

Different measurements have been used to assess the degree of scapula displacement. These measure the degree of external rotation and abduction of the humerus and the degree of scapula elevation (LEIBOVIC et al. 1990; NUALART et al. 1995). A clinical grading system has been developed to simplify active intervention (CAVENDISH 1972). Grade I, the shoulder joints are level and the deformity is invisible or almost so when the patient is dressed; Grade II, the shoulder joints are level or almost level but the deformity is visible when dressed; Grade III, the shoulder joint is elevated 2–5 cm and the deformity easily visible; Grade IV, considerable elevation of the shoulder. In correcting a Sprengel's deformity the aim is to abduct the scapula to cause its lateral border to be more parallel with the spine. Operative treatment should ideally be undertaken between the ages of 2-4 years old.

Scapula dysplasia mal-rotation and mal-position can also be evaluated using three-dimensional computed tomography (3D-CT) (CHO et al. 2000). The 3D-CT technique allows the shape, surface area of the scapula and the curvature of the supraspinatus portion and glenoid fossa to be assessed more accurately. The degree of rotation and supradisplacement can also be measured. Assessment of the omovertebral connection gives good correlation with operative findings. Most of the affected scapula were larger and had a decreased height-to-width ratio compared with the contralateral scapula.

7.4
Congenital Pseudoarthrosis of the Clavicle

Congenital pseudoarthrosis of the clavicle usually occurs in the middle third of the clavicle and is seen almost exclusively on the right side, with approximately 10% of cases being bilateral. It has been described on the left in association with dextrocardia (LLOYD ROBERTS et al. 1975). Other associations include cervical ribs and superior extension of the

first rib. The condition is usually sporadic, but a familial pattern has been reported (GIBSON and CARROLL 1970). The condition usually presents at birth with a lump or is noticed by the mother whilst breast-feeding. During childhood function is usually unaffected but there may be a degree of painless motion between the ends of the clavicle.

PA radiographs of the chest and clavicle show that the sternal fragment is larger and is elevated and displaced in front of the thinner, shorter lateral fragment which is depressed and posteriorly displaced. The bone ends are enlarged and there is no callus formation (ALLDRED 1963). Surgical findings show sclerotic cartilage capped bone (OWEN 1970; GIBSON and CARROLL 1970) (Fig. 7.4).

The lateral end of the medial fragment may become more prominent with drooping of the shoulder and asymmetry. Reduced ability to abduct the shoulder, increased swelling and aching of the shoulder have been reported (OWEN 1970).

The commonest differential diagnosis is from a birth fracture. With a fracture there is a periosteal reaction and callus formation with no enlargement at the separation site. The appearances of a birth fracture will change with repeat radiographs.

It is believed that the right side is most commonly affected due to the pressure in utero of the right subclavian artery, which lies in a lower position than on the left side. The subclavian artery is normally at a high level on the right side. Surgery is recommended only for those who have an unsightly lump, pain or shoulder weakness.

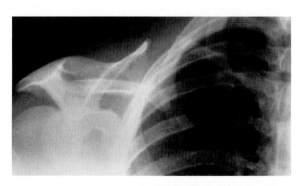

Fig. 7.4. AP radiograph of the right shoulder demonstrating a pseudoarthrosis of the clavicle. The medial/sternal component lies in the superior position. The humeral/lateral portion lies more inferiorly. There is no callus formation and the bone ends are well corticated

7.5
Congenital Absence of the Pectoralis Muscle and Poland's Syndrome

The congenital absence of the pectorals muscle may be a separate entity or be part of Poland's syndrome, where there is also syndactyly and hypoplasia of the ipsilateral upper extremity. Poland's syndrome is an autosomal recessive condition with an incidence of 1 in 30,000 live births (COBBEN et al. 1989). In all cases there is unilateral absence of the costal head of the pectorals major muscle, but additionally there may be absence of the pectoralis minor muscle, an abnormal clavicle, hypoplastic ribs and vertebral anomalies. Occasionally a fibrous remnant of the pectoralis muscle may require resection if it limits abduction or extension. Clinically the affected side has a flattened chest wall, which causes the nipple to be elevated, and causes relative hyper-translucency on PA chest radiograph. The scapula can be elevated and there may be a thoracic scoliosis. Axillary and breast alopecia have been described in Poland's syndrome (COBBEN et al. 1989; DARIAN et al. 1989; IRELAND et al. 1976).

7.6
Glenoid Fossa Abnormalities

7.6.1
Glenoid Version

Similar to the angle of femoral anteversion in the hip there is a dynamic process and change in the degree of glenoid version around the shoulder. The greatest degree of retroversion is at 2 years of age and this decreases with age so that by approximately 10 years of age it has reached the degree of adult glenoid version (MINTZER et al. 1996). Glenoid version is assessed from either an axial CT or MR image through the centre of the glenoid fossa and humeral head. Children with glenoid retroversion are more prone to shoulder instability.

7.6.2
Congenital Glenoid Dysplasia

Congenital glenoid dysplasia (CGD) or hypoplasia may be an isolated condition, form part of congenital syndrome or be a feature of a known skeletal dysplasia (CURRARINO et al. 1998; OWEN 1953) (Fig. 7.5). Known associations include fucosidosis (LEE et al.

1977), Grant syndrome (MACLEAN et al. 1986), TAR syndrome (HALL 1987) and Holt-Oram syndrome (POSNANSKI et al. 1970).

Isolated CGD is a relatively rare condition with a wide spectrum of deformity. Most cases are sporadic but a familial pattern and an autosomal dominant inheritance pattern has been described (KOZLOWSKI and SCOUGALL 1987; WEISHAUPT et al. 2000). Some cases have been associated with spina bifida, hemivertebrae and cervical ribs (BORENSTEIN et al. 1991; RESNICK et al. 1982). The defect may be due to the failure of the pre-cartilage of the inferior apophysis of the glenoid to form (KOZLOWSKI and SCOUGALL 1987) or alternatively it may be the result of failed ossification of the glenoid cartilage (CURRARINO et al. 1998). Clinically the condition usually presents in adulthood because, unlike the acetabulum, the shoulder joint is non-weight bearing and less stress is placed upon it during infancy. Asymptomatic cases may be discovered on routine chest radiographs in later life. Signs and symptoms may include stiffness, reduced movement, pain, early arthritis, joint subluxation and instability. Radiographic findings are usually bilateral and symmetrical. There is a shallow glenoid fossa with decreased ossification of the lower two thirds of the glenoid and adjacent scapula neck (Fig. 7.6). The joint surface is usually smooth but may be irregular and notched (dentate glenoid). There is apparent widening of the lower joint space (RESNICK et al. 1982). Hypoplasia of the scapula neck, prominence of the

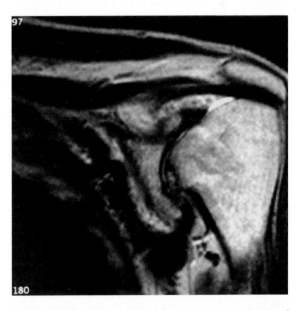

Fig. 7.5. Coronal T2-weighted magnetic resonance image of the left shoulder in an adult with multiple epiphyseal dysplasia. There is deformity of the humeral head, a shallow glenoid and loss of articular joint space

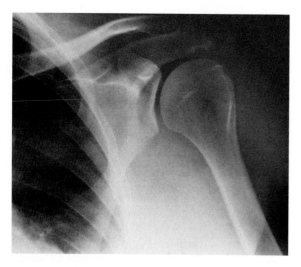

Fig. 7.6. AP radiograph of the left shoulder in an adult demonstrating glenoid hypoplasia

coracoid process and enlargement of the acromion have been described. The humeral head is flattened with varus angulation and the clavicle is bowed. There is general progression of severity with age.

Arthrography and MRI shows there is an enlarged and thickened articular cartilage that has a smooth outline and normal labrum. Capsular volume is decreased. An inferior notch within the joint capsule has been described in some cases (RESNICK et al. 1982; MANNS and DAVIES 1991; COLLINS et al. 1995).

CGD is described in numerous skeletal dysplasias including Apert's syndrome, bird-headed dwarfism, Cornelia de Lange syndrome, Holt–Oram syndrome, Grant syndrome and oculo-dental osseous dysplasia. A hypoplastic glenoid is a well-recognised feature of mucopolysaccharidoses and mucolipidoses. An abnormal shaped glenoid may be a unilateral feature of Erb's palsy, neuromuscular delay and reduced ossification of the humeral head.

7.6.2.1
Mucopolysaccharidoses

A spectrum of disorders relate to defects in the metabolism of complex carbohydrates. The inheritance, time of onset, radiological, biochemical and clinical features vary between the conditions. The eponymous names for the conditions are Hurler's disease (type IH), Scheie's syndrome (type IS/V), Hunter's disease (type II), Sanfilippo syndrome (type III), Morquio's syndrome (type IV), Maroteaux–Lamy syndrome (type VI) and Sly's disease (type VII).

There is a generalised osteopenia with areas of bone destruction. There is varus deformity of the

humeral neck. The scapula is hypoplastic and has a shallow glenoid fossa. The clavicles are short and broad (EGGLIS and DORST 1996).

7.6.2.2
Apert's Syndrome (Type I Acrocephalosyndactyly)

There is synostosis of the cranial sutures, abnormalities of the forehead, midface and orbits (hypertelorism). In the hands and feet there are accessory digits and fusion of the carpal and tarsal bones. Clinically patients have reduced mobility most marked in the shoulder and elbow which progresses with age.

Around the shoulder the glenoid is elongated and concave with irregularities in the centre. The humeral head becomes flattened with irregular lucencies in the proximal epiphysis and metaphysis. Progressive incongruity at the shoulder joint leading to subluxation and dislocation can occur. Overgrowth of the tuberosity can cause impingement on a prominent acromion resulting in limitation of abduction. Ossification of the humeral heads and greater trochanters can be delayed or be asymmetrical (WOOD et al. 1995).

7.6.2.3
Congenital Dislocation

Isolated congenital dislocation of the shoulder is rare. It presents at birth and there are no associated anomalies or injuries. Clinically the shoulder is small and unstable and there is usually evidence of abnormal intrauterine development causing absence or hypoplasia of the humerus, glenoid and acromion. Treatment is analogous to congenital dislocation of the hip, with immobilisation in reduction. Ossification of the humeral epiphysis is delayed and there is atrophy of the deltoid, pectoralis and rotator cuff muscles (HEILBRONNER 1990).

Dislocation or subluxation may be seen in association with brachial plexus injury, severe birth trauma or infection. In arthrogryposis, joint contractures, abnormal muscle bulk and fat deposits can cause instability and dislocation of the shoulder (AZOUZ and OUDJHANE 1998).

7.7
Hypoplasia of the Scapula

Scapula hypoplasia is a feature of a number of skeletal dysplasias and congenital syndromes. It is associated with Sprengel's deformity, the mucopolysaccharidoses, congenital glenoid dysplasia and long-standing Erb's palsy. It is also associated with those skeletal dysplasias that have a narrow thoracic cage, such as achondroplasia and pseudoachondroplasia. Scapula hypoplasia is particularly prevalent in those conditions that are characterised by poor thoracic cavity development, lung hypoplasia and abnormal ribs including, asphyxiating thoracic dysplasia (Jeune's syndrome), short rib polydactyly syndrome, diastrophic dysplasia, chondroectodermal dysplasia (Ellis–van Creveld syndrome), achondrogenesis, camptomelic dwarfism and thanatophoric dwarfism (KEATS et al. 1970; CORTINA et al. 1979; NAUMOFF et al. 1977; MORTIER et al. 1997). In many of these syndromes both the ribs and clavicles are thinned and ossification may be delayed.

7.8
Lateral Clavicle Hook

Lateral clavicle hook (or handlebar clavicle) describes a very angulated clavicle. The deformity may form part of a wider skeletal dysplasia or be an acquired defect. It is believed to be related to ipsilateral weakness and deformity of the upper arm that causes abnormal muscle contraction at the site of insertion on and around the clavicle.

The presence of any deformity is determined by measuring the lateral clavicle angle. The degree of angulation is expressed as an index obtained from measurements made on PA radiograph. The value of the index is obtained from the ratio of clavicle length (a straight line connecting the midpoints of the most cephalad and caudal points at either end of the clavicle (distance A) and from the distance of a point that connects the mid point of the clavicle from the site of greatest deviation from the line measuring

clavicle length (distance B). The index of angulation or normalised bending measure is distance B divided by distance A multiplied by 100. A value below 6 is regarded as normal while a value above 12 is regarded as abnormal (Fig. 7.7) (IGUAL and GIEDION 1979; OESTREICH 1981).

The anomaly has been described in Holt–Oram syndrome, trisomy 8, Cornelia de Lange syndrome, Pierre Robin syndrome, Fanconi pancytopenia, camptomelic dwarfism, Patau syndrome and VATER association (FINEMAN et al. 1975), and as an acquired defect in osteogenesis imperfecta and persisting brachial plexus injury (OESTREICH 1981).

7.9
Defects of Outer End of the Clavicle

Defects of the clavicle may result from either congenital or developmental causes or result from other acquired disorders of the post-traumatic, dietary or metabolic type. The more common non-congenital causes of defects of the clavicle include rickets, hyperparathyroidism, malignant disease, infection, inflammatory conditions and trauma. (For a discussion of mucopolysaccharidosis, please see Sect 7.5.2.1.)

7.9.1
Cleidocranial Dysostosis

Cleidocranial dysostosis is an autosomal dominant inherited condition that results in delayed, abnormal or absent ossification of cartilage that predominately affects midline membranous structures. There is a wide spectrum of abnormality around the shoulder joint ranging from simple loss of lateral aspect to complete absence of the clavicle (Fig. 7.8). The defect

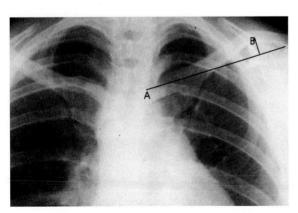

Fig. 7.7. AP radiograph of the left shoulder demonstrating the calculation of the lateral clavicle hook angle. Line A connects the mid points of the most cephalic and caudal points of the clavicle. Line B connects the mid point of the clavicle at its greatest deviation from Line A to Line A.

$$\text{The index of angulation} = \frac{\text{Distance A}}{\text{Distance B}} \times 100$$

A value below 6 is normal. Above 12 is abnormal

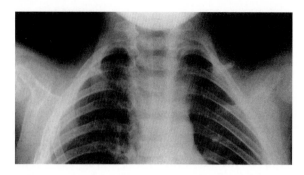

Fig. 7.8. AP radiograph in a 3-year-old girl demonstrating cleidocranial dysostosis. Both clavicles are hypoplastic

is bilateral in 82% of the cases (FAIRBANKS 1949). Other features include delayed closure of the cranial sutures and fontanelles and incomplete development of the pubis. Clinically patients have a large head, small face with a long neck and drooping shoulders. In the more severe cases there may be scoliosis with dental abnormalities, absence of the forearm bones and abnormally developed small bones of the hands and feet.

7.9.2
Pyknodysostosis

A short-limb dwarfism with some features very similar to cleidocranial dysostosis but there is generalised increase in bone density. There is widening of the skull sutures, hypoplastic mandible and resorption of the acromial end of the clavicles. There is narrowing of the thorax diameter and resorption of the distal ends of the distal phalanges. The bones are brittle and there is an increased propensity to fracture.

7.9.3
Progeria (Hutchinson-Gilford Syndrome)

This is a rare disease occurring in 1 in 8 million births. The classical presentation is the infant with an "old-man-appearance"; symptom onset is usually in the second year of life. There is generalised thinning of the skin, loss of subcutaneous fat, alopecia, delayed dentition, premature arteriosclerosis, hypertension and heart failure.

There is generalised skeletal hypoplasia and dwarfism particularly affecting the mandible and face. Overall bone density is reduced. The ribs, clavicles and long bones are thin and hypoplastic and the thorax is poorly developed. There may be bony reab-

sorption, particularly of the clavicles of the ribs. The distal phalanges are pointed due to acro-osteolysis (OZONOFF and CLEMETT 1967).

7.9.4
Mucopolysaccharidosis

For discussion of mucopolysaccharidosis see Sect. 7.5.2.1

7.10
Hypoplasia of the Clavicle (Clavicle Aplasia)

Hypoplasia of the clavicle can be an isolated condition or form part of wider group of skeletal and clinical abnormalities. A hypoplastic clavicle has been described in Edwards' syndrome, trisomy 13 (JAMES et al. 1969, 1971), Melnick–Needles syndrome (EGGLI et al. 1992), Goltz syndrome (GOLTZ et al. 1970), pyknodysostosis and fucosidosis.

7.10.1
The Short Clavicle Syndrome

Isolated congenital short clavicle is a rare disease where there is shortening of the clavicle that leads to forward rotation of the scapula that then becomes tangentially orientated to the chest wall and prominent posteriorly (BEALS 2000). Radiographically the medial borders of the scapula are widely spaced from the spine. The clavicle appears nearly horizontal but no other abnormalities are seen. There is normal appearance of the spine and skull. Clinically the major complaint is of abnormal posture but pain that limits movement has also been described.

7.10.2
Cleidocranial Dysostosis

For discussion of cleidocranial dysostosis see Sect. 7.9.1.

7.10.3
Progeria

For discussion of progeria see Sect. 7.9.3.

7.10.4
Holt-Oram Syndrome

Holt-Oram syndrome is a disorder exhibiting auto-somal dominant inheritance, with a female prepon-derance. Clinically there is an association of cardiac and skeletal abnormalities. The commoner cardiac abnormalities include atrial septal defects, ventricu-lar septal defects and abnormal orientation of the great vessels. The commonest skeletal abnormalities are hypoplasia of the upper arm structures, charac-teristically the radius and thumb, as well as carpal fusion. The features are usually symmetrical but if asymmetrical the left side is more often affected. The clavicles can be hypoplastic with a shallow glenoid fossa and voluntary dislocation of the shoulder can occur. Handlebar or lateral clavicle hook has been described. A contralateral pseudoarthrosis of the clavicle has been described in cases of lateral clavicle hook (POSNANSKI et al. 1970)

7.11
Broad or Thickened Clavicle

Thickening of the clavicle may be seen along with abnormalities of the ribs in the storage disorders; these include the mucopolysaccharidoses (see Sect. 7.5.2.1) the mucolipidoses, Winchester syn-drome and fucosidosis.

Some of the sclerotic bone dysplasia may cause thickening of the clavicle and these include Pyle's disease, pachydermoperiostosis, Menkes' syndrome and Van Buchem disease (BEIGHTON et al. 1984). A thickened clavicle may also be a feature of Holt–Oram disease.

7.11.1
Congenital Syphilis

Congenital syphilis is the result of transplacental acquired infection from the mother in the 2nd and 3rd trimesters, but skeletal changes may not occur until 8 weeks of age. Clinical manifestations include skin rash, anaemia, ascites, hepatosplenomegaly and nephrotic syndrome. Skeletal involvement is common occurring in 80% of cases. The characteristic features occur around the knee joint with the erosions of the proximal tibial metaphysis (Wimberger sign). Around the shoulder there is radiolucency or radio-opaque transverse bands of the proximal humeral metaphysis and the metaphysis may be fragmented. Lytic lesions occur in the flat bones including the clavicle and skull and there may be thickening of the sternal end of the clavicle. (LILIEN et al. 1977). Pathological fractures may occur with exuberant callus formation.

7.12
Infantile Cortical Hyperostosis (Caffey's Disease)

This disease was common in the 1950s being first described in 1945 (CAFFEY and SILVERMAN 1945), but its incidence is now very rare which raises the question of its aetiology. The disease occurs within the first 5 months of life but cases have been described in utero (LABRUNE et al. 1983). Clinically there is irrita-bility, fever, pallor and anaemia. There is significant soft tissue involvement and subcutaneous oedema. There may be a leucocytosis, and an elevated eryth-rocyte sedimentation rate; the differential diagnosis includes sepsis, trauma or neoplasm. Every bone of the body can be involved except the vertebrae and the small bones of the hands and feet. The mandible, clavicles and ribs are those most commonly involved. Radiographically there is increased bone density, cortical thickening, periosteal new bone formation predominantly along the diaphysis and tender soft tissue swelling. Scapula involvement is often isolated or asymmetrical but can cause a pseudoparalysis of the arm (HOULTSMAN 1972). The soft tissue involve-ment can be assessed on MR imaging (SANDERS and WEIJERS 1994). The clinical course is varied ranging from complete remission within weeks to a prolonged course over months. Steroid treatment may be of value in controlling the inflammatory response.

7.13
Epiphyseal Irregularities

Abnormal development and irregularity of ossification of the proximal humeral epiphysis may cause devel-opment abnormalities of the glenoid analogues to congenital dysplasia of the hip . A shallow glenoid and early arthritis is a feature of multiple epiphyseal dys-plasia. Hypothyroidism (CARSWELL et al. 1970), chon-drodysplasia punctata, hypophosphatasia (KOZLOWSKI et al. 1976) and warfarin embryopathy can also cause irregularity of the proximal humeral epiphysis.

7.14
Regional Limb Absence/Duplication

7.14.1
Congenital Bilateral Absence of the Acromion

This disorder shows bilateral absence of the lateral aspect of the scapula, spine and acromion. The lateral ends of the clavicle are hypertrophied, convex and blunted. There is no significant clinical dysfunction of the shoulder joint (KIMM and BINN 1994).

7.14.2
Scapula Duplication

Scapula duplication is a rare condition that may occur on either side of the body. There are associated abnormalities of the associated upper limb and spine. The craniomedially placed scapula usually articulates with the clavicle and the caudolateral one articulates with the humerus (STACY and YOUSEFZADEH 2000).

References

Alldred A (1963) Congenital pseudarthrosis of the clavicle. J Bone Joint Surg (Br) 45:312–319

Azouz EM, Oudjhane K (1998) Disorders of the upper extremity in children. MRI Clin North Am 6:677–695

Banagle RC, Kuhns LR (1983) Traumatic separation of the distal femoral epiphysis in the newborn. J Paediatr Orthop 3:396–398

Barrett WP, Almquist EA, Shaheli LT (1984) Fracture separation of the distal humeral physis in the newborn. J Paediatr Orthop 4:617–619

Banniza von Bazan U (1979) The association between congenital elevation of the scapula and diastematomyelia. A preliminary report. J Bone Joint Surg (Br) 61:59–63

Beals RK (2000) The short clavicle syndrome. J Paediatr Orthop 20:389–391

Beighton P, Barnard A, Hamersma H, van de Wouden A (1984) The syndromic status of sclerosteosis and van Buchem disease. Clin Genet 1984;25:175–181

Borenstein ZC, Mink J, Oppenheim W, Rimion DL, Lachman RS (1991) Case report 655. Skeletal Radiol 20:134–136

Broker FHL, Burbach T (1990) Ultrasonic detection of separation of the proximal humeral epiphysis in the newborn. J Bone Joint Surg (Am) 72:187–191

Caffey J, Silverman WA (1945) Infantile cortical hyperostosis: preliminary report of the new syndrome. AJR 54:1–16

Carson WG, Lovell WW, Whiteside TE (1981) Congenital correction of the scapula. Correction by the Woodward procedure. J Bone Joint Surg (Am) 63:1199–1207

Carswell F, Kerr MM, Hutchinson JH (1970) Congenital goitre and hypothyroidism produced by maternal ingestion of iodide. Lancet 1:1241–1243

Cavendish ME (1972) Congenital elevation of the scapula. J Bone Joint Surg (Br) 54:395–408

Cho TJ, Choi IH, Chung CY, Hwang JK (2000) The Sprengel deformity. Morphometric analysis using 3D CT and its clinical relevance. J Bone Joint Surg (Br) 82:711–718

Cobben JM, Robertson PH, van Essen AJ, van de Wiel Hl et al (1989) Poland anomaly in mother and daughter. Am J Med Genet 33:519–521

Collins JI, Colston WC, Swayne LC (1995) MR findings in congenital glenoid hypoplasia. J Comput Assist Tomogr 19:819–821

Conforty B (1979) Anomaly of the scapula associated with Sprengel's deformity. J Bone Joint Surg (Am) 61:1243–1244

Cortina H, Beltran J, Olague R, Ceves L, Alonso A, Lanuza A (1979) The wide spectrum asphyxiating thoracic dysplasia. Paediatr Radiol 8:93–99

Currarino G, Sheffield E, Twiklett D (1998) Congenital skeletal dysplasia. Paediatr Radiol 28:30–37

Darian VB, Argenta LC, Pasyk KA (1989) Familial Poland's syndrome. Ann Plastic Surg 23:531–537

Diaz MJ, Hedlund GL (1991) Sonographic diagnosis of traumatic separation of the proximal femoral epiphysis in the neonate. Paediatr Radiol 21:238–240

Eggli K, Giudici M, Ramer J, Easterbrook J, Madewell J (1992) Melnick needles syndrome 4 new cases. Paediatr Radiol 22:257–261

Egglis KD, Dorst JP (1996) The mucopolysaccharidoses and related conditions. Semin Rontegenol 21:275–294

Fairbanks TAH (1949) Cleidocranial dysostosis. J Bone Joint Surg (Br) 31:608–617

Fineman RM, Ablow RC, Howard RO, Albright J, Breg WR (1975) Trisomy 8 mosaicism syndrome. Pediatrics 56:762–767

Gibson DA, Carroll N (1970) Congenital pseudoarthrosis of the clavicle. J Bone Joint Surg (Br) 52:629–652

Goltz RW, Henderson RR, Hitch JM, Ott JE (1970) Focal dermal hypoplasia syndrome. A review of the literature and report of two cases. Arch Dermatol 101:1–11

Greenwald AG, Schute PC, Shiveley JL (1984) Brachial plexus birth palsy: a 10-year report on the incidence and prognosis. J Pediatr Orthop 4:689–692

Gudinchet F, Maeder P, Oberson JC, Schnyder P (1995) Magnetic resonance imaging of the shoulder in children with brachial plexus birth palsy. Pediatr Radiol 25S:125–128

Hall JG (1987) Thrombocytopenia with absent radius (TAR) syndrome. J Med Genet 24:79–83

Hamner DL, Hall JE (1995) Sprengel's deformity associated with multidirectional shoulder instability. J Pediatr Orthop 25:641–643

Heilbronner DM (1990) True congenital dislocation of the shoulder. J Pediatr Orthop 3:408–410

Hensinger RN (1986) Orthopedic problems of the shoulder and neck. Paediatr Clin North Am 33:1495–1509

Hernandez RJ, Dias L (1988) CT Evaluation of the shoulder in children with Erb's palsy. Pediatr Radiol 18:333–336

Houltsman D (1972) Infantile cortical hyperostosis of the scapula presenting as ipsilateral Erb's palsy. J Paediatr 81:785–788

Hunter JD, Franklin K, Hughes PM (1998) The ultrasound diagnosis of posterior shoulder dislocation associated with Erb's palsy. Pediatr Radiol 28:510–511

Igual M, Giedion A (1979) The lateral clavicle hook: its objective measurement and its diagnostic value in Holt-Oram syndrome, diastrophic dwarfism, thrombocytopenia-absent radius syndrome and trisomy 8. Ann Radiol (Paris) 22: 136–141

Ireland DCR, Takayama N, Flatt AE (1976) Poland's sydrome review of 43 cases. J Bone Joint Surg (Am) 58:52–58

James AE, Belcourt C L, Atkins L, Janower M L (1969) Trisomy 13–15. Radiology 92:44–49

James AE, Merz T, Janower M L, Dorst J P (1971) Radiological features of most common autosomal disorders. Clin Radiol 22:417–433

Jeannopoulos CL (1952) Congenital elevation of scapula. J Bone Joint Surg (Am) 34:883–892

Joseph PR, Rosenfeld W (1990) Clavicular fractures in neonates. Am J Dis Child 144:165–167

Keats TE, Riddervold HO, Michealis LL (1970) Thanatophoric dwarfism. AJR 108:473–480

Kimm SJ, Binn BH (1994) Congenital bilateral absence of the acromion a case report. Clin Orthop 300:117–119

Kozlowski K, Scougall J (1987) Congenital bilateral glenoid hypoplasia: a report of four cases. Br J Radiol 60:705–706

Kozlowski K, Sutcliffe J, Barylak A, Harrington G, Kemperdick H, Nolte K, Rheinwein H, Thomas PS, Uniecka W (1976) Hypophosphatsia. Review of 24 cases. Pediatr Radiol 5:103–107

Labrune M, Guedj G, Vial M, Bessis R, Roset M, Kerbrat V (1985) Caffey's Disease with antenatal onset. Arch Fr Pediatr 40:39–43

Lee FA, Donnell GN, Gwinn GI (1977) Radiographic features of fucosidosis. Pediatr Radiol 5:204–208

Leibovic SJ, Ehrlich MG, Zaleske DJ (1990) Sprengel deformity. J Bone Joint Surg (Am) 72:192–197

Lilien LD, Harris VJ, Pildes OS (1977) Congenital syphilis osteitis of scapulae and ribs. Pediatr Radiol 6:183–185

Lloyd Roberts GC, Appley AG, Owen R (1975) Reflections upon the aetiology of congenital pseudarthrosis of the clavicle. J Bone Joint Surg (Br) 57:24–29

Maclean JR, Lowry RB, Wood BJ (1986) The Grant syndrome. Persistent wormian bones, blue sclerae, mandibular hypoplasia, shallow glenoid fossa and campomelia – an autosomal dominant trait. Clin Genet 29:523–529

Manns RA, Davies AM (1991) Glenoid hypoplasia: assessment by computed tomographic arthrography. Clin Radiol 43: 316–320

Miller SF, Glasier CM, Griebel ML, Boop FA (1993) Brachial plexopathy in infants after traumatic delivery: evaluation with MR imaging. Radiology 189:481–484

Mintzer CM, Waters PM, Brown DJ (1996) Glenoid version in children. J Pediatr Orthop 16:563–566

Mortier GR, Rimoin DL, Lachman RS (1997) The scapula as a window to the diagnosis of skeletal dysplasias. Pediatr Radiol 27:447–451

Naumoff P, Young WLW, Mazer J, Amortegui AJ (1977) Short rib-polydactyly syndrome type 3. Radiology 122:433–447

Nualart L, Cassis N, Ocha R (1995) Functional improvement with sever L'Episcopo procedure. J Pediatr Orthop15: 637–640

Oestreich AE (1981) The lateral clavicle hook. An acquired as well as congenital anomaly. Pediatr Radiol 11:147–150

Owen R (1953) Bilateral glenoid hypoplasia, report of five cases. J Bone Joint Surg (Br) 35:262–267

Owen R (1970) Congenital pseudarthrosis of the clavicle. J Bone Joint Surg (Br) 52:644–652

Ozonoff MB, Clemett AR (1967) Progressive osteolysis in progeria. AJR 100:75–79

Pollock AN, Reed MH (1989) Shoulder deformities from obstetrical brachial plexus paralysis. Skeletal Radiol 18: 295–297

Poznanski AK, Gall JC, Stern AM (1970) Skeletal manifestations of Holt-Oram syndrome. Radiology 94:45–53

Resnick D, Walter RD, Crudale AS (1982) Bilateral dysplasia of the scapular neck Am J Radiol 139:387–389

Sanders DGM, Weijers RE (1994) MRI findings in Caffey's Disease. Pediatr Radiol 24:325–327

Stacy GS, Yousefzadeh DK (2000) Scapular duplication. Pediatr Radiol 30:412–414.

Weishaupt D, Zanetti M, Exner GU (2000) Familial occurrence of glenoid dysplasia; a report of two cases in two consecutive generations. Arch Orthop Trauma Surg 120: 349–351

Wood VE, Sauser DD, O'Hara RC (1995) The shoulder and elbow in Apert's syndrome. J Pediatr Orthop 15:648–651

8 Bony Trauma

B. J. Preston and L. Neumann

CONTENTS

The shoulder has five main compartments:
1. Glenohumeral joint
2. Acromioclavicular joint
3. Sternoclavicular joint
4. Subacromial space
5. Scapulothoracic space

The bones associated with the regions include:
1. Humerus
2. Clavicle
3. Scapula
4. Ribs and sternum

The majority of injuries are assessed and monitored by plain radiographs and in only a small percentage of cases is imaging such as computed tomography (CT), magnetic resonance imaging (MRI) and ultrasound required. Plain films usually allow an accurate diagnosis to be quickly made so that treatment can be commenced, and will also give guidance as to the necessity for and type of any specialised imaging.

A thorough knowledge of the radiographic views, normal appearances of the structures on plain films and the types of injuries which may be encountered is essential. Obtaining consistently good plain films is vital.

8.1 Introduction

Injuries to the shoulder are common and it is important to have a rational imaging strategy for assessment. The shoulder is however a complex region with its major axes lying obliquely to the body and thus even obtaining conventional films in two planes at right angles can be difficult.

B. J. PRESTON, MB, BS, FRCR
Consultant Radiologist, Department of Imaging, University Hospital, Queens Medical Centre, Nottingham, NG7 2UH, UK
L. NEUMANN, FRCS
Consultant Orthopaedic Surgeon, Nottingham Shoulder and Elbow Unit, City Hospital, Nottingham, NG5 1PB, UK

8.2 Glenohumeral Joint

8.2.1 Radiography

The basic views are discussed and the relevant anatomical detail is introduced in this section.

Anteroposterior View. The standard frontal projection is the anteroposterior view where the patient is rotated towards the affected side to bring the shoulder into contact with the cassette. If the humerus is externally rotated the greater tuberosity is profiled laterally with the line for the lesser tuberosity situated a little more medially (Fig. 8.1). If the humerus is internally rotated then the greater tuberosity is no longer profiled laterally (Fig. 8.2). With even more marked internal rotation the articular surface is directed posteriorly, is largely obscured and the proximal humerus has a circular appearance with a cortical rim (Fig. 8.3). The glenoid is seen as an ellipse with the anterior margin positioned a little more medially than the posterior lip of the glenoid. (Fig. 8.1). The anterior and posterior margins can be superimposed if the shoulder is more rotated and this is routinely employed for assessing the joint space.

"Lateral" Views. A variety of techniques have been described in order to obtain a second film of the shoulder at right angles to the anteroposterior view. It is necessary to know about views that can be done when the patient is severely injured and has to remain supine as well as those which can be done with the patient sitting or standing.

Axial Views. The axial view (Fig. 8.4) is normally obtained with the cassette in the axilla and the tube positioned superiorly. In the emergency room it is important to obtain any film with minimal disturbance of the injured patient and thus it may not be possible to perform the above technique. If, however, the arm is slightly abducted it may be possible to posi-

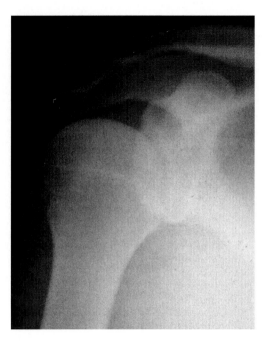

Fig. 8.2. Anteroposterior view. The humerus is internally rotated and the greater tuberosity is no longer profiled laterally

tion the X-ray tube between the trunk and the arm and have the cassette superiorly (Warwick 1948).

Alternative views may be necessary and those who are concerned with shoulder injuries should be aware of the techniques and be conversant with the resultant images. If the patient is sitting a lateral view of the scapula or a modified axial view can be employed. If, however, the patient is supine then the apical oblique view described by RICHARDSON et al. (1988) can be employed.

The transthoracic view is not a satisfactory substitute for the axial or lateral scapular view but is more suitable for imaging the upper humerus.

60° Anterior Oblique View (Scapular "Y" View or Lateral Scapular View). This view is taken with the beam in the direction of the main plane of the scapula. It is best done with the patient erect (sitting or standing), but can also be done with the patient supine with reversal of the tube and film. It is also known as the "Y" view because of the appearance at the junction of the spine and coracoid process with the blade of the scapula (Fig. 8.5). This view is good for detecting dislocations in addition to fractures.

If an additional and alternative view is required, we would recommend that described by WALLACE and HELLIER (1983).

Modified Axial View as Described by Wallace and Hellier (1983). This can be employed when the patient

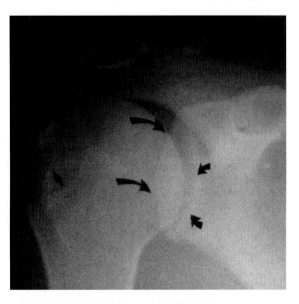

Fig. 8.1. Anteroposterior view. The humerus is externally rotated. The *small curved arrows* indicate the anterior glenoid rim and the *larger curved arrows* the posterior glenoid. The *straight arrow* indicates the lesser tuberosity

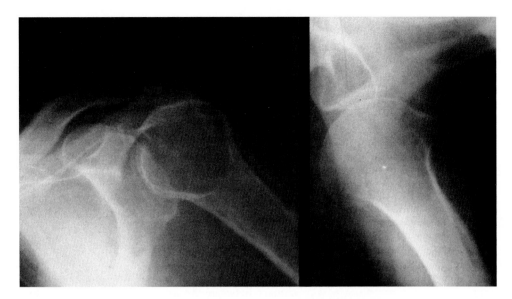

Fig. 8.3. Anteroposterior view with the humerus very markedly internally rotated and the humeral head has a circular appearance with a cortical margin. The glenohumeral distance is normal. An axial view shows the head is not dislocated

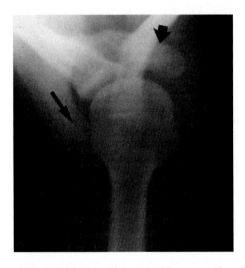

Fig. 8.4. Axial view. The coracoid process (*broad arrow*) is noted anteriorly and the acromion (*long arrow*) is posteriorly and laterally

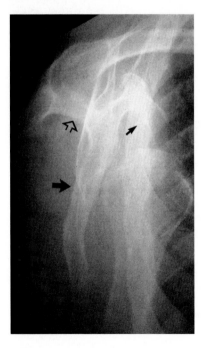

Fig. 8.5. A 60° anterior oblique (scapular Y or lateral) view. The blade of the scapula (*large arrow*), the coracoid process (*small arrow*) and the spine of the scapula (*open arrow*) converge on the glenoid producing a Y configuration. The humeral head is anteriorly dislocated

is capable of sitting. The body is rotated about 30° so that the scapula of the side under review is parallel to the edge of the film and the cassette is placed horizontally behind the humerus in contact with the arm. The X-ray tube is angled posteriorly 30° from the vertical and the centring point is the glenohumeral joint (Fig. 8.6). The structures appear magnified and slightly distorted on the film (Fig. 8.7), but nevertheless dislocations and fractures can be well demonstrated. It is an ideal view for assessing the post reduction status.

Apical Oblique View. The patient is invariably supine for this view and the method for obtaining it has been described by RICHARDSON et al. (1988) and is depicted in Fig. 8.8.

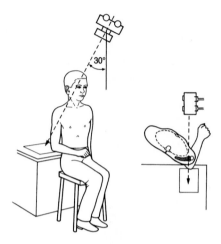

Fig. 8.6. Position of patient, film and tube angulation for the modified axial view described by Wallace and Hellier

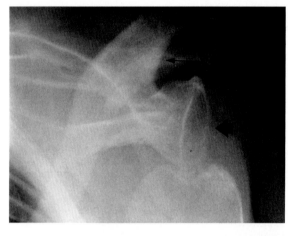

Fig. 8.7. Modified axial view. The acromion process (*long arrow*) is seen posteriorly to the glenoid (*large arrow*). The humeral head is dislocated anteriorly

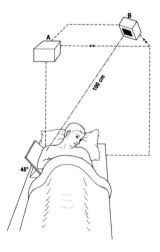

Fig. 8.8. Method of obtaining an apical oblique view in a supine patient

8.2.2
Dislocations

It is vital to have two views at right angles to assess and detect dislocations and, depending on the clinical situation, the films will be taken with the patient standing, sitting or supine.

According to ROWE (1968), approximately 85% of dislocations of the shoulder occur at the glenohumeral joint whilst 12% are at the acromioclavicular joint and 3% at the sternoclavicular joint.

Shoulder instability may be classified by the degree, direction, mechanisms and whether voluntary or involuntary. The emphasis in this section is on those lesions seen in the emergency room and they are usually dislocations, which are acute. A dislocation is identified when there is no significant contact between the articulating surfaces. Subluxation is where there is some contact of the articulating surfaces and is usually a transient episode. It must be remembered that translation of up to 50% of the humeral head in relation to the glenoid can be normal. The following types of dislocation may be seen at the glenohumeral joint:
1. Acute
2. Chronic
3. Recurrent
4. Pathological
5. Multi-directional
6. Congenital

Acute dislocations can de classified into:
1. Anterior
2. Posterior
3. Inferior, luxatio erecta
4. Superior

Approximately 95% of acute dislocations are anterior, 4% are posterior and the others are only rarely encountered.

8.2.2.1
Anterior Dislocation

This is easily recognisable on routine views because of the complete lack of congruity at the joint with obvious displacement of the humeral head even on the anteroposterior view as well as the lateral projection. On the anteroposterior view the humeral head usually appears externally rotated.

Depending on the position of the humeral head the type of anterior dislocation is further categorised (Fig. 8.9) as follows:

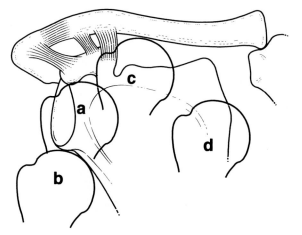

Fig. 8.9. Position of the humeral head and thus types of anterior dislocation. *a*, Subcoracoid; *b*, subglenoid; *c*, subclavicular; *d*, intrathoracic

1. Sub-coracoid: the humeral head is inferior to the coracoid process; this is the commonest type (Fig. 8.10a).
2. Sub-glenoid: the humeral head is anterior and inferior to the glenoid and the humerus is directed downwards (Fig. 8.10b).
3. Sub-clavicular: the humeral head is medial to the coracoid process and just inferior to the lower border of the clavicle.
4. Transthoracic: the head of the humerus lies between the ribs in the thoracic cavity (BROGDON et al. 1995).

The common complications of a dislocation are axillary nerve damage, tear of the rotator cuff and recurrence

8.2.2.2
Posterior Dislocation

This may occur from either significant direct trauma or secondary to electric shocks or convulsions and they may be bilateral. Nocturnal epileptic fits may cause a dislocation which can be 'silent'.

Posterior dislocations of the humerus are frequently missed because the injury is not common, the clinical findings are not appreciated, the abnormalities on the anteroposterior view are difficult to detect, an associated fracture is thought to account for all the symptoms and a lateral film is not obtained (ARNDT and SEARS 1965).

On the anteroposterior view the two most important signs of a posterior dislocation are a circular appearance of the humeral head due to marked internal rotation and a widened joint space. The appearance of the humeral head has been likened to a light bulb and is known by many as the 'light bulb sign'. The joint space is measured from the anterior lip of the glenoid to the medial point of the proximal humerus and if this is more than 6 mm then there is a high suspicion of a posterior dislocation (Fig. 8.11). A narrow joint space with abnormal overlap of the humeral head and glenoid may occur if there is an accompanying fracture. In this situation there may also be an associated trough line on the medial aspect of the humeral head (Fig. 8.12).

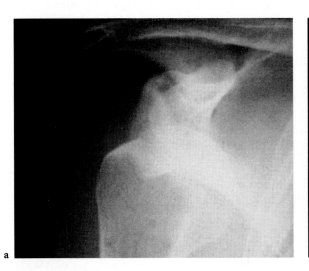

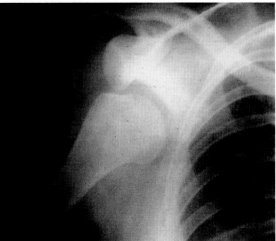

a   b

Fig. 8.10a, b. Anterior dislocations. **a** Sub-coracoid: the humerus is medial to the glenoid, inferior to the coracoid and is externally rotated. **b** Sub-glenoid: the humerus is inferior to the glenoid, externally rotated and directed downwards

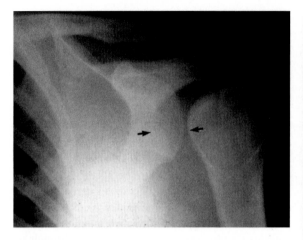

Fig. 8.11. Anteroposterior view of posterior dislocation. The humerus is markedly internally rotated producing a circular appearance (light bulb sign) and there is widening of the distance (*arrows*) between the anterior lip of the glenoid and the medial aspect of the humerus

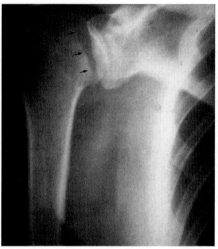

Fig. 8.12. Posterior dislocation with overlap of the glenoid and humerus and an associated compression fracture shown by a trough line (*arrows*) on the medial aspect of the humerus

Posterior dislocations are easily identified on the axial, lateral scapular view (Fig. 8.13a) and the modified axial view (Fig. 8.13b).

8.2.2.3
Inferior Dislocation: Luxatio Erecta

In this type of dislocation which is also known as luxatio erecta the humerus is directed superiorly and the head is situated inferiorly below the glenoid (Fig. 8.14).

8.2.2.4
Superior Dislocation

This type of dislocation occurs when an upward force is exerted on an adducted arm and the humeral head

comes to overlie the acromion or clavicle (DOWNY et al. 1983).

8.2.2.5
Chronic Dislocation

A dislocation which has been present for more than 2–3 weeks can be termed chronic. The importance of recognising a chronic dislocation is because of the increased possibility of producing a fracture of the humerus and soft tissue damage with a closed reduction. The history will be vital in determining the duration of a dislocation but it might be suspected on radiographic findings alone if there is a periarticular osteoporosis suggesting disuse and the presence of callus in relation to any associated fracture.

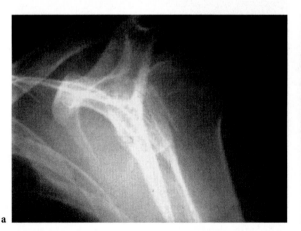

a

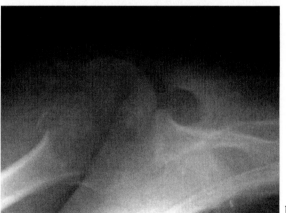

b

Fig. 8.13a, b. Posterior dislocation. **a** Lateral scapular view. **b** Modified axial view

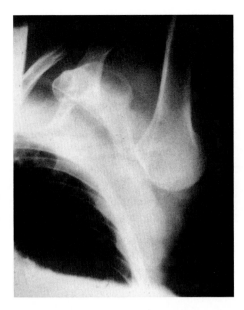

Fig. 8.14. Inferior dislocation, also known as luxatio erecta. The humeral head is beneath the glenoid and the humerus is directed upwards

8.2.2.6
Recurrent Dislocation

The glenohumeral joint is the most mobile joint in the body and it is not surprising that dislocations occur and that the injury may be repeated. Each subsequent dislocation usually requires less force as each further dislocation produces more tissue damage. The immediate role of radiology in a patient with recurrent dislocation is to ascertain the diagnosis, direction and monitor the relocation.

8.2.2.6.1
Recurrent Anterior Dislocation

In recurrent dislocations bony and soft tissue lesions occur and it is the bony lesions that can be detected on the plain radiographs. It is important to recognise these as they are an indicator of a dislocation and its direction having been present. The bone abnormalities that may be seen include:

1. Humeral Head Defect: This lesion is an impaction fracture of the articular surface of the posterolateral aspect of the humeral head on the anterior rim of the glenoid and according to ADAMS (1950) it was first described by Curling, a surgeon from the London Hospital in 1837. It is commonly called the Hill-Sachs lesion following the publication on the topic by HILL and SACHS (1940). It tends to be larger in cases where the shoulder is

dislocated for a longer period of time and when there are multiple recurrences of the dislocation. The defect may not always be visible on the routine anteroposterior and "lateral" views but it might be suspected if a line of bony condensation is seen extending distally on the anteroposterior view from the top of the humerus at the subchondral bone near the lateral aspect (Fig. 8.15). It is known as a trough line and can be differentiated from the margins of the bicipital groove because it commences at a higher level. As it is not always easily demonstrated a variety of special radiographic techniques have been described and ROCKWOOD and WIRTH (1996a) have listed eight views. However, it is best to become conversant with just one or two views and we have found it appropriate to use the anteroposterior view with the humerus internally rotated 65° (Fig. 8.16) as described by ADAMS (1950), or the Stryker notch view (Figs. 8.17 and 8.18) (HALL et al. 1959). On CT images the defect can be well demonstrated and it is identified on the images at the level of the coracoid process (Fig. 8.19).

2. Glenoid rim fractures: these occur at the anteroinferior aspect and may be obvious on the routine anteroposterior (Fig. 8.20) and axial views. Some are difficult to detect and with this in mind a further modified axial view, the so-called West Point view has been described (Fig. 8.21) by ROKOUS et al. (1972). These fractures can however be easily seen on CT.

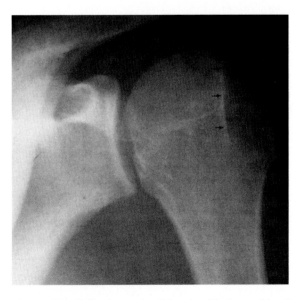

Fig. 8.15. Trough line in anterior dislocation. The humeral head defect in recurrent anterior dislocation recognised as a sclerotic line of bone (*arrows*) seen on the lateral aspect of the humeral head extending to the articular surface

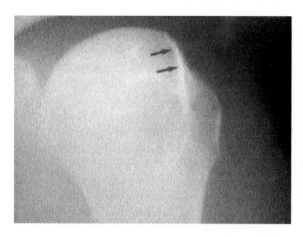

Fig. 8.16. Humeral head defect (*arrows*) of recurrent anterior dislocation profiled by internally rotating the humerus

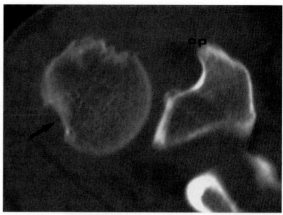

Fig. 8.19. Computed tomography of humeral head defect (*arrow*) on posterolateral aspect of the humeral head at the level of the coracoid process (*cp*)

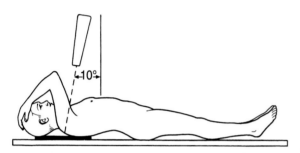

Fig. 8.17. Stryker notch view: position of patient, film and tube angulation

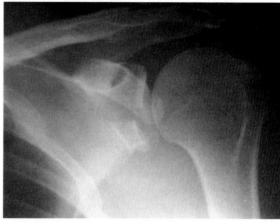

Fig. 8.20. Anterior glenoid rim fracture. The anteroinferior glenoid margin is disrupted and the bone fragment has been displaced medially

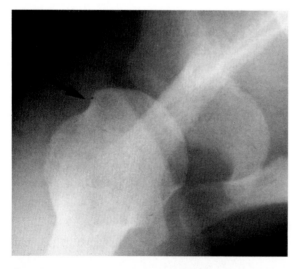

Fig. 8.18. Stryker view showing the humeral head defect (*arrow*) on the posterolateral aspect of the humeral head

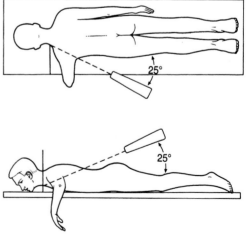

Fig. 8.21. West Point view: position of patient, film and tube angulation

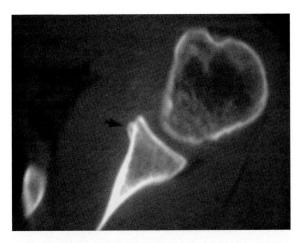

Fig. 8.22. Computed tomography showing periosteal new bone (*arrow*) at the antero-inferior aspect of the glenoid following a previous anterior dislocation

The anteroinferior glenoid defects and ectopic bone formation are known as the osseous Bankart lesion (BANKART 1923).

A combination of a humeral head defect and a glenoid abnormality increases the risk of a further recurrence.

4. Loose bodies: these can be seen on plain films but along with all the above bony lesions they are better demonstrated by CT. (Fig. 8.23a, b).

Three dimensional CT images allow graphic visualisation of all the abnormalities (STEVENS et al. 1999) and usually only two 3D images (Fig. 8.23a, b) are required to demonstrate all the information.

8.2.2.6.2
Recurrent Posterior Dislocation

Similar but reverse bony changes are seen in recurrent posterior dislocation as to those with recurrent anterior dislocation. A humeral head defect (Fig. 8.24a,) due to a compression fracture from the posterior lip of the glenoid can be seen but it is on the anteromedial aspect of the humeral head. It might be suspected on the anteroposterior view if a sclerotic line of bone condensation (Fig. 8.25) is seen on the medial aspect of the humerus extending from the articular surface. It is known as a trough line and has been described by CISTERNINO et al. (1978). Fractures of the posterior lip of the glenoid rim may also occur as well as loose bodies.

8.2.2.7
Pathological Dislocation

This is where a dislocation occurs at an abnormal joint subjected only to normal stress. Conditions causing this type of dislocation are rheumatoid arthritis (Fig. 8.26), infective arthritis and neuroarthropathy.

8.2.2.8
Multi-direction Dislocation

Abnormal muscle balance or laxity in this condition produces a dislocation or subluxation. The modified axial view can be useful in the detection of anterior or posterior shift of the humeral head as the episode may only be transient and difficult to visualise by fluoroscopy and other imaging modalities.

8.2.2.9
Congenital Dislocation

This is a dislocation occurring at birth and is fortunately a rare phenomenon. It may not be detected until later in life.

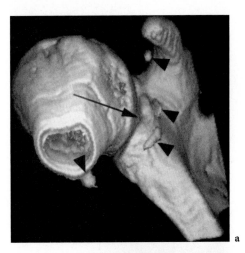

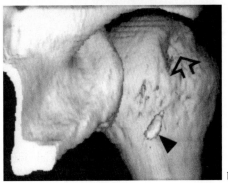

Fig. 8.23a, b. Three-dimensional computed tomography images. **a** Antero-inferior view showing loose bodies (*arrowheads*) and defect in anterior glenoid with periosteal new bone (*arrow*). **b** Posterior view showing humeral head defect (*open arrow*) and loose body (*arrowhead*)

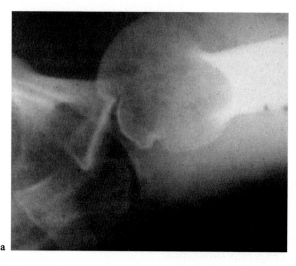
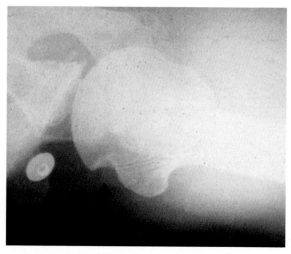

a   b

Fig. 8.24a, b. Axial views of a posterior dislocation showing the glenoid impinging upon the anterior aspect of the humeral head producing a compression fracture (**a**) and post-reduction film showing the defect (*arrow*) (**b**)

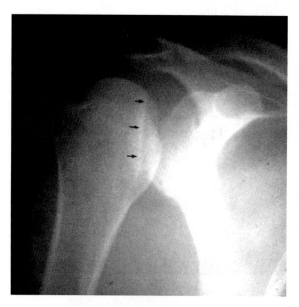
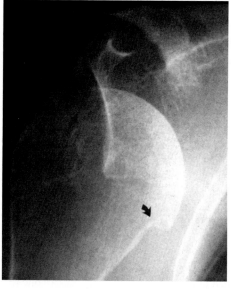

Fig. 8.25. Trough line (*arrows*) on medial aspect of humeral head due to defect produced by a posterior dislocation

Fig. 8.26. Pathological dislocation in rheumatoid arthritis. Note the erosions (*arrows*) in the humeral head

8.3
Acromioclavicular Joint

The acromioclavicular joint is a synovial joint within a capsule which is strengthened by superior, inferior, anterior and posterior ligaments of which the superior ligament which is the strongest. The joint space normally measures 3–5 mm and a difference of more than 2 mm between the two sides should indicate an abnormality. The alignment at the joint is judged by observing the inferior aspects of the clavicle and the acromion process and they are normally congruent, but PETTRONE and NIRSCHL (1978) found this to be present in only 81% of patients. A recent article by KEATS and POPE (1988) reemphasised that the clavicle may be superior or inferior to the acromion and that this normal variant should not be mistaken for subluxation. Comparison with the opposite uninjured side and weight bearing films may be of value.

The coracoclavicular ligament is the prime suspensory ligament of the upper limb and its fibres pass from the outer inferior aspect of the clavicle to the base of the coracoid process. It has two components, namely the conoid and trapezoid ligaments (Fig. 8.27). The ligament is not visible on plain films but if torn calcification and ossification may develop in its bed and this is readily identified (Fig. 8.28). The normal distance between the inferior aspect of the clavicle and superior aspect of the coracoid is 1.1–1.3 cm.

On some radiographs the appearances would suggest that there is a joint between the clavicle and coracoid process. This articulation is recognised by a downward bony outgrowth with a smooth cortical margin projecting from the clavicle towards the coracoid process leaving a small gap between the two bones (Fig. 8.29).

8.3.1
Dislocations

A classification for acromioclavicular dislocations has been proposed by Rockwood et al. (1996) and this is depicted in Fig. 8.30.

In type I injury, which is essentially a sprain, the radiographs appear normal except for possibly some soft tissue swelling, whilst in type II injury there is subluxation shown by widening of the joint space and superior displacement of the clavicle but the coracoclavicular distance is normal or only minimally increased.

In type III injury dislocation is seen with the clavicle being displaced above the superior border of the acromion (Fig. 8.31) and the coracoclavicular distance is increased. Type IV injury is similar to type III but there is a posterior displacement of the clavicle and this is best appreciated on an axial view of the shoulder (Fig. 8.32).

In type V injury there is marked separation between the clavicle and scapula with the coracoclavicular distance increased by two to three times and the scapula is displaced inferiorly. The deltoid and trapezius are detached from the clavicle.

Type VI injury is rare and the clavicle is dislocated inferiorly to the acromion. The coracoclavicular distance is decreased if the clavicle is subacromial in position or reversed if the clavicle is dislocated to a subcoracoid position.

8.4
Sternoclavicular Joint

This is a gliding joint which contains an intra-articular disc and the shoulder is anchored to the chest

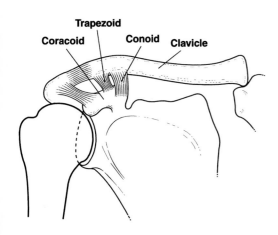

Fig. 8.27. Conoid and trapezoid components of the coracoclavicular ligament

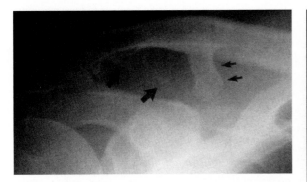

Fig. 8.28. Ossification in the conoid (*small arrows*) and the trapezoid (*large arrows*) components of the coracoclavicular ligament

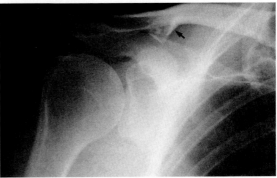

Fig. 8.29. Coracoclavicular articulation: downward bony projection (*arrow*) from clavicle towards the coracoid process

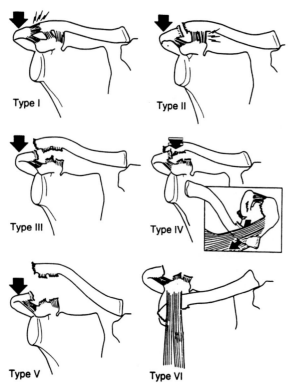

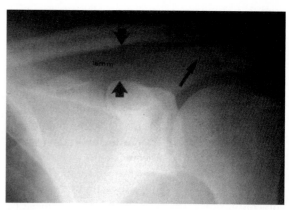

Fig. 8.31. Acromioclavicular dislocation (*long arrow*) with widened coracoclavicular distance (*broad arrows*) indicating rupture of the ligaments (Type III)

Fig. 8.30. *Types I*: a sprain, normal appearances except for soft tissue swelling; *Type II*: acromioclavicular (ac) joint is widened; *Type III*: ac joint widened and coracoclavicular (ccl) distance increased; *Type IV*: the lateral end of the clavicle is posterior and this is best seen on an axial view, the ac joint may be narrowed; *Type V*: clavicle very elevated with the ac joint and coracoclavicular distances increased, and the scapula is depressed; *Type VI*: clavicle is inferiorly displaced. (From ROCKWOOD et al. 1996, reprinted with permission)

wall through this joint. The ligaments supporting the capsule are the anterior and posterior sternoclavicular, a very strong costoclavicular ligament and an interclavicular ligament.

8.4.1
Radiography

Anteroposterior and oblique views are used most frequently. Lateral as well as the "serendipity" views are also employed. This latter projection was developed by CHARLES ROCKWOOD and has been described by ROCKWOOD and WIRTH (1996b) and is obtained with

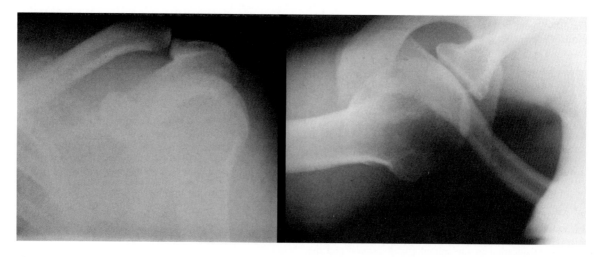

Fig. 8.32. Posterior dislocation of clavicle at the acromioclavicular joint (Type IV). The axial view shows the clavicle is posterior and overlying the acromion and the joint space is narrowed on the anteroposterior view

a 40° cephalad angulation. However, CT is the imaging modality which can very quickly and easily provide an accurate analysis of dislocations and fractures in this region and should be readily employed.

8.4.2
Dislocations

Patients with acute dislocations are usually in severe pain which is increased with any movement of the arm. This pain is also more severe with posterior dislocations and the displaced medial end of the clavicle can cause breathing difficulties, shortness of breath, choking sensation and venous congestion due to the medial end of the clavicle pressing on vital structures.

The diagnosis of a dislocation is made when there is displacement of the medial end of the clavicle. On the serendipity view the clavicle is displaced higher than the normal side with an anterior dislocation and conversely with a posterior dislocation it will not be projected so high as the normal side. However, CT is undoubtedly the best imaging modality in this clinical situation and can be used as a first time investigation.

8.5
Subacromial Space

This space is situated between the inferior aspect of the acromion and the superior part of the humeral head and contains the subacromial bursa and superior part of the rotator cuff which is the supraspinatus tendon. The region is seen on the routine anteroposterior film of the shoulder and whilst there are specific views designed to show this area these are not employed in the acute situation. Injuries and diseases can be reflected by radiological changes in this region. The acromiohumeral distance, that is the distance between the inferior aspect of the acromion and the superior aspect of the humeral head, should be at least 6 mm. The most common abnormal radiological signs seen at this region are widening, narrowing and abnormal contents.

Abnormal widening of the subacromial space is usually due to the inferior subluxation of the humerus (Fig. 8.33) and this can be due to traumatic and non traumatic causes. The commonest cause is trauma and is usually a fracture of the proximal humerus but may also be seen in association with other fractures

around the shoulder. It is noted in patients with brachial plexus injuries and haemarthrosis. It is a benign condition (COPE and SLATTERLEE 1992) and invariably resolves spontaneously. Non-traumatic causes are stroke with hemiplegia, brachial neuritis (LEV-TOAFF et al. 1984), nerve injury and septic arthritis. Subluxation can in itself be a cause of pain.

Narrowing of the subacromial space can occur as a result of fractures of the adjacent bone, commonly the acromion process (Fig. 8.34) and greater tuberosity of the humerus. However, the commonest cause of reduction of the space is degeneration and tears of the rotator cuff.

Abnormal contents other than bone fragments may be seen and in the acute situation calcification in the supraspinatus tendon (Fig. 8.35) or bursa is

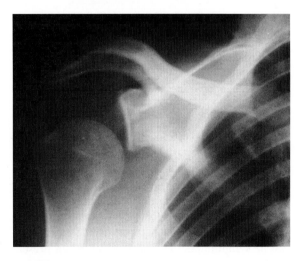

Fig. 8.33. Inferior subluxation of the humeral head with a widened acromiohumeral distance

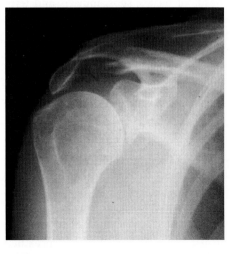

Fig. 8.34. Narrowed subacromial space due to a fracture of acromion process (*arrow*) with inferior displacement

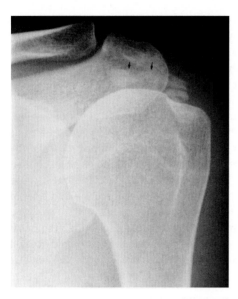

Fig. 8.35. Calcification (*arrows*) in supraspinatus tendon

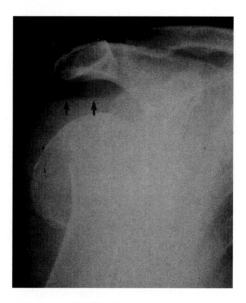

Fig. 8.36. Fat-fluid level (*arrows*) indicating a lipohaemarthrosis due to a fracture of the humerus

the commonest. The symptoms of pain and reduced function can be quite severe mimicking a fracture or septic arthritis and patients frequently attend for emergency treatment. The opacity is due to calcium hydroxyapatite and the condition is known as hydroxyapatite deposition disease (HADD) but is also called calcific tendonitis or calcific periarthritis. In the very acute stage the calcification appears less pronounced and has an indistinct margin, whilst in the chronic stage the calcification can appear more dense with a sharp margin. It can also be present and not be symptomatic. The calcification when present is observed in the supraspinatus tendon in 52% of cases but can also be seen in the infraspinatus, long and short heads of biceps, subscapularis and teres minor muscles (BROWER 1997). Calcification in the rotator cuff can rupture into the subacromial bursa.

Occasionally a lipohaemarthrosis (Fig. 8.36) can be seen in the subacromial space and this usually follows a fracture of the proximal humerus.

8.6
Fractures of the Proximal Humerus

Injuries in this region are more common in elderly persons with a higher incidence in women and usually occur due to a direct blow or falling onto the outstretched hand. Fractures of the proximal humerus tend to occur along the approximate lines of epiphyseal union and can thus be separated into

four distinct fragments, namely the greater and lesser tuberosities, the humeral head and shaft.

Anteroposterior and lateral views usually enable a diagnosis of a fracture to be made, although in some circumstances where the displacement is minimal MRI (Fig. 8.37) or CT may be required to demonstrate the lesion. Both anteroposterior and lateral projections such as the axial, modified axial, scapular Y, or transthoracic view will be required for a full analysis of the injury to be made and it is the lateral projection which frequently shows most angulation and displacement (Fig. 8.38). CT scanning with sagittal, coronal and three-dimensional reconstructions can be of great

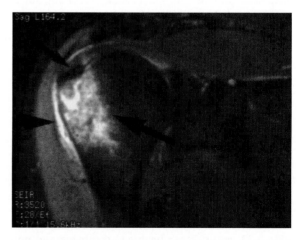

Fig. 8.37. Magnetic resonance imaging (STIR sequence) showing fracture (*superior arrow*) of greater tuberosity of the humerus with bruising in the soft tissues (*lateral arrow*) and bone (*medial arrow*)

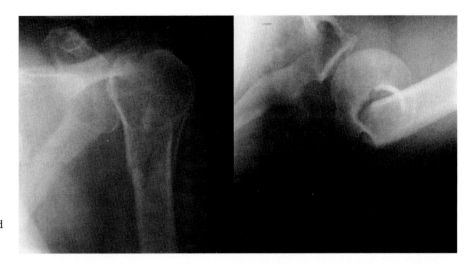

Fig. 8.38. Fracture of the proximal humerus and it is the axial projection which reveals the marked displacement at the surgical neck

value in assessing displacement, comminution and associated glenoid fractures in complex injuries.

A total of 85% of proximal humeral fractures are minimally displaced and thus only a small proportion have significantly displaced fragments but it is these that provide a formidable therapeutic challenge. Several classifications have been devised and it is the NEER (1970) and AO systems that are the most frequently used, although the reliability of both have been questioned (KRISTIANSEN et al. 1988). The Neer classification, probably the most popular, is related to the four distinct bone fragments and their displacement (Fig. 8.39). The fragments are either undisplaced or displaced and for a fragment to be considered displaced there has to be separation of 10 mm or more or angulation greater than 45°. Undisplaced fractures regardless of the number of fracture lines are classified as one part fractures.

Displaced two part fractures may involve the anatomical or surgical neck or one of the tuberosities when one fragment is displaced according to the above definition.

Three part fractures result from a displaced fracture of the surgical neck in combination with a displaced fracture of either a displaced fracture or the greater or lesser tuberosities.

A four part fracture is identified when there is a fracture of the surgical neck and both tuberosities.

Any fracture pattern may be associated with dislocation at the glenohumeral joint whilst head splitting and compression fractures are special cases.

The AO/ASIF classification relates to the vascular supply of the articular segments and the severity of the injury but it is not widely employed. The major sub-groups are Type A where the fracture is extracapsular and involves two of the four primary frag-

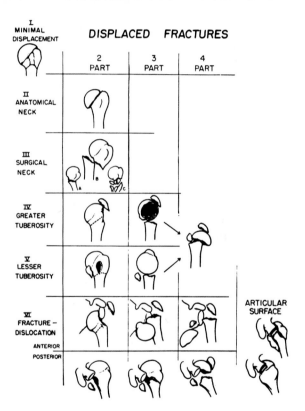

Fig. 8.39. The Neer four-part classification of displaced fractures of the proximal humerus. Fractures are considered to be displaced if they are separated by more than 1 cm or angulated by more then 45°. Displaced fractures are thus two-, three- or four-part and they may be associated with a dislocation. An impression fracture of the articular surface may also be seen with a dislocation. (From NEER 1970, reprinted by permission)

ments, Type B where the fracture is intracapsular and three major segments are involved and Type C where there is total isolation of the articular segment. The risk of avascular necrosis is minimal in Type A, low in Type B and high in Type C.

Compression impression fractures of the articular surface are classified as small if less than 20% of the humeral head is involved and large if involvement is more than 50%.

Isolated avulsion fractures of the lesser tuberosity have been documented (EARWAKER 1990) but they may be associated with posterior dislocation of the humerus.

Common complications are axillary nerve injury which can occur at the time of the injury or be delayed, malunion, non-union and avascular necrosis.

8.7
Proximal Humeral Fractures in Children

Fractures in children are described according to the location and displacement with also an assessment of the stability. The majority of fractures involve the growth plate and are categorised according to the Salter-Harris classification (Fig. 8.40).

In neonates Salter-Harris Type 1 fractures are the most common injury encountered, whilst in adolescents it is Type 2. The other types are rarely encountered. Great potential for remodelling is present at fractures of the immature proximal humerus.

The normal epiphyseal line in an adolescent can be mistaken for a fracture (Fig. 8.41). It can be recognised by being sinuous and having slightly sclerotic margins.

Pathological fractures of the proximal humerus can occur at any age and a full account of these is not within the remit of this chapter. It is however worth mentioning a fracture through a simple bone cyst which is encountered in children in the proximal

humerus. The cysts are a membrane lined cavity containing a clear fluid and normally develop in patients under 10 years of age. They usually start in the metaphysis and extend into the diaphysis thus growing away from the epiphyseal plate. The cysts are recognised as a central radiolucency with a well defined margin and sharp demarcation between abnormal and normal bone. There is no periosteal reaction unless there is an associated fracture. A diagnostic radiological sign of a cyst is the 'fallen fragment' (KILLEEN 1998; STRUHL et al. 1989) which occurs when there is a fracture and a bone flake descends through the fluid to a dependent portion (Fig. 8.42a,) and this, of course, cannot occur in the case of a solid tumour.

8.8
Fractures of the Clavicle

The clavicle is one of the commonest bones to be fractured occurring in both children and adults. Fractures are usually easily clinically detected because

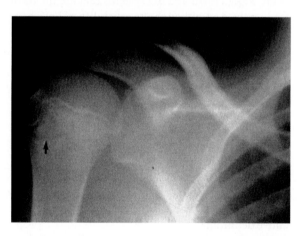

Fig. 8.41. Pseudofracture. Line (*arrow*) due to upper humeral epiphysis simulating a fracture

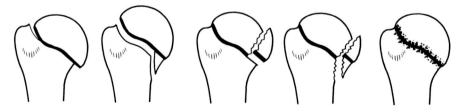

Fig. 8.40. Salter-Harris classification of epiphyseal injuries. Type I: separation; Type II: a fragment from the metaphysis accompanies the displaced epiphysis; Type III: a vertical fracture through the epiphysis and along the growth plate; Type IV: a vertically orientated fracture through the epiphysis, growth plate into the metaphysis; Type V: crushing of the growth plate

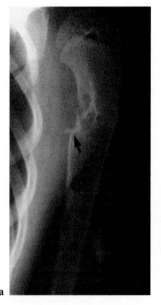 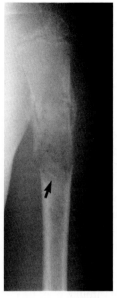

a   b

Fig. 8.42a, b. Fallen fragment sign. **a** Fracture through a cyst with a small bone fragment (*arrow*) at the level of the fracture. **b** Radiograph 2 weeks later showing bone fragment (*arrow*) fallen through the cyst

of its subcutaneous position and the majority are revealed on frontal projections, but for the detection of some and a more accurate evaluation of fragment position views with tilt of the X-ray tube may be required. The tube angulation can vary and be as much as 30–45°.

Fractures of the clavicle are classified according to their anatomical site.

8.8.1
Group I: Middle Third Fractures

Fractures of the middle third of the clavicle account for approximately 80% of the injuries and are usually due to a fall onto the outstretched hand or onto the shoulder.

8.8.2
Group II: Distal Third Fractures

These fractures account for approximately 15% of injuries and are related to a force driving the scapula and humerus downwards. They are further sub-classified according to the positions of the fracture in relation to the coracoclavicular ligament.

Three major types of these fractures have been described. Type I is where the fracture occurs lateral

to the coracoclavicular ligament and thus superior displacement of the clavicle is minimal. Type II is where there is significant displacement (Fig. 8.43) as the fracture is either medial to the ligament which is intact, sub-type A or where the fracture is interligamentous, sub-type B, and the conoid ligament is torn. Type III fractures are those involving the articular surface but there is no disruption of the coracoclavicular ligament. This classification has been developed by CRAIG (1996). Type IV occurs in children and there is a displacement of the proximal fragment but the ligaments are still attached to the periosteum. In Type V the fracture is comminuted with the coracoclavicular ligament attached to the inferior surface.

8.8.3
Group III: Medial Third Fractures

The incidence of fractures in this region is approximately 5%. Some of the fractures may be difficult to detect even on views of the sternoclavicular joints and thus CT should be readily employed for detection and evaluation. The fractures are subdivided and the integrity of the ligaments is the defining factor. If the costoclavicular ligament is intact there is little displacement. Five main types have been described (CRAIG 1996) and they are namely minimal displacement, significant displacement with disruption of ligaments, intra-articular, epiphyseal separation and comminuted.

Stress fractures may also be encountered in the clavicle.

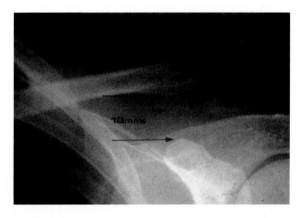

Fig. 8.43. Type II fracture (*arrowhead*) of the distal third of the clavicle with the coracoclavicular distance abnormally increased. A bone fragment (*short arrow*) has been avulsed from the inferior surface of the clavicle

Fractures of the middle third of the clavicle may be associated with neurovascular injury but fortunately this is rare. Other complications are non- and malunion, and osteoarthritis of the acromioclavicular joint if the fracture has involved the joint.

8.8.4
Congenital Pseudarthrosis

Most pseudarthroses are due to non-union of a fracture but in the clavicle a congenital cause is encountered. The discontinuity of the bone is in the middle third and callus is not present. It is considered to be due to failure of the medial and lateral ossification centres and is perhaps also related to underlying subclavian artery pulsation. It is usually on the right side but if there is a dextrocardia it is on the left side.

8.9
Fractures of the Scapula

The basic radiographic views to assess the scapula are anteroposterior and lateral views such as the 60° anterior oblique (scapula Y) and axial. If difficulty is encountered obtaining these views or a more detailed analysis is required prior to surgery then CT should be employed and three dimensional, oblique coronal and oblique sagittal reconstructions should be made.

Fractures of the scapula can be divided into four main categories depending on the anatomical position; the regions include: (1) the glenoid and neck, (2) coracoid, (3) acromion and (4) body. Combinations of the fractures may frequently be encountered.

8.9.1
Glenoid and Neck

The classification of IDEBERG et al. (1995) is the one most frequently employed and the five patterns are described (Fig. 8.44). Type I is a fracture of the anterior margin of the glenoid (Fig. 8.45) and in over 50% of cases is associated with an anterior dislocation of the humerus. This fracture is caused by indirect violence to the shoulder whilst the four other types are caused by direct violence.

In Type II fractures the fracture line is orientated transversely or obliquely at the inferior aspect of the glenoid and a triangular fragment of the neck is taken with the injury. Inferior subluxation of the humerus may be associated.

Type III fractures pass across the glenoid to about the middle of the superior margin of the scapula. This injury may be combined with fractures of the acromion and clavicle and even dislocations at the acromioclavicular joint.

Type IV fractures extend horizontally through the glenoid across the blade to the medial border. Severe displacement may occur. Type V fracture is a combination of Type IV with a further fracture of the neck which separates the inferior part of the glenoid.

8.9.2
Coracoid Process

Isolated fractures of the coracoid are rare but can be caused by direct trauma or avulsion. The fractures are frequently more easily seen on the axial or scapula Y view than the anterior projection. According to EYRES et al. (1995) the fractures are classified

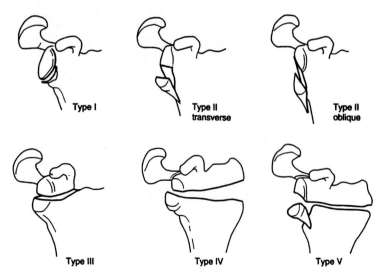

Fig. 8.44. Ideberg classification of fractures of the glenoid. (From IDEBERG et al. 1995, reprinted by permission)

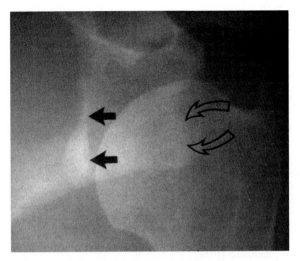

Fig. 8.45. Anterior glenoid fracture with an associated anterior dislocation. The *open curved arrows* indicate the deficient glenoid while the *solid arrows* point to the displaced bone fragments

according to their anatomical position and this is as follows : Type 1, coracoid tip or apophysial fracture; Type 2, mid process; Type 3, base; Type 4, involvement of superior part of the glenoid; Type 5, extending into the glenoid fossa.

8.9.3
Acromion Process

Fractures of the acromion may be isolated or part of a more extensive fracture pattern. They are frequently seen in the anteroposterior view but an axial or scapula Y view will be of value for further analysis. Depressed fractures will encroach on the subacromial space (Fig. 8.34) and may lead to impingement. The os acromiale is a separate bone due to persistence of the secondary centre of ossification for the acromion process and this can be mistaken for a fracture. However, the bone fragments have sclerotic edges and rounded anterior and posterior margins.

8.9.4
Body of Scapula

Fractures of the body are frequently comminuted and associated with rib fractures. They are invariably treated conservatively as the thin blade is not amenable to internal fixation.

8.9.5
Avulsion Fractures

Fractures of the scapula are usually due to direct trauma but fractures at certain anatomical locations related to muscle attachments and the absence of a history of direct violence would indicate an avulsion type injury. This type of injury has been reported and reviewed by Heyse-Moore and Stoker (1982). The common sites for these avulsion fractures of the scapula are the tip and base of the coracoid, acromion process, infraglenoid tubercle, the lateral and superior borders and inferior angle. The main mechanics for these injuries are uncoordinated muscle contracture due to electric shock, convulsions or resisted muscle pull due to trauma or unusual exertion, or avulsion of a ligamentous attachment. Stress fractures have also been recorded (Brower et al. 1977).

8.10
Scapulothoracic Compartment

Movement occurs between the scapula with its muscles and the thoracic cage. Fractures of the scapula or ribs may affect motion at this compartment.

8.10.1
Scapulothoracic Dissociation

This is a very severe injury leading to lateral displacement of the scapula with associated fracture of the clavicle and soft tissue damage to such structures as the brachial plexus, arteries and veins. The diagnosis can be made by comparing the lateral displacement of the scapula from the midline with that of the opposite side on a straight radiograph of the chest.

8.10.2
Floating Shoulder

This is where there is a fracture of the neck of the scapula combined with a fracture of the ipsilateral clavicle or separation at the acromioclavicular joint. It will cause the weight of the arm and the muscles acting on the humerus to pull the glenoid distally and anteromedially resulting in reduced function of the glenohumeral joint.

8.11
Pathological and Insufficiency Fractures

A fracture through a localised destructive bone lesion is not uncommon in the bones of the shoulder and the usual underlying cause is a metastasis, lymphoma or myeloma, but even primary bone tumours and infection are possible causes. Radiation osteonecrosis is also another cause which has to be listed.

Insufficiency fractures may also be encountered and should not be confused with an acute fracture. They are recognised as a radiolucent band and are commonly seen on the lateral border of the scapula and occasionally in the clavicle. There is usually no history of trauma.

References

Adams JC (1950) The humeral head defect in recurrent dislocation of the shoulder. Br J Radiol 23:151–156

Arndt JH, Sears AD (1965) Posterior dislocation of the shoulder. AJR 94:639–645

Bankart ASB (1923) Recurrent or habitual dislocation of the shoulder joint. BMJ ii:1132–1133

Brogdon BG, Crotty JM, MacFeely L, McCann SB, Fitzgerald M (1995) Intrathoracic fracture-dislocation of the humerus. Skeletal Radiol 24:383–385

Brower AC (1997) Arthritis in black and white, 2nd edn. Saunders, Philadelphia

Brower AC, Neff JR, Tillema DA (1977) An unusual scapular stress fracture. AJR 129:519–520

Cisternino SJ, Rogers LF, Bradley C, Stufflebam C, Kruglik GD (1978) The trough Line: a radiographic sign of posterior shoulder dislocation. AJR 130:951–954

Cope R, Satterlee CC (1992) The drooping shoulder: clinical presentation, causes and management. J Southern Orthop Assoc 1:72–78

Craig EV (1996) Fractures of the clavicle. In: Rockwood CA, Green DP, Bucholz RW, Heckman JD (eds) Fractures in adults, vol 2, 4th edn. Lippincott-Raven, Philadelphia

Downey EF Jr, Cartes DJ, Brower AC (1983) Unusual dislocations of the shoulder. AJR 140:1207–1210

Earwaker J (1990) Isolated avulsion fracture of the lesser tuberosity of the humerus. Skeletal Radiol 19:121–125

Eyres KS, Brook A, Stanley D (1995) Fractures of the coracoid process. J Bone Joint Surgery (Br) 77:425–428

Hall RH, Isaac F, Booth CR (1959) Dislocation of the shoulder with special reference to accompanying small fractures. J Bone Joint Surg (Am) 41:489–494

Heyse-Moore GH, Stoker DJ (1982) Avulsion fractures of the scapula. Skeletal Radiol 9:27–32

Hill HA, Sachs MD (1940) The grooved defect of the humeral head. A frequently unrecognised complication of dislocations of the shoulder joint. Radiology 35:690–700

Ideberg R, Grevsten S, Larsson S (1995) Epidemiology of scapular fractures. Incidence and classification of 338 fractures. Acta Orthop Scand 66:395–397

Keats TE, Pope TL (1988) The acromioclavicular joint: normal variation and the diagnosis of dislocation. Skeletal Radiol 17:159–162

Killeen KL (1998) The fallen fragment sign. Radiology 207:261–262

Kristiansen B, Andersen ULS, Olsen CA, Varmarken J (1988) The Neer classification of fractures of the proximal humerus. Skeletal Radiol 17:420–422

Lev-Toaff AS, Karasick D, Rao VM (1984) Drooping shoulder nontraumatic causes of glenohumeral subluxation. Skeletal Radiol 12:34–36

Neer CS (1970) Displaced proximal humeral fractures. Part 1. Classification and evaluation. J Bone Joint Surg 52:1077–1189

Pavlov H, Warren RF, Weiss CB, Dines DM (1985) The roentgenographic evaluation of anterior shoulder instability. Clin Orthop 194:153–158

Pettrone FA, Nirschl RP (1978) Acromioclavicular dislocation. Am J Sports Med 6:160–164

Richardson JB, Ramsay A, Davidson JK, Kelly IG (1988) Radiographs in shoulder trauma. J Bone Joint Surg (Br) 70:457–460

Rockwood CA, Wirth MA (1996a) Subluxations and dislocations about the glenohumeral joint. In: Rockwowod CA, Green DP, Bucholz RW, Heckman JD (eds) Fractures in adults, vol 2, 4th edn. Lippincott-Raven, Philadelphia

Rockwood CA, Wirth MA (1996b) Injuries to the sternoclavicular joint. In: Rockwood CA, Green DP, Bucholz RW, Heckman JD (eds) Fractures in adults, vol 2, 4th edn. Lippincott-Raven, Philadelphia

Rockwood CA, Williams GR, Young DC (1996) Injuries to the acromioclavicular joint. In: Rockwood CA, Green DP, Bucholz RW, Heckman JD (eds) Fractures in adults, vol 2, 4th edn. Lippincott-Raven, Philadelphia

Rokous JR, Feagin JA, Abbot HG (1972) Modified axillary roentgenogram. A useful adjunct in the diagnosis of recurrent instability of the shoulder. Clin Orthop 82:84–86

Rowe CR (1968) An atlas of anatomy and treatment of midclavicular fractures. Clin Orthop 58:29–120

Stevens KJ, Preston BJ, Wallace WA, Kerslake RW (1999) CT imaging and three-dimensional reconstructions of shoulders with anterior glenohumeral instability. Clin Anat 12:326–336

Struhl S, Edelson H, Seimon LP, Dorfman HD (1989) Solitary (unicameral) bone cyst. The fallen fragment sign revisited. Skeletal Radiol 18:261–265

Wallace WA, Hellier M (1983) Improving radiographs of the injured shoulder. Radiography 49:229–233

Warrick CK (1948) Posterior dislocation of the shoulder. J Bone Joint Surg (Br) 30:651–655

9 Impingement and Rotator Cuff Disease

A. STÄBLER

CONTENTS

A. STÄBLER, MD
Institute for Radiologic Diagnostic, Klinikum Grosshadern, Ludwigs-Maximilians University, Marchioninistrasse 15, 81377 Munich, Germany

Shoulder pain and chronic reduced function are frequently heard complaints in an orthopaedic outpatient department. The symptoms are often related to the unique anatomic relationships present around the glenohumeral joint (URI 1997). Impingement of the rotator cuff and adjacent bursa between the humeral head and the coracoacromial arch are among the most common causes of shoulder pain. NEER noted that elevation of the arm, particularly in internal rotation, causes the critical area of the cuff to pass under the coracoacromial arch. In cadaver dissections he found alterations attributable to mechanical impingement including a ridge of proliferative spurs and excrescences on the undersurface of the anterior margin of the acromion (NEER 1972). Thus it was NEER who introduced the concept of an impingement syndrome continuum ranging from chronic bursitis and partial tears to complete tears of the supraspinatus tendon, which may extend to involve other parts of the cuff (NEER 1972; MATSEN 1990).

The muscles of the rotator cuff, the deltoid muscle, and the muscles inserting at the proximal humerus, including the thoracodorsalis muscle, and the pectoralis muscles, control the shoulder joint. Without muscle control, a relatively free subluxation of the humeral head in anterior, posterior or inferior direction is possible despite intact glenohumeral ligaments and muscles. The deltoid muscle, the pectoralis major muscle, and parts of the rotator cuff muscles center the humeral head under the coracoacromial arch by pulling the humeral head upwards. This force is counteracted only by downward directed gravitation, and muscles with an inferior insertion at the humeral head or proximal humerus.

Rotator cuff disease is related to various factors. A dominant mechanism seems to be upward centering of the humeral head with a failure to stabilize the shoulder against this muscle action. Stiffness of the posterior capsule or increased muscle tension in the posterior located cuff muscles may aggravate the impingement process by forcing the humeral head upwards against the anteroinferior acromion as the arm is elevated (Fig. 9.1) (MATSEN 1990).

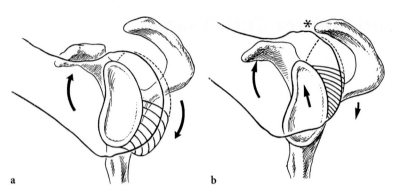

Fig. 9.1a, b. Stiffness of the posterior glenohumeral capsule or increased muscle tension is frequently associated with signs of impingement. A normally lax posterior capsule allows downward shift during flexion of the arm (**a**). Stiffness of the posterior capsule or increased muscle tension force the humeral head upwards, causing narrowing of the supraspinatus outlet near the anterior tip of the acromion (**b**). (Adapted from Matsen 1990)

a   b

Anatomic variants in the shape of the acromion, degeneration of the rotator cuff tendons with or without calcifying deposits, repetitive or severe trauma, chronic overuse due to occupation or sports activities, contribute to the development of rotator cuff pathology by increasing friction and wear against the acromion and the coracoacromial arch (Bigliani et al. 1991; Bigliani and Levine 1997; Hijioka et al. 1993). An increase in volume of the soft tissue in the subacromial space, for example due to swelling from mucoid degeneration of a tendon, compromises the subacromial space and symptoms of impingement appear because of the unyielding nature of the coracoacromial ligament (Uthoff et al. 1988).

Others believe that the pathogenesis of most rotator cuff tears is an intrinsic degenerative process of the rotator cuff, because they observed such degenerative changes at the undersurface of the acromion in the absence of tears (Ogata and Uhthoff 1990), or found specimens that had a partial tear of the rotator cuff on the articular side with an usually intact undersurface of the acromion (Ozaki et al. 1988).

9.1
Definition of Impingement Syndrome

Subacromial impingement syndrome is a painful compression of the supraspinatus tendon, the subacromial–subdeltoid bursa, and the long head of the biceps tendon between the humeral head and the anterior portion of the acromion occurring during abduction and forward elevation of the internally rotated arm (Neer 1972). The test injection is used to prove the presence of impingement syndrome. Impingement syndrome is present in a painful shoulder when subacromial infiltration with an anesthetic agent results in pain relief, while provoking pain with the arm elevated (Kessel and Watson 1977; Watson 1989; Neer 1995).

Any abnormality that disturbs the relationship of the subacromial structures may lead to impingement (Bigliani et al. 1991; Bigliani and Levine 1997). Several forms of impingement have been differentiated. Causes leading to impingement can be classified as intrinsic (intratendinous) or extrinsic (extratendinous). Impingement is further characterized as primary or secondary to another process, such as instability. Impingement of the supraspinatus tendon can be caused by a primary narrowing of the supraspinatus outlet or by secondary subacromial bone apposition (osteophytes), bone apposition at the greater tuberosity, glenohumeral instability, including superior labrum anterior posterior (SLAP) lesions, muscle imbalance with increased forces centering the humeral head under the coracoacromial arch, and supraspinatus hypertrophy due to occupation or sports activities.

Impingement of the supraspinatus tendon and the greater tuberosity occurs primarily against the acromial end of the coracoacromial ligament and the anterior tip of the acromion during stretching of the ligament, which explains the presence of traction osteophytes on the anterior acromion (Burns and Whipple 1993). Biceps tendon impingement occurs predominantly against the lateral free edge of the coracoacromial ligament (Burns and Whipple 1993).

Coracoid impingement is a painful compression of the subscapularis tendon between the anterior portion of the humeral head at the level of the lesser tuberosity and the coracoid process. The glenoid rim impingement occurs from repetitive posterior and cranial subluxation of the humeral head in throwers or tennis players with compression of the posterior superior labrum and subsequent degeneration of the labrum, frequently followed by ganglion cyst formation. This form of impingement is better classified as instability.

Impingement, which ultimately results in degeneration of the rotator cuff tendons, is a combined interaction of several elements including vascular, degenerative, traumatic, and mechanical or anatomic factors. These elements are interrelated, and each affects the tendons in a manner that contributes to tendon weakening (NEVIASER and NEVIASER 1990).

9.2
Stages of Impingement

The changes in the supraspinatus tendon from normal to complete rupture are classified according to NEER in three stages (NEER 1977, 1983). The first stage of impingement syndrome is *edema and hemorrhage* in the distal part of the tendon close to the insertion at the greater tuberosity. In this area, called the critical zone, the nutrition of the avascular tendon is limited because of the distance from the vascularized bone and the vascularized supraspinatus muscle. Unfortunately, this zone is also exposed to the pressure between the upward centered humeral head and the anterior portion of the acromion. Stage I is found in persons younger than 25 years, may result from excessive overhead use in sports or work, and can be reversible.

Repetitive mechanical trauma and stress causes *fibrosis and thickening* of the subacromial–subdeltoid bursa and tendonitis in the supraspinatus tendon, indicating the second stage of impingement syndrome. On histopathology degeneration rather than inflammation is present. Stage II is frequently seen in patients 25–40 years at age. The shoulder functions satisfactorily for light activity but becomes symptomatic after vigorous overhead use.

The third stage is represented by progressive impairment due to degeneration and rupture of the supraspinatus tendon. With further impingement wear, incomplete or complete tears of the rotator cuff and biceps lesion occur. In general affected patients are older than 40 years. This stage is associated with osseous changes at the undersurface of the acromion with bone appositions directed anteriorly inside the coracoacromial ligament, laterally, and caudally and changes at the greater tuberosity with cyst formation, bone apposition, and increased bone sclerosis. Later bone changes include narrowing of the acromiohumeral distance and ascent of the humeral head in relation to the glenoid (NEER 1972).

PANNI et al. determined the prevalence of rotator cuff pathologies in 80 shoulder specimens obtained from 40 cadavers. The mean age at death was 58.4 years. The rotator cuff was normal in 82.5% (66 shoulders); an articular-side partial tear was present in 5% (four cuffs); a bursal-side partial tear was seen in 7.5% (six cuffs); and a full-thickness tear was found in 5% (four cuffs) (PANNI et al. 1996).

9.3
Imaging of Impingement Syndrome: Imaging Modalities

For imaging impingement syndrome and rotator cuff pathologies, radiographs, ultrasound, arthrography, computed tomography (CT), magnetic resonance imaging (MRI) and magnetic resonance (MR) arthrography are used. Three radiographs comprising 'true' anteroposterior (AP) outlet-view and 'Rockwood' projection are obtained routinely. Ultrasound is used frequently to get an overview of the rotator cuff pathology. Arthrography is only rarely used as a single method. When available, a combination of MRI following the distension of the joint capsule with fluid is a widely used practice.

9.3.1
Radiography

Imaging of the shoulder should start with radiographs. Three projections are routinely obtained: A 'true AP' view is needed with 30° rotation of the opposite shoulder away from the screen holder and 10°–15° caudal angulation of the tube. This view provides a tangent projection of the glenoid. The angulation of the tube compensates for the downsloping of the acromion in dorsal direction, the rotation for the anterior angulation of the glenoid (Figs. 9.2, 9.3).

Deltoid contraction, as well as the muscles of the rotator cuff, center the humeral head under the coracoacromial arch. The subacromial space, measured by the acromiohumeral interval (AHI), closely reflects the thickness of the rotator cuff tendons. The normal acromiohumeral interval measures 9–10 mm with a range from 8 to 12 mm. It is significantly greater in men, and shows a slight reduction with age (PETERSSON and REDLUND-JOHNELL 1984). An acromiohumeral interval of less than 7 mm indicates pathologic thinning of the supraspinatus tendon due

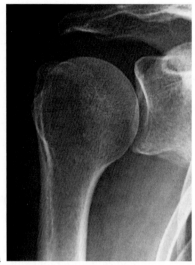

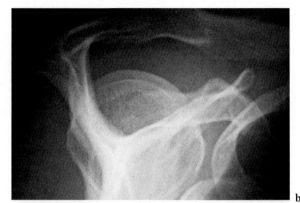

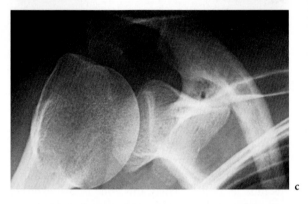

Fig. 9.2a–c. The subacromial space is visible without superimposition on the 'true' AP projection. The acromiohumeral interval can be measured. In this patient with long-standing impingement syndrome a lateral acromial spur with bone appositions is seen with sclerosis of the undersurface of the acromion (**a**). The outlet view displays the anteroposterior extent of the caudally orientated bone proliferations at the undersurface of the acromion (**b**). The Rockwood projection delineates the anterior overhanging of the acromion and the secondary hook (**c**)

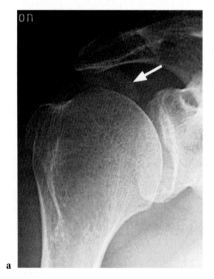

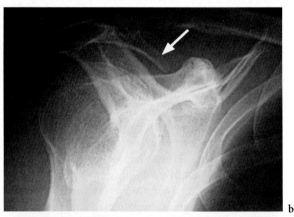

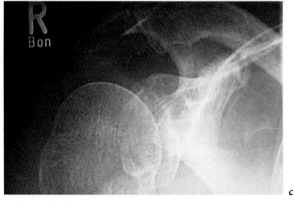

Fig. 9.3a–c. The three standard radiographic projections in a patient with long-standing impingement syndrome, 'true' anteroposterior, outlet view and 'Rockwood' view, is displayed (**a–c**). A marked enthesophyte with outgrowth of bone is present at the anterior acromion, projecting mainly anteriorly, following the course of the coracoacromial ligament

to degeneration, or partial or small full thickness tear. When the acromiohumeral interval is 5 mm or less, this usually indicates that the tear has reached such an extent that reconstructive surgery for the supraspinatus tendon is associated with poor results. In cases with progression to rupture of the long head of the biceps tendon, the mean AHI is 2.2 mm (HAMADA et al. 1990).

With a 'true ap' view, the bone appositions under the acromion, the position, and lateral orientation of the coracoid process and lateral superacromial osteophytes can be evaluated (Figs. 9.2–9.4). The AP view also provides information regarding the relationship of the humeral head to the glenoid. In the presence of thinning of the rotator cuff tendons, the muscles subluxate the humeral head in cranial direction and place the humeral head off-center under the acromion. With the progressive upward migration of the humeral head in patients with chronic complete

and massive tears, an acromiohumeral articulation occurs with concave remodeling of the acromial undersurface.

A lateral view of the acromion for evaluation of the acromial shape is possible with an 'outlet view,' a modified transscapular lateral view at a 5°–10° caudal angle of the central beam to compensate for the down slope of the acromion from medial to lateral (KILCOYNE et al. 1989). To obtain high quality projections, an experienced technician must adapt the angulations according to the individual position of the scapula in every patient. The 'outlet view' demonstrates the bone appositions at the undersurface of the acromion, the AP extension of those appositions and the congruity of the relation of the coracoacromial arch and the humeral head (Figs. 9.2–9.4).

The 'Rockwood' view is an anteroposterior projection at a 30° caudal angle of the X-ray beam (KILCOYNE

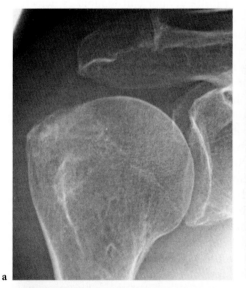

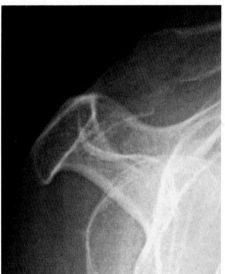

a

b

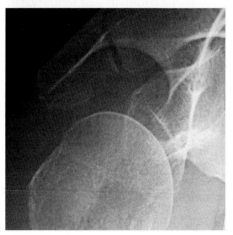

c

Fig. 9.4a–c. A patient with long-standing impingement syndrome, 'true' AP, outlet view, and 'Rockwood' projection. Bone proliferations at the undersurface of the acromion are present, with a concave appearance and sclerosis on the AP projection. There are also irregularities, sclerosis, and bone appositions at the greater tuberosity visible (a). On the outlet view bone proliferations are located predominantly under the middle and anterior third of the acromion with a remodeling of the acromion from a more flat to a curved appearance (b). The extension of the bone formations towards anterior is visible on the 'Rockwood' projection (c)

et al. 1989; KITCHEL et al. 1984; ROCKWOOD and LYONS 1993). The anterior extension of bone apposi-tions at the anterior acromion are best seen on this view. This projection outlines the down-bowing curvature of the lateral clavicle and the acromio-clavicular joint from an anterosuperior point of view. A tangent line is drawn caudally along the cortex of the clavicle from medial to lateral. The normal acromion does not override the lateral extension of this line. Enthesophytes in patients with chronic impingement syndrome form convex hook-like and sometimes bizarre bone appositions at the anterior acromion. Frequently, the presence of such bone appositions is appreciated well in one of these three projections, but no prediction can be made in which particular projection these will be seen best. The combination of the 'true AP' view, the 'Rockwood' view with 30° caudal angulation of the central ray, and outlet view provides a near-orthogonal projection of the anterior third of the acromion and the acromioclavicular joint (GOLD et al. 1993).

9.3.2
Ultrasound

Ultrasound is widely used for the evaluation of the rotator cuff, but is largely operator-dependent (GOLD et al. 1993). Proper positioning of the patient is criti-cal for the performance of shoulder Ultrasound. The examination is performed with the patient seated. Imaging begins with the patient's arm adducted and in the neutral position, and continues as the arm is internally rotated and placed behind the back. In this position the extent of the rotator cuff that is exposed laterally to the acromion is increased (SOBLE et al. 1989; SEIBOLD et al. 1999). This investigation ter-minates after the arm is elevated laterally and then anteriorly (GOLD et al. 1993). Transducers with a frequency rage of 9–13 MHz are used, providing an in-plane resolution of 200–400 μm and a section thickness of 0.5–1.0 mm.

Major diagnostic criteria for rotator cuff tears are a well-defined discontinuity within the normal echogenic cuff substance, which is usually visible as a hypoechoic focus within the cuff, absence or nonvisualization of the cuff, indicating a large tear, and an echogenic focus within the cuff (SOBLE et al. 1989; CRASS and CRAIG 1988). Ultrasound can detect increased fluid in the subacromial subdeltoid bursa, which is normally thinner than two millimeters and is usually poorly seen in its nondistended state (BRETZKE et al. 1985).

Rotator cuff ultrasound was reported to be less reliable than MRI and to have a limited role in the evaluation of rotator cuff pathologies (BRANDT et al. 1989; NELSON et al. 1991). With recent sonographic technical advances, SWEN et al. (1999) found a sen-sitivity for the detection of full thickness tears of the rotator cuff of 0.81, and a specificity of 0.94. The results for ultrasound were equal to or better than MRI in this study. Ultrasound should be the primary diagnostic method in screening shoulder pain because it is economical and fast (BACHMANN et al. 1997).

9.3.3
Arthrography

Shoulder arthrography with injection of contrast media is an indirect method for the evaluation of the glenohumeral joint. Only the filling of partial or com-plete defects in the rotator cuff tendons is detected when the defects originate from the articular side. Partial tears of the bursal surface and intrasubstance changes are not detectable. Soft tissue pathologies, including muscle atrophy and hypertrophy, inflam-matory or stress related reactions in the bursae, the tendons, the labrum or in the bone, are also not visu-alized on arthrograms.

If possible, an arthrogram should be followed by an MRI study. The distension of the joint capsule and the fluid in the joint cavity enhances the sensitivity and specificity of MRI, especially in the evaluation of partial and full thickness tendon tears. We recom-mend using a mixture of 0.2 ml of a gadolinium-con-taining contrast medium and 15 ml of a non-ionic iodinated water-soluble contrast agent for MRI.

Double-contrast shoulder arthrography was rec-ommended for the evaluation of rotator cuff tears because of its exquisite sensitivity and accuracy. The site of disruption has been reported to be directly visible in 93% of cases (MINK et al. 1985). For dem-onstration of the precise site of rotator cuff defects digital arthrography has also been recommended (STILES et al. 1988). Due to side effects of magnetic susceptibility, double contrast arthrography is not suitable for MRI. If MRI is available, arthrography as a stand-alone investigation is no longer performed and single contrast arthrography is used to prepare the patient for MRI.

9.3.4
Magnetic Resonance Imaging

MRI is an ideal imaging modality for pathologies of the shoulder and significantly influences the clinicians' diagnostic confidence for lesions of the shoulder (BLANCHARD et al. 1997). Soft tissue structures, including the tendons and muscles of the rotator cuff, the glenoid labrum, the long head of the biceps tendon, fluid collections and edema in bone and soft tissue are all well displayed. With MRI, there is free access to the imaging plane, and with technical developments including suppression of the fat signal, extension of the matrix to 512, and increasing imaging speed, sensitivity and specificity of MRI of the shoulder is unsurpassed by other imaging modalities.

For MRI of the shoulder, a relaxed placement of the patient inside the gantry is important. The arm should rest in a neutral position without internal or external rotation beside the body. Imaging in internal rotation produces overlap of the supraspinatus and infraspinatus tendon with soft tissue interposition or apparent discontinuity of the tendon and should be avoided (DAVIS et al. 1991). Placing the forearm on the abdomen can result in motion artifacts due to breathing. Most MRI studies are performed without provocative positioning with the arm in neutral position and display only secondary findings of shoulder impingement syndrome. It was shown that supraspinatus impingement is best seen at 60° forward flexion, 60° abduction, and internal rotation and proposed that the shoulder be imaged in different positions to additionally detect dynamic aspects of shoulder impingement syndrome (BROSSMANN et al. 1996).

We suggest that routine MRI protocols for unenhanced shoulder studies begin with an axial T2-weighted gradient-recalled echo sequence from the acromion to the axillary recess. This sequence, predominately necessary to show the labrum in patients with suspected instability, also displays the oblique course of the supraspinatus muscle.

This sequence should be followed by oblique coronal T1-weighted images and a short inversion time inversion recover (STIR) sequence in the same imaging plane. The angulation of this plane should be adapted to the anatomical course of the supraspinatus tendon (SEEGER 1989). Instead of a STIR sequence, one can use a proton density or T2-weighted fat saturated sequence which provides similar contrast with high sensitivity to water protons. However, occasionally an inhomogeneous saturation of the fat signal can occur when using a frequency selective fat suppression sequence. This problem does not occur with STIR sequences. The supraspinatus muscle and tendon are displayed in their complete course (VAHLENSIECK 2000).

Sagittal images are equally important and are performed perpendicular to the oblique coronal images. They should also be aligned to the course of the glenoid. A T2-weighted fast spin-echo (FSE) sequence is preferred to a fat saturated sequence as the high signal intensity of the marrow fat from the acromion and the humeral head serves as a good contrast for the low signal intensity of the cortical bone and the tendons of the rotator cuff. Using perfectly fat-suppressed sequences can make the differentiation of the tendons from the bone difficult. The images must be obtained from the most outer part of the supraspinatus tendon, including the fibroosseous junction, and the greater tuberosity to at least the middle part of the muscle belly of the supraspinatus muscle. These images through the supraspinatus fossa are mandatory for evaluation of the muscle quality and for quantification of supraspinatus atrophy.

Most important for imaging rotator cuff pathologies are the oblique coronal STIR sequence and the oblique sagittal T2-weighted sequence. Criteria to look for include fluid collections in the subacromial subdeltoid bursa; the thickness of the rotator cuff tendons and muscles, especially thinning or thickening of the supraspinatus tendon; bone marrow edema at the greater tuberosity and the acromioclavicular joint; cyst formation in the posterior upper part of the humeral head; the shape of the acromion, including bone appositions underneath the acromion and at the anterior or lateral border of the acromion; and fluid collections in the tendons of the rotator cuff with focus to the supraspinatus tendon.

9.3.4.1
Sequences

For T2-contrast, FSE techniques perform equally well compared to conventional spin-echo sequences and include time-saving benefits (SONIN et al. 1996; CARRINO et al. 1997). Adding fat-suppression techniques increases overall image quality and visualization of the supraspinatus tendon or any abnormality (CARRINO et al. 1997). Fat suppression reduces respiratory artifacts due to the reduction of signal intensity of the subcutaneous fat. Fat suppression also results in improved soft-tissue contrast by expansion of the dynamic image display, and eliminates chemical misregistration artifacts. Finally, sensitivity for pathologic fluid collections and areas of edema are enhanced greatly with fat suppression techniques (MIROWITZ 1991). Fat-saturation FSE imaging can effectively replace conventional FSE imaging for the detection of rotator cuff pathology and tends to perform better in the diagnosis of partial tears (REINUS et al. 1995; QUINN et al. 1995; SINGSON et al. 1996; NEEDELL and ZLATKIN 1997).

T2*-weighted gradient-recalled echo (GRE) sequences have also been proposed as an alternative method for rotator cuff evaluation (HOLT et al. 1990; RESENDES et al. 1991; KAPLAN eta l. 1992; VAHLEN-SIECK et al. 1993; TUITE et al. 1994). T2*-weighted sequences can shorten scan time and improve the signal-to-noise ratio. Unfortunately T2*-weighted images tend to be less sensitive and specific compared to standard T2-weighted images and with the availability of fast spin-echo techniques with or without fat-suppression, gradient-recalled echo sequences are no longer used for imaging rotator cuff pathologies (PARSA et al. 1997). However, these sequences are still in use for axial imaging of the glenoid labrum.

9.3.4.2
Gadolinium

Intravenous contrast material (gadolinium) is not applied routinely. In cases with calcifying tendinitis the inflammatory fibrovascular tissue adjacent to the calcium deposits can be displayed with i.v. contrast. Synovial enhancement in patients with adhesive capsulitis, rheumatoid arthritis, or non-specific synovitis is also well delineated with i.v. contrast. Enhancement can be found in fibrovascular tissue in partial or complete rotator cuff tears, although STIR images also delineate the pathologic changes with increased signal intensity.

With the i.v. administration of gadolinium, an indirect arthrographic effect by enhancement of joint fluid can be produced (WINALSKI et al. 1993). It has been proposed that the patient should exercise the shoulder for 10–20 min after the contrast injection based on findings by VAHLENSIECK who reported a four times greater signal intensity in joints that were exercised before imaging than in joints that had not been exercised (VAHLENSIECK et al. 1993). Because exercise may be problematic in patients with rotator cuff pathologies, indirect arthrography of the unexercised shoulder in patients with rotator cuff tears was evaluated (ALLMANN et al. 1999). ALLMANN found 120% enhancement after 4 min and 145% enhancement after 8 min without exercise of the shoulder, which lead him to suggest this method as a less time-consuming alternative to indirect arthrography after joint exercise. The limits of indirect arthrography include the lack of active distension of the joint capsule and the inability of patients with shoulder pathology to exercise the affected shoulder properly for 15–20 min.

9.3.4.3
MR Arthrography

MR arthrography enhances the accuracy of MRI in the evaluation of rotator cuff tendons (FLANNIGAN et al. 1990; HODLER et al. 1992). Conventional MRI of the shoulder is limited in depicting intraarticular structures when insufficient fluid is present to outline their structure. Fat-suppressed sequences further improve the diagnostic performance of MR arthrography, especially in the differentiation of partial from full-thickness cuff tears and in the detection of small partial tears of the inferior tendon surface (PALMER et al. 1993).

MR arthrography should be performed with a 20-gauge needle under fluoroscopic control. The technique performing shoulder arthrography usually involves an anterior approach for needle placement regardless of the presenting history and symptoms. Tailoring the arthrographic technique by using a posterior approach if patients present with a history of anterior instability or anterior symptoms can help to avoid damage to anterior structures including the capsulolabral complex (Chung et al. 2000). The intraarticular position of the needle can be confirmed by injecting 1 ml of iodinated contrast material. There have been attempts to puncture the glenohumeral joint with MR guidance (PETERSILGE et al. 1997; TRATTNIG et al. 1997). The additional time required for the puncture in the MR unit is 10–21 min.

The joint should be distended with a total of 12–14 ml of fluid. If a gadolinium solution is used, 1 ml gadopentetate dimeglumine are diluted in 100–250 ml of saline (BRENNER et al. 2000; BINKERT et al. 2001a). Exercise, usually included in conventional shoulder arthrography protocols, has no beneficial or detrimental effect on image quality or on the depiction of rotator cuff or labral tears (BRENNER et al. 2000). If a combination of iodinated contrast material and gadolinium is used, the addition of 1 ml of gadopentetate dimeglumine to 10 ml of iodinated contrast material is recommended (KOPKA et al. 1994).

Controversies related to the non-defined legal status of intraarticular gadolinium-based solutions have resulted in increased interest in alternative contrast materials. BINKERT et al. (2001a) compared two concentrations of gadoteridol with Ringer solution as contrast material for MR arthrography of the glenohumeral joint. MR arthrograms of the shoulder obtained with gadoteridol and those obtained with Ringer solution provided equivalent diagnostic accuracy. The authors, however, preferred the image quality of the gadoteridol-enhanced arthrograms.

A routine protocol uses fat-suppressed T1-weighted images at a 3-mm slice thickness in all three planes (coronal oblique, sagittal oblique, and axial) post-injection, if gadolinium is added to the injected fluid (STOLLER 1997). If only saline is injected, proton density-weighted images with fat-suppression are acquired. Three-dimensional (3D) gradient echo acquisitions with T2 contrast and fat-suppression have also proved to be very useful (Fig. 9.5).

The ABER position, in which the patient's arm is abducted and externally rotated, is reported to enhance the detectability of partial thickness tears of the undersurface of the rotator cuff, especially in the infraspinatus tendon during MR arthrography (TIRMAN et al. 1994). This position is easily achieved in an open magnet, but is problematic in high field strength magnets and dedicated shoulder coils. The ABER position and external rotation alone has been shown to optimize the visualization of the biceps–labral complex and glenohumeral ligaments (KWAK et al. 1998). The ABER position should be included in the imaging protocol in athletes suffering shoulder pain from throwing (ROGER et al. 1999).

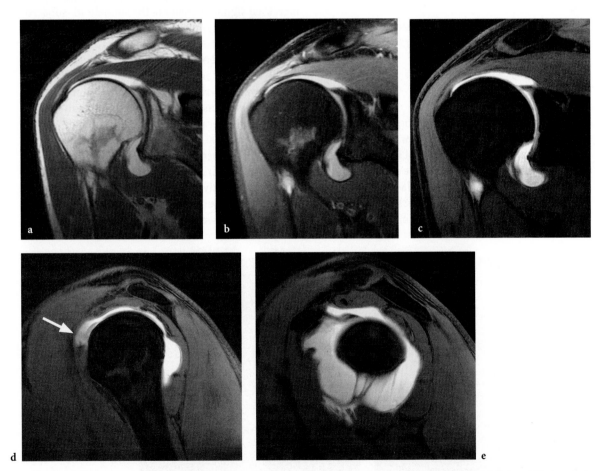

Fig. 9.5a–e. Magnetic resonance arthrogram with a combination of iodinated contrast material and gadolinium. The supraspinatus muscle and tendon is outlined by the positive contrast of the injected fluid. The joint cavity has high signal intensity from the added gadolinium (**a**). Proton density fat-suppressed image (**b**) and fat-suppressed gradient echo three-dimensional image (Flash) (**c**) have high signal-to-noise ratios due to the high signal intensity of fluid in the joint space (**b, c**). Magnetic resonance arthrography, sagittal fat-suppressed gradient echo three-dimensional FLASH images, calculated slice thickness 1.8 mm (**d, e**). The only 2-mm thick capsule of the rotator interval and the grayish ovoid biceps tendon passing through the joint are seen (*arrow*) (**d**). A more medially located cut displays the superior glenohumeral ligament inserting at the biceps anchor. Also, the inferior humeral insertion of the middle and inferior glenohumeral ligaments are visible (**e**)

Patient discomfort during MR arthrography of the shoulder has been assessed. Arthrography-related discomfort was well tolerated, often less severe than anticipated, and rated less severe than MRI-related discomfort (BINKERT et al. 2001b). In a study to establish whether patients prefer arthrography or MRI, anxiety, pain, and preferences of the patients were evaluated. Mean levels of anxiety were slightly higher, but not statistically significant different, for patients undergoing MRI than those having arthrography. Also, no significant differences were found regarding whether patients would prefer MRI or arthrography on the basis of past or current experience (BLANCHARD et al. 1997).

9.4
Imaging Findings in Impingement Syndrome and Rotator Cuff Tears

9.4.1
Bursal Effusion

The subacromial bursa is located between the acromion and coracoacromial ligament superiorly, and the rotator cuff and rotator interval inferiorly, medially reaching the undersurface of the acromioclavicular joint. The subdeltoid bursa is placed between the deltoid muscle and the lateral aspect of the humeral neck. Both bursae communicate in 95% with each

other, forming the so-called subacromial–subdeltoid bursa, which does not communicate with the glenohumeral joint (VAHLENSIECK 2000; MELLADO et al. 2002). Fluid distending the subacromial–subdeltoid bursa is a non-specific finding, as it may be encountered in association with subacromial impingement, partial or complete rotator cuff tears, and calcifying tendinitis (Fig. 9.6).

During impingement of the supraspinatus tendon the subacromial–subdeltoid bursa becomes compressed between the greater tuberosity of the humeral head and the anterior portion of the acromion. This chronic compression can result in an inflammatory reaction of the bursal synovium and secretion of fluid into the bursa. Fluid is not detected in the normal bursa (BUREAU et al. 1996). Fluid in the bursa is recognized on T2-weighted images by the increased signal intensity of the subdeltoid–subacromial bursa which indicates local bursal inflammation (SCHRANER and MAJOR 1999). Imaging of patients with impingement syndrome must be sensitive to the detection of fluid collection in the bursa, which is achieved by the use of highly water-sensitive sequences, such as STIR sequences or proton-density fat signal suppressed sequences.

TASU et al. (2001) evaluated MR criteria in patients with impingement syndrome in comparison to normal volunteers. The patients had a type III acromion significantly more often. The acromiohumeral distance in patients was significantly decreased to 4.9 mm compared to 6.0 mm, and the coracohu-

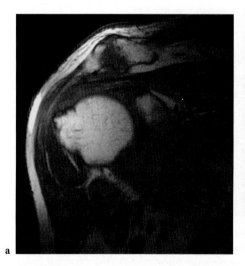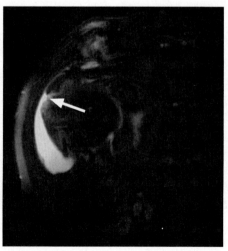

a   b

Fig. 9.6a, b. Tendinosis and partial thickness tear of the supraspinatus tendon with bursal effusion. The peripheral part of the supraspinatus tendon is thickened and signal intensity on T1-weighted image is increased (**a**). On the fat-suppressed T2-weighted image a large bursal effusion has high signal intensity (**b**). Near the greater tuberosity a partial, bursa-sided tear is seen. The bone marrow edema in the degenerated acromioclavicular joint and the bone appositions at the undersurface of the acromion are associated findings in chronic impingement syndrome

meral distance was also significantly decreased to 7.9 mm compared to 8.9 mm in asymptomatic volunteers. Finally, the anterior covering of the humeral head by the acromion was significantly reduced in the impingement group. All these factors reflect a decrease in the acromiohumeral space except for the anterior covering of the humeral head, which is probably due to anterior instability.

9.4.2
Imaging Following Impingement Test Injection

KIEFT et al. (1988) noted large areas of increased signal intensity on the T2-weighted images at the side of injection. Two studies had been conducted to determine the appropriate minimum waiting time between an impingement test with subacromial injection and subsequent MRI to avoid misinterpretation if the injected fluid is still present (WRIGHT et al. 1998; BERGMAN and FREDERICSON 1998). WRIGHT et al. (1998), who imaged their patients every 12 h until the fluid disappeared, recommended that MRI should be delayed a minimum of 24 h after subacromial injection. BERGMAN and FREDERICSON (1998) on the other hand, recommended a delay of 3 days. They had their first control examination of their six patients at day three after the test injection test.

9.4.3
Tendinosis

There was early evidence that MRI is well suited for evaluation of the rotator cuff because MR is the only imaging modality capable of direct visualization of the rotator cuff tendons, the subacromial subdeltoid bursa, and the biceps tendon (HOLT et al. 1990; REEDER and ANDELMAN 1987; SEEGER et al. 1988). A normal supraspinatus tendon should exhibit low signal intensity on all pulse sequences. There is general agreement that a focal area of increased signal intensity on a T1-weighted image without increased signal intensity on a T2-weighted image and without thickening or thinning of the tendon is due to the magic angle artifact or is without clinical relevance.

Mucoid degeneration of a rotator cuff tendon, a finding frequently present in the anterior portion of the supraspinatus tendon near the insertion at the greater tuberosity, is the initial finding in subacromial impingement (TASU et al. 2001). This peripheral part of the tendon is called the critical zone because of its lack of nutritial vessels, which extend from the

proximal muscle belly and the distal fibro-osseous junction partly into the tendon, leaving a part of the tendon free from vessels.

In addition to the lack of nutritial vessels, this part of the tendon is mechanically exposed to increased loading due to the deviation of the tension forces during activation of the supraspinatus tendon while elevating the arm. The tendon is not only exposed to tension forces but also to an increased pressure load against the humeral head while changing the direction of the tension forces downwards to the greater tuberosity.

Stress to the peripheral part of the supraspinatus tendon near the insertion is also produced by friction forces occurring between the subacromial bone surface and the supraspinatus tendon during elevation of the arm and gliding of the tendon underneath the coracoacromial arch. If there is increased muscle tone centering the humeral head under the coracoacromial arch, the friction between the supraspinatus tendon and the anterior acromion is increased. At this point occupational and socio-cultural influences in the etiology of impingement syndrome may exist.

A tendon with focal or diffuse increased signal intensity on proton density-weighted images without further increase of signal intensity on T2-weighted images and an indistinct margin at the articular side of the supraspinatus tendon corresponds to eosinophilic, fibrillar, and mucoid degeneration and scarring. Tendons with areas of increased signal intensity on T2-weighted images are associated with severe degeneration and disruption of the supraspinatus tendon (KJELLIN et al. 1991) and have increased signal intensity also on STIR and T1-weighted images (Fig. 9.7). No focal or linear area of water-equivalent signal intensity is seen. Frequently in cases of focal or diffuse regions of increased signal intensity or in cases with a nonhomogenous pattern of increased signal intensity, a thickening of the degenerated part of the tendon with enlargement is present (RAFII et al. 1990).

Tendinosis in many cases is a result of impingement syndrome. Fluid collections can be present in the subacromial subdeltoid bursa, findings similar to that of inflammation (Fig. 9.8). This early stage of rotator cuff disease is frequently called tendinitis. The histologic data reported in the study of KJELLIN et al. (1991) were not those of active inflammation but rather tendon degeneration. Contrast enhancement, if present, is related to fibrovascular tissue and not due to inflammation. Therefore, the term tendinitis should not be used to describe tendinosis in the early stages of rotator cuff disease.

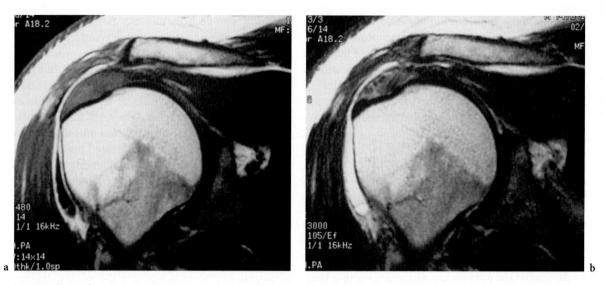

Fig. 9.7a, b. Tendinosis in impingement syndrome. The supraspinatus tendon is thickened, signal intensity is increased on the T1-weighted (**a**) and T2-weighted image (**b**). Bursal effusion predominantly seen lateral to the greater tuberosity. Capsular thickening and a small osteophyte is seen at the undersurface of the lateral clavicle, probably in part responsible for the impingement syndrome

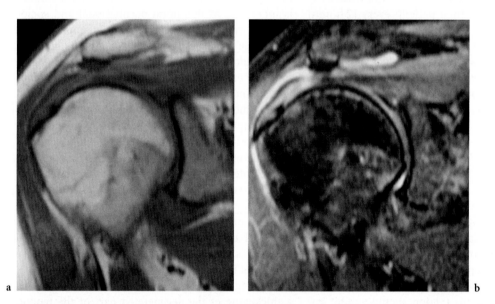

Fig. 9.8a, b. Tendinosis in chronic impingement syndrome. The supraspinatus tendon exhibits increased signal intensity on the T1-weighted image (**a**) and fat-suppressed T2-weighted image (**b**). The peripheral part of the mucoid degenerated tendon is thickened and effusion in the subacromial–subdeltoid bursa is present. Note also the marked bone apposition at the undersurface of the acromion, impinging upon the supraspinatus tenon

To determine if supraspinatus pathology as defined by MRI is associated with clinical signs of impingement, FROST et al. (1999) obtained MRIs of the shoulder in 42 workers with and 31 age-matched workers without signs of impingement. In all, 55% of the subjects in the impingement group and 52% of the subjects in the control group had a pathologic supraspinatus tendon. These findings lead FROST et al. (1999) to conclude that supraspinatus tendon pathology is related to age rather than to clinical signs of impingement.

Others have also noted a high prevalence of rotator cuff tears and tendon and peritendinous and bone abnormalities in an asymptomatic population (NEUMANN et al. 1992, 1996; SHER et al. 1995). The prevalence of rotator cuff tears is 34% in a population with an average age of 53 years (19–88 years), with 15% having full thickness rotator cuff tears, and 20% having partial-thickness tears (SHER et al. 1995). The frequency of tears increased significantly with age (SHER et al. 1995). The presence of subacromial spurs was 37% and was correlated closely with MR-evident tendon abnormalities. The prevalence of spurs was 11% in subjects with a normal tendon, 33% in those with MR-evident tendinopathy, 68% in those with MR-evident partial tears, and 79% in those with MR-evident complete tears. Humeral head cysts were found in 24% of asymptomatic subjects (NEEDELL et al. 1996).

In 89%–95% of asymptomatic shoulders, the supraspinatus tendon shows a focal, linear, or diffuse increased signal intensity on proton density-weighted images without abnormalities on T2-weighted images (NEUMANN et al. 1992; LIOU et al. 1993). The peribursal fat plane is poorly defined or absent (focally obliterated) in 49%–95% of asymptomatic shoulders, and fluid in the subacromial–subdeltoid bursa is found in 20% (NEUMANN et al. 1992; LIOU et al. 1993).

Increased signal intensity within the distal portion of the supraspinatus tendon in healthy subjects can also be caused by the magic-angle effect (TIMINS et al. 1995). ERIKSON et al. described a markedly increased intratendinous signal intensity observed at the 'magic angle' of 55°, intermediate signal intensity was observed at 45° and 65°. Tendon orientation in relation to the static magnetic field greatly affects the signal intensity of the tendon during MRI (ERICKSON et al. 1991, 1993). Although VAHLENSICK et al. (1993) recognized two segments

of the supraspinatus muscle, an anterior fusiform portion that contains the dominant tendon and a strap-like posterior portion, they concluded that the zone of increased signal intensity seen near the insertion is related to tendon orientation in the magnetic field ('magic angle') and not explained by fat or partial volume averaging.

9.4.4
Partial Thickness Tears

Defects of the fibers of a rotator cuff tendon can include only parts of the tendon without penetrating the full thickness of the tendon. These partial defects are located either on the articular surface at the synovial reflection (rim rents), within the central portion of the tendon or outside the joint along the bursal aspect of the tendon (CODMAN and AKERSON 1931).

Rim rents (partial tears at the articular surface) develop frequently at the point of attachment immediately adjacent to the articular surface of the humeral head, but can also occur distant from this attachment (Fig. 9.9). The prevalence of these partial thickness supraspinatus ruptures is reported to be 32%–37% and increase with age, most often seen in the sixth and seventh decades (ELLMAN 1990; LOHR and UHTHOFF 1987). Partial tears occurring in the bursal surface are less commonly reported. The defects appear to be the result of friction of the acromion (Fig. 9.10) (CODMAN and AKERSON 1931). Tears can develop from within 1 cm of the insertion and can vary from superficial flap to nearly full-thickness. At the distal stump hypervascularity has been

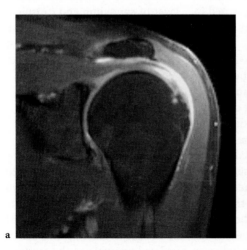 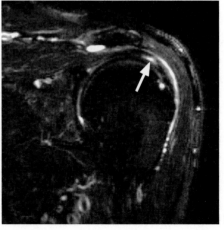

a   b

Fig. 9.9a, b. Articular-sided partial supraspinatus tear. Bursal effusion and fluid in the partial defect in the mid-substance of the supraspinatus tendon is seen well on both the proton-density fat-suppressed image (**a**) and the STIR image (**b**). There is also a small cyst present in the greater tuberosity at the fibro-osseous junction of the supraspinatus tendon

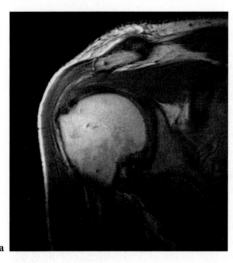 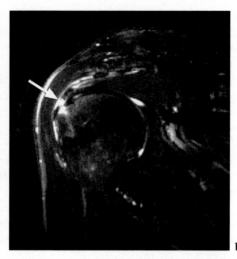

a   b

Fig. 9.10a, b. Bursa-sided partial thickness tear with bone marrow edema in greater tuberosity. This case combines a classic combination of imaging findings in long-standing impingement syndrome including fibrillation and thickening of the peripheral part of the supraspinatus tendon, bursal effusion, remodeling of the undersurface of the acromion with bone apposition, bone marrow edema at the fibro-osseous junction at the greater tuberosity, and partial thickness tear in this area (*arrow*)

observed in several cases on histology (Fig. 9.11) (FUKUDA et al. 1990). Rim rent tears can be mistaken for a intratendinous signal, and should be carefully looked for in younger patients with shoulder pain (TUITE et al. 1998).

Isolated intratendinous tearing of the supraspinatus tendon is rare, and most cases are associated with bursal or joint side cuff tears (FUKUDA et al. 1994). Usually they are located in the mid-layer of the tendon and extend parallel to the axis of the tendon. These partial mid-substance tears frequently reach the enthesis and show local disruptions there. If fluid is present, water equivalent signal intensity is seen in the area of the defect. Partial thickness tears are usually circumscribed and rarely exceed 10 mm measured in the AP or sagittal direction. They can be missed by MRI and arthrography (FUKUDA et al. 1996).

Consistent differentiation of tendinosis, partial thickness tears and full-thickness tears of the rotator cuff tendons is more difficult on non-enhanced MR images when no fluid is present in the joint cavity or in the bursa (ROBERTSON et al. 1995). Partial thickness tears or a horizontal splitting of the tendon beginning from the joint surface or the bursal surface is only detectable if there is fluid signal present in the defect or between the tendon layers. Frequently this fluid is absent and sensitivity for partial thickness tears of non-enhanced MR imaging of the shoulder is low. The reported sensitivities and specificities for the detection of partial thickness tears ranges between 15% and 92%, and 85% and 99%, respectively. In a large series of 222 patients with 26 partial and 45 full-thickness tears the sensitivity ranged from 35% to 44% and the specificity ranged from 85% to 97% (REINUS et al. 1995; QUINN et al. 1995; SINGSON et al. 1996; IANNOTTI et al. 1991; BALICH et al. 1997).

MR arthrography can solve the problem of partial thickness tears originating from the joint surface of the tendon. Unfortunately partial thickness tears originating from the bursal surface of the tendon are still missed, as long as there is no communication of the joint cavity with the bursa, allowing for the injected contrast medium or the fluid to fill the bursa and the partial thickness tear. Rare cases of partial thickness tears that progressed to full-thickness tears of the supraspinatus tendon, leaving a very thin layer of synovium and capsule intact, can be missed in arthrography and even in MR arthrography, but can be suspected due to the substance loss on nonenhanced MR images (BLANCHARD et al. 1998).

9.4.5
Full-Thickness Tears

A complete or full-thickness tear of a rotator cuff tendon involves all fibers of the tendon from the joint surface to the bursal surface (Fig. 9.12). A full thickness tear always creates a communication between the joint cavity and the bursa. A total of 78% of all tendon tears involve the supraspinatus muscle, isolated ruptures of the tendon of the infraspinatus muscle and the subscapularis muscle are relatively rare. If present, they frequently occur in combina-

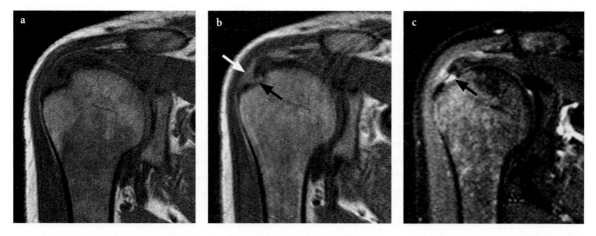

Fig. 9.11a–c. Bursa-sided partial thickness tear. Oblique coronal non-enhanced T1-weighted image (**a**), T1-weighted image following gadolinium application (**b**), and STIR image (**c**). The supraspinatus tendon is thickened (**a**) and there is marked enhancement visible in the subacromial–subdeltoid bursa and in the gap of the partially ruptured tendon (*arrow*) (**b**). Here, fluid with high signal intensity is present (*arrow*) (**c**)

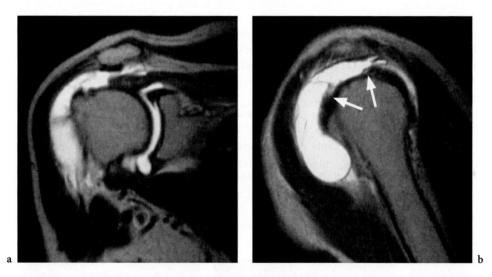

Fig. 9.12a, b. Large full-thickness supraspinatus tendon tear, oblique coronal and oblique sagittal T2-weighted magnetic resonance arthrography arthrograms. Between the dark cortex of the humeral head and the low signal intensity bone apposition at the undersurface of the acromion only the bright signal from fluid is seen (**a**). On the oblique sagittal image complete absence of tendon tissue is visible from the rotator interval anteriorly to the anterior aspect of the infraspinatus tendon (*arrow*) (**b**)

tion with a supraspinatus tendon lesion. A rupture of the teres minor muscle tendon does not occur under normal circumstances. Tears are centered in the anterior half of the rotator cuff in 79% of patients younger than 36 years old, and in 89% of the patients older than 36 years (TUITE et al. 1998).

The prognosis of a full-thickness supraspinatus tear is influenced by several factors. Most important is the size of the tear. A focal defect of only a few millimeters in size can be responsible for significant clinical complaints. These defects are relatively easily excised and repaired. The larger the defect becomes

in the AP diameter, the greater the possibility that parts of the ruptured tendon fibers can retract, which can also increase the size of the defect in the mediolateral direction. Retraction of the tendon stumps increases the difficulties associated with intraoperative reinsertion of the tendon into the bone at the greater tuberosity and facilitates the development muscle atrophy, a sign related to a poor outcome of supraspinatus repair surgery.

The imaging criteria of a full-thickness tear include discontinuity of the cuff with water equivalent signal intensity on T2-weighted or STIR images within the musculotendinous gap and extending from the low intensity cortical bone of the humeral head to the cortical bone of the undersurface of the acromion or to the undersurface of the deltoid muscle (from the bursal to the joint surface of the tendon) (Fig. 9.13) (REINUS et al. 1995; KNEELAND et al. 1987; EVANCHO et al. 1988; BURK et al. 1989). No residual fibers are present in a localized area in the subacromial space. A diagnosis of a full-thickness tear of a rotator cuff tendon only refers to the communication of the joint cavity with the bursa, without giving the information as to whether the tear is large or small. Reported values for sensitivities and specificities in the detection of full-thickness rotator cuff tears are high and range from 84% to 100% and 93% to 100%, respectively (QUINN et al. 1995; SINGSON et al. 1996; IANNOTTI et al. 1991; BALICH et al. 1997; BURK et al. 1989).

Full-thickness tears are associated with fluid collections in the subacromial subdeltoid bursa, which is the most common finding in full-thickness rotator cuff tears (93%) (FARLEY et al. 1992). Interruption of tendon continuity is the most specific finding in full-thickness tears (FARLEY et al. 1992).

When describing a full-thickness rotator cuff tendon tear, the exact extension of the tear in the oblique AP and oblique sagittal directions should be measured. In 1990, PATTE (1990b) introduced a classification system of rotator cuff lesions from a clinical point of view. This system helps when comparing studies reporting the outcome of surgical repairs and describing rotator cuff lesions radiologically. The following factors are classified within this system: *Extent of tear*; *topography of tear in sagittal plane*; *topography of tear in frontal plane*; *quality of muscle*; and *state of the long head of biceps tendon* (LHB). Sub-classifications of the extent of the tear include partial tears, full-thickness tears measuring less than 1 cm in the sagittal diameter at the bony detachment, full-thickness tears of the entire supraspinatus, full-thickness tears involving more than one tendon, massive tears with a secondary osteoarthritis. Topography of tear in the sagittal plane specifically classifies subscapularis tears, coracohumeral ligament tears (rotator interval), isolated supraspinatus tears, tears of entire supraspinatus and one-half of infraspinatus, tears of supraspinatus and infraspinatus, tears of subscapularis, supraspinatus, and infraspinatus (Fig. 9.14) (PATTE 1990b).

It is important to provide the orthopaedic surgeon a most detailed description of the morphology and extent of the rotator cuff lesion as outcome is closely related to the size and position of the defect preoperatively (WATSON 1985). Also, to monitor nonoperative management of full-thickness rotator cuff tears makes a precise description mandatory (GOLDBERG et al. 2001).

9.4.5.1
Subacromial Distance

The subacromial distance, like on radiographs, correlates to the presence of rotator cuff tears and also to the size of the tear. A total of 71% of shoulders with a full-thickness rotator cuff tear have a subacromial distance of 5 mm or less, 71% of control shoulders show more than 6 mm subacromial distance

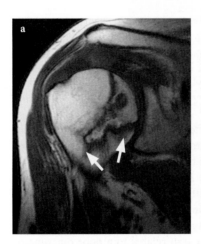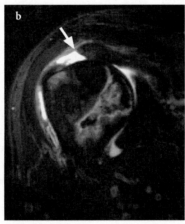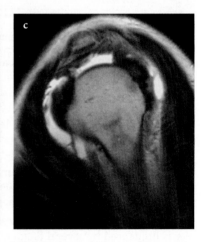

Fig. 9.13a–c. Full-thickness supraspinatus tendon tear; oblique coronal T1-weighted and STIR images, as well as an oblique sagittal T2-weighted image. The tendon defect is difficult to appreciate on T1-weighted image (**a**). On the STIR image the stump of the torn supraspinatus tendon is visible (*arrow*) (**b**). A small area of bone marrow edema is also present in the greater tuberosity. For assessment of the AP extent of the tendon defect oblique sagittal images are necessary (**c**). The bone marrow infarction also seen on the images is not related to the full-thickness tear (*arrows*)

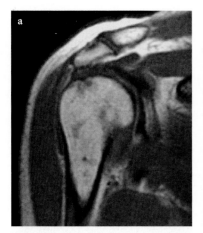
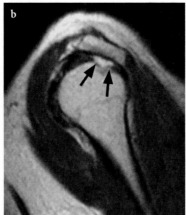
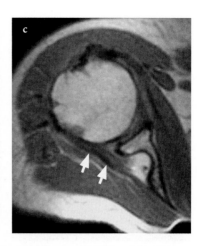

Fig. 9.14a–c. Full-thickness infraspinatus tendon tear; oblique coronal T1-weighted image, oblique sagittal T2-weighted image, and axial T1-weighted image. Signs of chronic cuff pathology are obvious: subacromial bone remodeling and bone apposition, full-thickness rotator cuff tear (**a**). The defect is located posterior under the mid-substance of the acromion in the infraspinatus tendon (*black arrows*)(**b**). Infraspinatus atrophy is seen posterior from the scapula; the anterior located subscapularis muscle is normal (*white arrow*) (**c**)

(KANEKO et al. 1994). An acromiohumeral distance of 5 mm or less indicates a poor prognosis if an operation will be performed.

9.4.5.2
Peribursal Fat Plane

On radiographs and MR images, a fat plane lines the subacromial-subdeltoid bursa. This curvilinear fat is located extrasynovial and 1–2 mm thick. A focal or complete obliteration of this fat plane is seen in partial or complete tears of the rotator cuff or other bursal or soft tissue abnormalities of the shoulder, including calcified tendinitis and rheumatoid arthritis (MITCHELL et al. 1988; ZLATKIN et al. 1989). Discontinuity or obliteration of the subacromial–subdeltoid bursal fat is an unreliable diagnostic sign, since the fat plane is often focally absent in normal shoulders (MIROWITZ 1991; KAPLAN et al. 1992).

9.4.5.3
Intramuscular Cysts

Cystic lesions that arise adjacent to the shoulder include paralabral cysts associated with a tear of the glenoid labrum with possible extension into the suprascapular or spinoglenoid notch and acromioclavicular cysts in association with massive tears of the rotator cuff. Recently, a series of 13 cases of intramuscular cysts of the rotator cuff were identified (SANDERS et al. 2000). Intramuscular cysts of the rotator cuff are associated with small, full-thickness tears or partial undersurface tears of the rotator cuff.

These cysts are relatively small and are contained within the facial sheath or in the substance of the muscle (Fig. 9.15). They are unilocular or multilocular oblong-shaped fluid masses, paralleling the long axis of the involved rotator cuff muscle (SANDERS et al. 2000).

9.4.6
Massive Tears

Small full-thickness tears will enlarge over time. When the tear is only a few millimeters, the humeral head remains in place and keeps its relationship to the glenoid. In tears greater than 10 mm in diameter the humeral head is slowly moved upward by those shoulder muscles centering the humeral head underneath the coracoacromial arch. In cases of massive tears, which exceed 20 mm in diameter, the infraspinatus tendon in addition to the supraspinatus tendon, and in rare cases, the subscapularis tendon, become torn and insufficient (Fig. 9.16). The humeral head migrates upward and finally articulates with the undersurface of the acromion (Fig. 9.17). With time the undersurface of the acromion becomes remodeled with resorption of the central bone and formation of a concave aspect of the inferior acromion. This process is appreciated roentgenographically as acromial acetabulization (HAMADA et al. 1990). In this late phase of impingement syndrome with chronic, massive rotator cuff rupture and joint remodeling, the acromioclavicular joint is also frequently severely damaged.

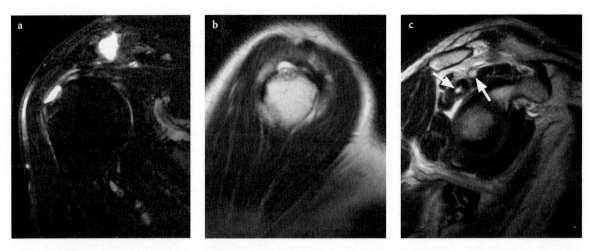

Fig. 9.15a–c. Full-thickness infraspinatus tendon tear, cyst in the infraspinatus muscle; oblique coronal T2-weighted fat-suppressed image (**a**), oblique sagittal T2-weighted image (**b, c**). In addition to a full-thickness infraspinatus tendon tear a small cyst is seen inside the infraspinatus muscle and at the posterior aspect of the supraspinatus muscle (*arrows*). Instability is present in the acromioclavicular joint indicated by fluid in the joint space

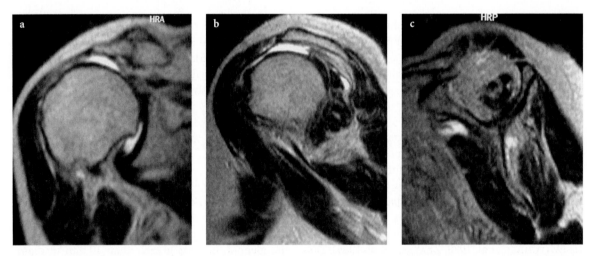

Fig. 9.16a–c. Massive rotator cuff tear, oblique coronal (**a**), and oblique sagittal (**b, c**) T2-weighted images. The complete supraspinatus and parts of the infraspinatus tendon are ruptured. Severe atrophy of the supraspinatus and infraspinatus muscle is seen on the sagittal image through the supraspinatus fossa (**c**)

9.4.6.1
Acromioclavicular Cyst

Acromioclavicular cysts can be an unusual occurrence with rotator cuff tears (CRAIG 1986). In the presence of a massive cuff tear, the chronic friction between the humeral head and the acromioclavicular joint leads to mechanical wear of the articular capsule in the undersurface of this joint. This allows synovial fluid to leak and accumulate into the acromioclavicular joint with free communication of the glenohumeral joint with the subdeltoid subacromial bursa, the acromioclavicular joint and the soft tissue cranial of the acromioclavicular joint (Fig. 9.18) (POSTACCHINI et al. 1993).

During arthrography with injection of contrast material a rapid flow of contrast medium is observed into a fluid-filled mass above the acromioclavicular joint. These acromioclavicular cysts are rare conditions usually occurring in the presence of a wide communication between glenohumeral and acromioclavicular joints in patients with a massive rotator cuff tear (POSTACCHINI et al. 1993). The fluid passes from the glenohumeral joint through the rotator cuff tear and the subacromial bursa, through the acromioclavicular joint into a cyst-like recess above the acromioclavicular joint. This finding is called the Geyser phenomenon, a sign without clinical significance (SCHWEITZER et al. 1994). It only indicates

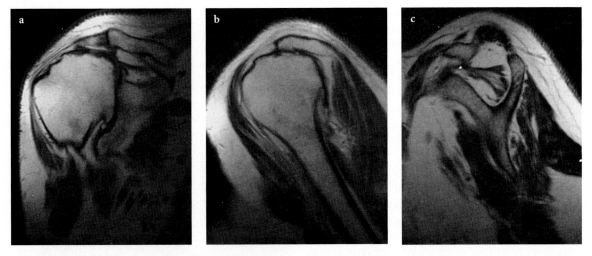

Fig. 9.17a–c. Massive tear of the rotator cuff. Cranial dislocation of the humeral head with remodeling of the glenohumeral joint is seen on oblique coronal T1-weighted image (**a**). All tendons of the rotator cuff are torn, and bone contact exists between the humeral head and the acromion (**b**). Severe atrophy of all muscles of the rotator cuff had occurred including atrophy of the deltoid muscle (**a–c**)

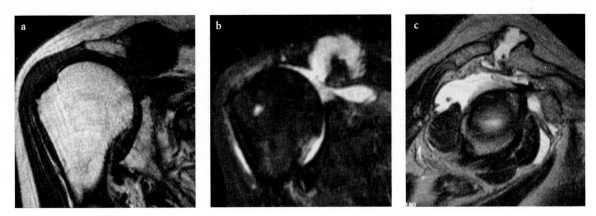

Fig. 9.18a–c. Massive tear of the rotator cuff with acromioclavicular cyst. Oblique coronal T1-weighted image (**a**) and STIR image (**b**), oblique sagittal T2-weighted image (**c**). Cranial dislocation of the humeral head. The acromioclavicular joint is disrupted with fluid extending from the glenohumeral joint through the acromioclavicular joint into a cyst cranial to the acromioclavicular joint

a chronic, long-standing, generally extensive tear of the rotator cuff. Generally, these tears should not be operated on because they are associated with a poor prognosis due to the severe retraction and atrophy of the supraspinatus muscle.

9.4.7
Rotator Cuff Muscles

Severe muscle atrophy is common in patients with large rotator cuff tears (SEEGER et al. 1988; IANNOTTI et al. 1991; ZLATKIN et al. 1989). The postoperative function of the shoulder with a torn rotator cuff is dependent on the degree of residual function of atrophic cuff muscles (NAKAGAKI et al. 1995). The degree of supraspinatus muscle atrophy and fatty degeneration serves as an indirect sign for rotator cuff pathology (THOMAZEAU et al. 1996). Tendinosis and partial thickness rotator cuff tendon tears can cause pain during elevation of the arm but the transmission of force is preserved and significant muscle atrophy cannot occur. In cases of small full-thickness tears, the torn fibers are still in contact with intact fibers, preventing retraction of the torn fibers. With increasing size of the defect the possibility for retraction of the tendon increases, contractile activity decreases, and muscle contractions become useless,

finally ending with atrophy of the muscle (BJORKEN-
HEIM 1989). A direct correlation between the size of
the tendon rupture and the extent of the atrophy
of the rotator cuff muscles as measured on oblique
coronal or parasagittal MR images has been proven
(NAKAGAKI et al. 1994; ZANETTI et al. 1998a).

Atrophy is characterized by a loss of muscle
volume and fatty degeneration. The degree of atrophy is significantly correlated to the degree of fatty
degeneration (FUCHS et al. 1999). Fatty degeneration of the supraspinatus muscle is correlated and
associated with the size of the cuff defect and the
degree of retraction of the tendon fibers (NAK-
AGAKI et al. 1996). Bands of bright signal within
the muscle belly on T1-weighted and T2-weighted
images are indicative of muscular fiber fatty degeneration (NAKAGAKI et al. 1995; BJORKENHEIM 1989).
NAKAGAKI and coworkers (1994, 1995) assessed the
muscle volume of the supraspinatus on oblique coronal images and calculated a supraspinatus muscle
belly ratio from the greatest width of the muscle
belly to the distance from the greater tuberosity to
the proximal end of the supraspinatus muscle. Fatty
infiltration is analyzed on T1-weighted images.
Linear bright bands and variation in signal intensity are indicative of fatty replacement and are classified into three grades: Grade 1, no linear bands,
homogenous muscle belly; Grade 2, presence of one
or two narrow bands, or one or two variegated areas
in muscle, excluding linear bands; Grade 3, presence
of three or more narrow linear bands, or one or two
thick linear bands, three or more variegated areas
in muscle excluding linear bands (NAKAGAKI et al.
1995).

The volume of the rotator cuff muscles is difficult
to assess on oblique coronal images. Exact measurement of the muscle volume is possible on oblique
sagittal MR images obtained parallel to the plane of
the glenoid fossa medially from the coracoid process
through the supraspinatus fossa, called the Y-shaped
view (Fig. 9.19) (THOMAZEAU et al. 1996). THOM-
AZEAU et al. (1996) correlated the area covered by the
muscle to the area of the supraspinatus fossa and calculated this ratio. An easier and more practical way
is suggested by ZANETTI et al. (1998a), who introduced the 'tangent sign'. For supraspinatus muscle
volume quantification a midsagittal image through
the supraspinatus fossa is selected in which bony
boarders are present anteriorly and posteriorly, and
a tangent line drawn from the superior aspect of the
scapula to the superior aspect of the scapular spine. A
normal supraspinatus muscle always extends above
this tangent line. If surgery is to be successful, the

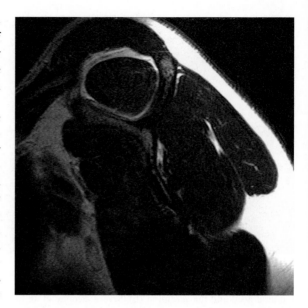

Fig. 9.19. Sagittal T2-weighted image. Normal muscles of the
rotator cuff

muscle belly must reach the tangent line or should
stay only a few millimeters beneath it. If fat surrounds
the supraspinatus muscle and the muscle is several
millimeters below that line, atrophy is advanced and
restitution of the rotator cuff with reinsertion of the
supraspinatus tendon is not promising (Fig. 9.20).
For measuring the infraspinatus muscle, a tangent
line is drawn from the posterior aspect of the spina
scapulae to the inferior boarder of the scapula. The
normal infraspinatus muscle overrides this line by
several millimeters.

9.4.8
Rotator Interval Tears

The triangular region between the superior border of
the subscapularis tendon and the anterior border of
the supraspinatus tendon with its base at the coracoid
process and its apex at the intertubercular sulcus is
called the rotator cuff interval (CHUNG et al. 2000;
NOBUHARA and IKEDA 1987). Through the rotator
interval the long head of the biceps tendon passes
from the bicipital groove into and through the shoulder joint to its anchor at the superior glenoid. The
rotator interval is composed of parts of the supraspinatus, subscapularis, coracohumeral ligament,
superior glenohumeral ligament, and glenohumeral
joint capsule. A medial part is composed of an inferior and an superior element and distinguished from
a more lateral part. The superior layers of the lateral

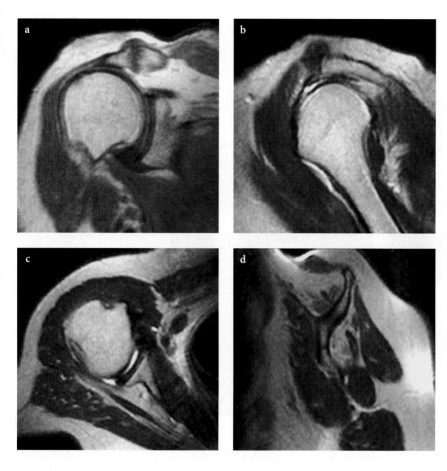

Fig. 9.20a–d. Massive tear of the rotator cuff with long-standing complete tear of the supra- and infraspinatus tendon (**a, b**). Severe atrophy of these muscles had occurred. In the fossa of the supra- and infraspinatus muscle large amounts of fat are seen, only few residual muscle fibers are detectable (**c, d**). Infraspinatus muscle atrophy is also well appreciated on an axial image with the muscle almost missing posterior to the glenoid and the scapula (**c**)

part form a fibrous plate (Jost et al. 2000). The lateral part is strengthened by the semicircular humeral ligament and the anterior fibers of the supraspinatus tendon (Kolts et al. 2002). The superior elements of the medial part are the coracohumeral and coracoglenoid ligament, the inferior element is reinforced by the superior and medial glenohumeral ligaments. The rotator interval is a complex network of ligamentous structures (Kolts et al. 2002).

The rotator cuff interval capsule is best evaluated after MR arthrography in the sagittal plane. The width of the rotator cuff interval capsule is 1.8 mm (rage 1.7–2.0 mm) on MR images (Chung et al. 2000). Tears of the rotator interval can increase the distance of the subscapularis and supraspinatus tendon and muscle on oblique sagittal images. Lesions of the rotator interval can be missed during conventional MRI unless fluid is present in the subacromial–subdeltoid bursa (Fig. 9.21). Interval lesions are frequently associated with tears of the subscapularis tendon, and dislocations or subluxations of the biceps tendon out from the bicipital groove can occur. In 47% of subscapularis tears the superior glenohumeral ligament (SGHL)/coracohumeral liga-

ment (CHL) complex is also involved. A total of 10% of supraspinatus tears involve also the lateral coracohumeral ligament (Bennett 2001). Tears of the rotator interval are often associated with subcoracoid effusions (Grainger et al. 2000). Because of a complete absence of rotator interval tissue in several fetal specimens, rotator interval defects may also be congenital (Cole et al. 2001).

9.4.9
Incomplete and Complete Subscapularis Tears and Biceps Tendon Lesions

Three types of subscapularis tendon lesions are described: (1) the isolated subscapularis tendon tear, (2) the involvement of the subscapularis in large rotator cuff tears, (3) and the anterosuperior lesions of the rotator cuff (Pfirrmann et al. 1999). Patients present with a characteristic clinical syndrome with a pathological 'lift-off test' and increased passive external rotation. In cases of a torn subscapularis tendon, full internal rotation cannot be maintained in hyperextension, documented by the patient's inability to

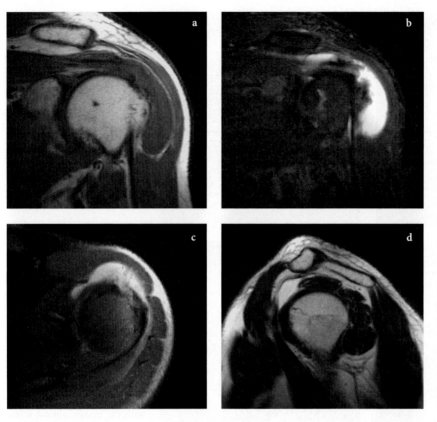

Fig. 9.21a–d. Rotator interval lesion. Oblique coronal T1-weighted (**a**) and STIR image (**b**), proton density-weighted fat-suppressed axial (**c**), and T2-weighted oblique sagittal image (**d**). In the area of the rotator interval, the rotator cuff tendons are thickened and show increased signal intensity (**a**). There is marked distension of the subdeltoid bursa by effusion. This fluid outlines the bursa-sided defect in the rotator interval (**b**). The fraying of the fibrous capsule of the rotator cuff interval is well appreciated on the axial image (**c**)

lift the hand off the back (GERBER and KRUSHELL 1991; GERBER et al. 1996).

Only 2% of rotator cuff tears predominantely or exclusively involve the subscapularis tendon (Fig. 9.22) (LI et al. 1999). Isolated rupture of the tendon of the subscapularis muscle is rare and is usually posttraumatic. In 45 evaluated subscapularis tears, 35 (78%) extended from the supraspinatus and 25 (56%) also involved the infraspinatus (Fig. 9.23). Two (4%) also extended into the teres minor. Only 9 (20%) isolated subscapularis tears were observed (LI et al. 1999). The anterosuperior rotator cuff tear, a combination of a subscapularis tear and a supraspinatus tear, with or without an infraspinatus tendon tear, represents a separate classification of rotator cuff injuries. Because the majority of cases are related to trauma, delay in diagnosis carries a poor prognosis, operative treatment is more extensive and outcome after surgical repair is inferior to posterosuperior rotator cuff tears (WARNER et al. 2001).

If an isolated subscapularis tear is present, communication to the subacromial subdeltoid bursa can be misinterpreted as a supraspinatus tear on an AP arthrogram. CT arthrography will show communication with air reaching from the glenohumeral joint to the bicipital groove. A medial dislocation of

the biceps tendon is indicative of a complete rupture of the subscapularis tendon (Fig. 9.24). Along with the coracohumeral and transverse humeral ligaments, which are parts of the rotator cuff interval, the subscapularis tendon is a major stabilizer of the long biceps tendon. Degeneration or disruption of the subscapularis tendon has been reported to be a common predisposing factor to medial dislocation of the biceps tendon (CHAN et al. 1991; CERVILLA et al. 1991; PETERSSON 1986; PATTEN 1994). In an autopsy study from PETERSSON (1986), medial displacement of the biceps tendon was found in five of 77 subjects, always in connection with a full-thickness supraspinatus tear. The tendon slips medially to the lesser tuberosity under the subscapularis tendon, which is partially internally ruptured (PETERSSON 1986).

On MRI, in the presence of a tear of the subscapularis tendon, the contours of the tendon are poorly defined and of abnormally high signal on T2-weighted images. Discontinuity and frank retraction is seen in 78% of patients. Subscapularis tears are well detected in the sagittal oblique plane with the deltoid muscle seen in direct apposition to the anterior humerus and the lesser tuberosity (LI et al. 1999).

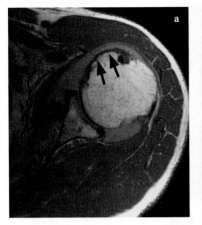
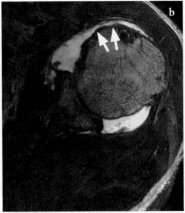
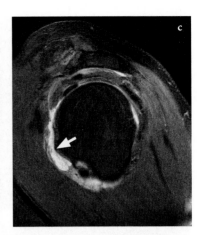

Fig. 9.22a–c. Magnetic resonance arthrogram of complete avulsion and rupture of the subscapularis tendon without luxation of the biceps tendon. Axial T1-weighted (**a**) and DESS image (**b**), sagittal FLASH fat-saturated image (**c**). The fluid freely passes from the anterior part of the glenohumeral joint across the lesser tuberosity (**a, b**). On T1-weighted axial image fatty infiltrates and atrophy is visible in the subscapularis muscle anterior to the scapula (**a**). On the oblique sagittal image fluid is seen anterior to the lesser tuberosity and without joint distension the deltoid muscle comes in contact with the anterior humerus (**c**). The supraspinatus, infraspinatus, and teres minor tendons including the intraarticular biceps tendon are normal

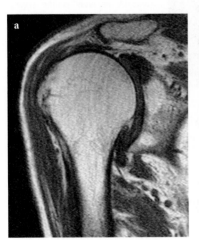
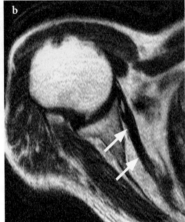
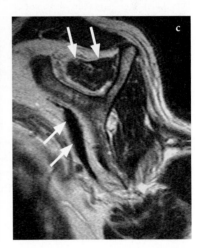

Fig. 9.23a–c. Massive tear of the rotator cuff with long-standing complete tear of the supraspinatus and subscapularis tendon (**a**). Severe atrophy of these muscles had occurred (**b, c**). In the supraspinatus fossa the muscle is surrounded by fat and does not reach a tangent line to the superior bony boarders of the fossa (*arrows*) (**c**). Subscapularis muscle atrophy is depicted on axial and sagittal image with the muscle almost missing anterior to the glenoid and the scapula (*arrows*) (**c**)

MR arthrography criteria for the evaluation of subscapularis lesions include leakage of intraarticular contrast medium under the insertion of the subscapularis tendon onto the lesser tuberosity on axial and parasagittal images (GERBER and KRUSHELL 1991; WALCH et al. 1994), presence of fatty infiltration (FARLEY et al. 1992; GOUTALLIER et al. 1994; ZANETTI et al. 1998b), and abnormalities in the course of the long biceps tendon, either subluxation or dislocation (CHAN et al. 1991; CERVILLA et al. 1991; ZANETTI et al. 1998b). Axial MR images are sensitive in detecting subscapularis tendon abnormalities. The specific-

ity of findings on axial images can be improved by including ancillary signs and findings from parasagittal images (PFIRRMANN et al. 1999).

Abnormalities of the biceps tendon are commonly recognized in subscapularis tendon lesions (PATTEN 1994). Subcoracoid effusion, either in the bursa or the subscapularis recess, is often associated with anterior rotator cuff tears, including tears of the rotator interval (GRAINGER et al. 2000). Long-standing tears of the subscapularis tendon result in fatty degeneration and substantial loss of volume of the subscapularis muscle (GERBER et al. 1996).

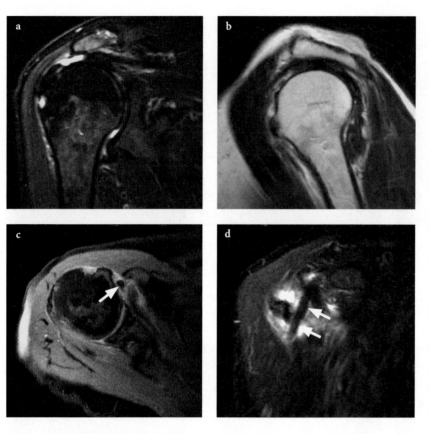

Fig. 9.24a–d. Complete rupture of the subscapularis tendon with medial luxation of the biceps tendon. Oblique coronal STIR images (**a, d**), oblique sagittal T2-weighted image (**b**), axial proton density-weighted fat-suppressed image (**c**). Bright fluid signal from the cortical bone of the humeral head to the acromion indicates a full-thickness tendon rupture (**a**). At the anterior aspect of the humerus no tendon tissue is visible between the deltoid muscle and the lesser tuberosity (**b**). On the axial image the empty bicipital sulcus and the medial dislocated long head of the biceps tendon (*arrow*), as well as the stump of the subscapularis tendon, is visible (**c**). The strait downward orientated biceps tendon on oblique images is characteristic for biceps tendon luxation (*arrow*) (**d**)

Incomplete tears of the subscapularis tendon occur in conjunction with small or medium-size tears of the supraspinatus tendon. This combination is common in older patients, and most subscapularis lesions are incomplete tears on the articular side (SAKURAI et al. 1998).

9.4.10
Adhesive Capsulitis

The clinical presentation of adhesive capsulitis with pain and severely decreased joint motion ("frozen shoulder") is nonspecific and often mimics several other shoulder disorders (NEVIASER and NEVIASER 1987). Adhesive capsulitis is caused by thickening and contraction of the joint capsule, the coracoacromial ligament, and the rotator cuff interval due to inflammation of the joint capsule and synovium (NEVIASER 1945; OZAKI et al. 1989). The characteristic MRI finding of adhesive capsulitis is thickening of the capsule and synovium of more than 4 mm. Mean thickness of the capsule in patients with adhesive capsulitis is 5.2 mm, in asymptomatic volunteers 2.9 mm (EMIG et al. 1995). In contradiction to arthrography, the volume of articular fluid seen on MR images is not significantly diminished in patients with adhesive capsulitis (EMIG et al. 1995).

9.4.11
Coracoid Impingement

Coracoid impingement, also called subcoracoid, anteromedial subcoracoid, or coracohumeral impingement, is an uncommon, but well-described, cause of anterior shoulder pain (PATTE 1990a; DINES et al. 1990). Impingement of the subscapularis muscle and tendon occurs between the lateral aspect of the tip of the coracoid process and the lesser tuberosity (Fig. 9.25). On CT scans, GERBER and coworkers (1985) determined the normal distance of the coracoid tip to the humeral head to be 8.6 mm. This distance decreases to 6.7 mm in patients with coracoid impingement. There is a dull pain in front of the shoulder, frequently extending to the front of the upper arm or to the forearm (GERBER et al. 1985). Pain is exacerbated by the coracoid impingement test with forward elevation, internal rotation, and cross-arm adduction (DINES et al. 1990; PAULSON et al. 2001). Injection of anesthetics between the coracoid process and the humeral head can help in making the diagnosis.

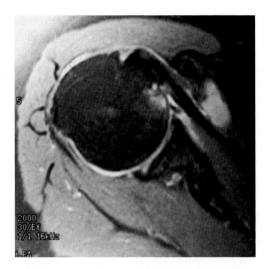

Fig. 9.25. Coracoid impingement. The subscapularis tendon becomes impinged between the coracoid process and the medial humeral head. Bone marrow edema is present medial to the lesser tuberosity

9.5
Acromion: Anatomic Variations and Associated Changes in Rotator Cuff Disease

Although acute exacerbations with pain, restricted motion, and impaired function of the shoulder play a major role in the clinical appearance, impingement syndrome is a chronic process with repetitive stress to the supraspinatus tendon being impinged between the anterior inferior border of the acromion and the upward moving humeral head with the eccentric greater tuberosity rotating inwards into the subacromial space.

These repetitive microtraumas to the anterior inferior border of the acromion induces the formation of bone at the under surface of the anterior acromion. These degenerative changes are limited to the anterior third of the acromion (EDELSON and TAITZ 1992). Involvement of the middle and posterior areas is limited to severe massive and chronic tears of all parts of the rotator cuff with formation and remodeling of a nearthrosis between the humeral head and the undersurface of the acromion.

Two types of degenerative changes of the acromion are described: a traction spur at the anterior edge of the acromion and a "facet-type" degeneration with a development of a eburnated pseudoarticular surface for the humeral head (EDELSON and TAITZ 1992). In the first instance, the bone apposition is predominately orientated anteriorly described as enthesophyte on the basis of chronic pathologic traction on the coracoacromial ligament, giving the appearance of an anterior subacromial spur or hook. The bone appositions can also develop as a plate of bone with an appearance similar to a horseshoe in the true AP radiograph and on oblique coronal MR images, giving the appearance of a pseudoarticular surface (Fig. 9.26). The slowly evolving bone appositions at the under surface of the acromion gradually decrease the subacromial space, subsequently increasing the impingement on the supraspinatus tendon.

a

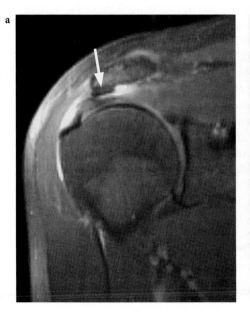

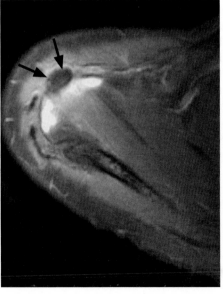

b

Fig. 9.26a, b. Subacromial bone proliferation and spur formation (*arrows*). Bursal effusion and a small partial, bursa-sided tear of the supraspinatus tendon is visible on the proton density-weighted fat-suppressed oblique coronal and axial image (**a, b**)

9.5.1
Acromial Shape

BIGLIANI and coworkers' (1986) classification system has become the accepted method for the evaluation of acromial morphology based on outlet view radiographs in patients with rotator cuff disease. He described three different acromial shapes in correlation to full-thickness rotator cuff tears (Fig. 9.27) (BIGLIANI et al. 1986). An acromion Type I has a flat undersurface and no relationship to impingement. Type II acromion is characterized by a curved undersurface and type III acromion has an anterior hook (hooked acromion). A fourth type of acromion shape was added that has a convex undersurface (FARLEY et al. 1994). BIGLIANI et al. (1986) found a type III acromion in 70% of cadavers with rotator cuff tears, whereas only 3% of type I acromion were associated with a tear. In the entire sample of 140 cadavers a type I (flat) acromion was present in 17%, type II (curved) in 43%, and type III (hooked) in 39% (BIGLIANI et al. 1986, 1991). Bursal-side partial tears or full-thickness tears of the rotator cuff are always associated with severe degenerative changes in the acromion, but degenerative changes in the undersurface of the acromion can be present when the rotator cuff is normal (PANNI et al. 1996).

Acromial morphology on outlet view radiographs is in general independent of age and seems to be a primary anatomic characteristic (NICHOLSON et al. 1996; GETZ et al. 1996), but the shape of the acromion can be modified by secondary bone apposition predominantly at the anterior inferior aspect of the acromion. This spur formation is an age-related change and is one of the most important factors in progression of impingement syndrome to rotator cuff rupture. Enthesophytes are most common in type III acromions. Therefore, the hooked acromion can be congenital or acquired (BIGLIANI et al. 1986). Acromial morphology in general is symmetrical. A type III acromion is more frequently found in men than in women (GETZ et al. 1996).

The determination of the real frequency of the different types of acromions is difficult. EDELSON (1995) examined 750 scapular dry bone specimens and 80 cadavers and did not find a hooking of the acromion under the age of 30 years. The hooked configuration developed at later ages in an increasing proportion of subjects as a result of calcification of the acromial attachment of the coracoacromial ligament (EDELSON 1995). To increase the reliability of the classification of the acromial shape, a method to calculate the anterior slope was described (BIGLIANI et al. 1986). A line through the mid-substance of the acromion is drawn from the posterior aspect of the acromion anteriorly. A second line is then drawn through the point of deflection in the acromion. The angle created at the intersection of the two lines is considered to be the angle of deflection of the anterior acromion. In general, 0°–15° is consistent with Type I, 16°-30° with type II, and >30° with type III.

With age, a consistent and gradual transition from a flat to a more hooked acromion is seen (MACGILLIVRAY et al. 1998). Using MRI, SCHIPPINGER et al. (1997) did not find a single hooked acromion in a young and symptomless population (mean 32 years) and concluded that the hooked acromion is acquired by chronic upward migration of the humeral head. Also using MRI, EPSTEIN and coworkers (1993) confirmed a significant correlation between type III (hooked) acromion and the presence of rotator cuff tears (62% vs 13%, $p<.0001$). He reported that there exists a tendency for the increased prevalence of type III acromion in patients with impingement syndrome (30%, $p= .17$).

In most shoulders of patients with impingement syndrome, a curved acromion was recorded, with a high concomitance of acromial spurs (PANNI et al. 1996; MAIER et al. 2001). Unfortunately the reliability of the radiographic evaluation for acromial morphology is low. By using outlet view radiographs, values for interobserver reliability and intraobserver repeatability are weak and more definite criteria are needed to distinguish and classify the acromion (BRIGHT et al. 1997).

Similar to outlet view radiographs, the acromial shape can be determined on oblique sagittal MR images. The assessment of the acromial shape on oblique sagittal MR images is frequently confusing and dependent on the location of the evaluated

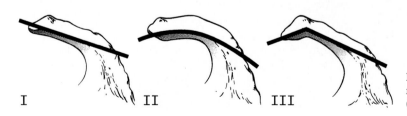

Fig. 9.27. Bigliani classification of acromial types: *I*, flat; *II*, curved; *III*, hooked. (From GETZ et al. 1996)

image. Only a few millimeters difference in slice position can alter the shape and undersurface of the acromion from flat to curved or even hooked. The evaluated slice has not only to lie lateral to the acromioclavicular joint but must cover the peripheral third of that part of the acromion (PEH et al. 1995). Although sagittal oblique MR images are significantly more likely than conventional radiographs to be considered diagnostic, interobserver agreement for MR examinations is poor (HAYGOOD et al. 1994).

9.5.2
Acromial Slope

The lateral acromial angulation in the coronal plane can be classified as type A (neutral, 0°–10°) or type B (downward sloping, >10°) (Fig. 9.28) (MACGILLI-VRAY et al. 1998). To define lateral acromial angulation, a line is drawn through the mid-substance of the acromioclavicular joint, and a second line is drawn through the mid-substance of the acromion (AOKI et al. 1986).

A different way of determination of lateral acromion down slope is to calculate the lateral acromion angle (LAA) as described by BANAS et al. (1995). The lateral acromion angle is formed by intersection of a line parallel to the undersurface of the acromion and a second line parallel to the most lateral extension of the superior and inferior bony glenoid (Fig. 9.29). The average LAA was 78°, with a range of 64°–99°. A significant correlation exists between increased downward sloping of the acromion on coronal MR scans (decreased acromion angle) and rotator cuff tears (BANAS et al. 1995). A total of 85% of patients with a downward sloping of the acromion had stage II or III impingement in a study by MACGILLIVRAY et al. (1998) (Fig. 9.30). BANAS et al. (1995) also found increasing age to be correlated with rotator cuff pathology, whereas MACGILLIVARAY et al. (1998) found a tendency towards increased incidence of lateral downsloping with age.

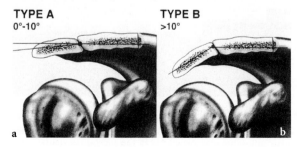

TYPE A
0°–10°

TYPE B
>10°

Fig. 9.28a, b. Calculation of the lateral acromion angulation according to MACGILLIVRAY et al. (1998)

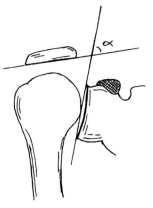

Fig. 9.29. Calculation of the lateral down slope of the acromion (lateral acromion angle) according to BANAS et al. (1995). The lateral acromion angle is formed by the intersection of a line parallel to the acromion undersurface and a line parallel to the farthest lateral extension of the superior and inferior bony glenoid

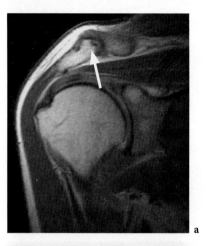

a

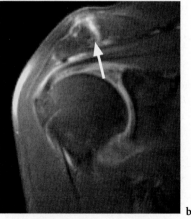

b

Fig. 9.30a,b. Lateral down sloping of the acromion in a patient with impingement syndrome. Oblique coronal T1-weighted (a) and proton density weighted fat suppressed images (b). Fluid is present in the subacromial–subdeltoid bursa and in an acromioclavicular joint with degenerative changes (*arrows*). A prominent coracoacromial ligament is visible at the undersurface of the acromion, probably also playing a part in the impingement process in this patient

9.5.3
Os Acromiale

The acromion arises from two or sometimes three distinct and separate centers of ossification called the pre-acromion, meso-acromion, and meta-acromion (LIBERSON 1937; MUDGE et al. 1984; EDELSON et al. 1993). These centers of ossification are usually united by 22–25 years of age. When these centers fail to unite, the ununited portion is called an os acromiale. The incidence of os acromiale is 8.2% in specimens and 2.7% when evaluating axial radiographs (LIBERSON 1937; EDELSON et al. 1993). In most cases, the free fragment is approximately one third of the overall length of the acromion, and includes the acromioclavicular facet and the principal areas of attachment of the coracoacromial ligament (LIBERSON 1937).

There are reports of an association of os acromiale and impingement syndrome and rotator cuff tears (MUDGE et al. 1984; EDELSON et al. 1993; PARK et al. 1994). In ten patients with os acromiale who underwent MRI, all ten had rotator cuff disease, four with tendinosis and six with tendon tears (Figs. 9.31, 9.32). Frequently osteophytic lipping at the margins of the acromial gap in os acromiale is present, indicating instability (MUDGE et al. 1984; EDELSON et al. 1993; PARK et al. 1994). An os acromiale can present with a "double joint appearance" representing the junction

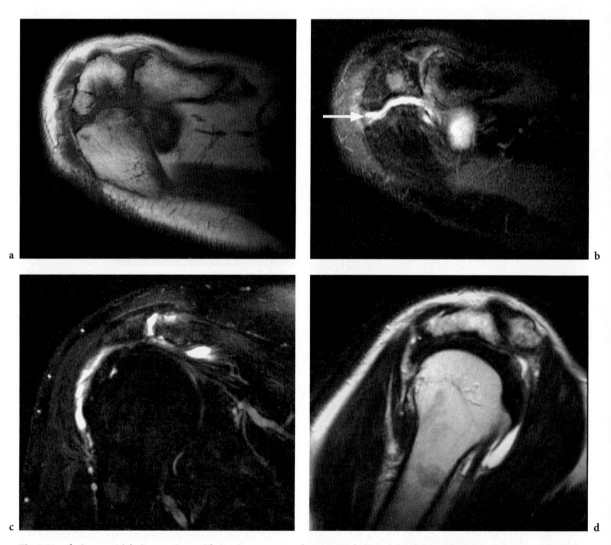

Fig. 9.31a–d. Os acromiale in a patient with impingement syndrome. Axial T1-weighted (**a**) and proton density-weighted fat-suppressed image (**b**), oblique coronal STIR image (**c**), and oblique sagittal T2-weighted image (**d**). Fluid signal in the fibrous gap between the acromion and the anterolateral located os acromiale and bone marrow edema in the acromioclavicular joint indicates mechanical alteration (*arrow*) (**a, b**). Fluid collection in the subacromial–subdeltoid bursa and the hooked acromion are signs of impingement syndrome (**c, d**)

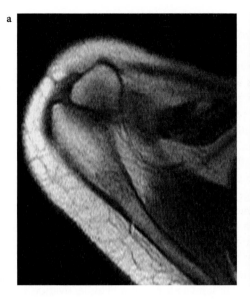

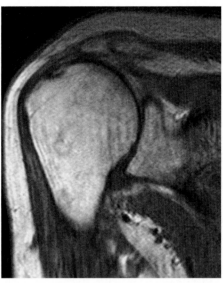

Fig. 9.32a, b. Os acromiale in a patient with massive tear of the rotator cuff. Axial (**a**) and oblique coronal (**b**) T1-weighted image

of the os acromiale with the acromion posteriorly, and with the clavicle anteriorly on oblique sagittal images (Park et al. 1994; Uri et al. 1997). This appearance is only present in 18% of cases (Uri et al. 1997).

The "pseudo acromioclavicular joint" is often noted to lie in a more posterior location than expected for the true AC joint on oblique sagittal images, using the vertical line sign (Uri et al. 1997). Identification of an os acromiale is frequently difficult on oblique coronal images. Correct identification of an os acromiale is more reliably achieved by identifying the coracoacromial ligament that has no clavicular insertion. In questionable cases, a ligament seen to insert on the anterior osseous structure identifies an unfused os and not the distal clavicle (Uri et al. 1997).

9.5.4
Coracoacromial Ligament

The coracoacromial ligament consists of a triangular fibrous sheet, 3–5 cm in length, flattened from above downward, and is seen on MR images as a low signal intensity structure originating at the undersurface of the acromion (Fig. 9.33). Its apex is attached to the apex of the acromion and extends to the inferior aspect of the acromion with different modes of attachment: attachment to the apex with an irregular appearance of the inferior aspect of the arch (8.7%), attachment to the apex of the acromion with a regular inferior aspect (49%), attachment to the acromion and the inferior aspect

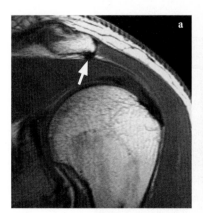

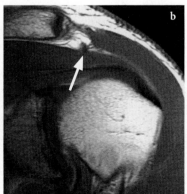

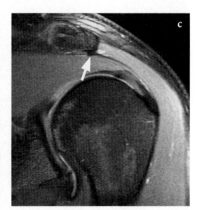

Fig. 9.33a–c. Prominent coracoacromial ligament. The ligament is seen on T1-weighted images as low intensity structure passing from the anterior undersurface of the acromion anteriorly with contact to the rotator cuff (*arrow*) (**a, b**). Corresponding proton density-weighted fat-suppressed image (**c**)

in 21.5%, and attachment only to the inferior aspect of the acromion (22.2%) (Fig. 9.34) (Gagey et al. 1993; Gallino et al. 1995). Its base is attached to the entire lateral boarder of the coracoid process. The thickness is not uniform and varies from 2 to 5.6 mm: its medial and lateral portions are condensed into thick bands; its middle portion is membranous and the lateral band is thicker than the medial band.

In patients with impingement syndrome the coracoacromial ligament shows degenerative changes with fibrillation of the collagen fibers, microtears, and fatty infiltration in the substance of the ligament (Uhthoff et al. 1998). Lesions in the ligament such as fibrin extravasation, degenerative changes in the matrix, and proliferation of metabolic organelles in some cells probably reflect a process of irritation caused by a sustained strain. This strain is most likely produced by the subacromial space. Thus the coracoacromial ligament does not appear to be primarily responsible for initiation of the impingement process (Sarkar et al. 1990).

A low signal intensity structure can be seen projecting inferolaterally from the undersurface of the acromion on coronal MR images in asymptomatic volunteers with normal shoulders; this structure can simulate a subacromial "pseudo"-spur. Unless proven on sagittal images and on radiographs, this structure is related to the coracoacromial ligament and to the normal inferior tendon slip of the deltoid muscle attachment to the acromion (Kaplan et al. 1992).

9.5.5
Acromioclavicular Joint

During elevation of the arm the eccentric greater tuberosity has to move under the acromion. The humeral head has not only to rotate but also to glide in the caudal direction along the glenoid fossa to give space for the inward moving greater tuberosity. Increased tension in those muscles centering the humeral head underneath the coracoacromial arch, or weakness of the muscles resisting this upwardly directed force result in impingement of the supraspinatus tendon.

This mechanism creates a lateral load upon the acromion and the acromioclavicular joint. Stress to the acromioclavicular joint results in bone marrow edema of the peripheral end of the clavicle and the adjacent acromion, and fluid collections in the acromioclavicular joint can be seen. This activation of the acromioclavicular joint in patients with impingement syndrome is frequently not clinically relevant and the patients do not complain (Fig. 9.35) (Fiorella et al. 2000). Bone marrow edema at the acromioclavicular joint is significantly associated with impingement syndrome and can lead to a diagnosis of impingement syndrome (Fig. 9.36). It is not well recognized that both bone marrow edema around the acromioclavicular joint and acromioclavicular joint effusions are not symptomatic by themselves. As bone marrow edema and effusions do not occur in asymptomatic volunteers, they can indicate the presence of impingement syndrome and rotator cuff tears (Schweitzer et al. 1994).

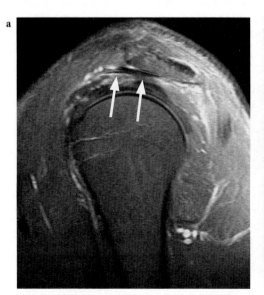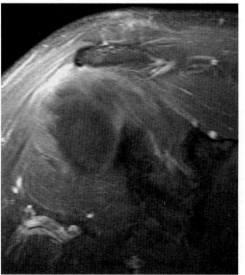

Fig. 9.34a, b. Thickened coracoacromial ligament (*arrows*) with attachment to the inferior aspect of the acromion. Oblique sagittal (**a**) and oblique coronal (**b**) proton density-weighted fat-suppressed image

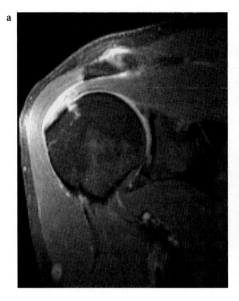
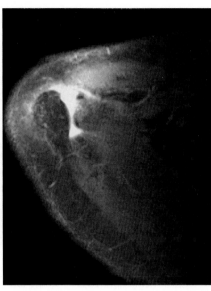

Fig. 9.35. Synovitis and fibrovascular tissue in the subacromial–subdeltoid bursa and the acromioclavicular joint. T1-weighted fat-suppressed coronal (a) and axial (b) images after gadolinium application. Mechanical stress in subacromial impingement is translated to the acromioclavicular joint

Degeneration of the acromioclavicular joint is in most cases not a primary, extrinsic factor for impingement syndrome, but a secondary change as a result of long-standing impingement syndrome. On MR images of a painful shoulder, osteophytes and capsular hypertrophy at the inferior boarder of the acromioclavicular joint are frequently seen. Those changes appear to impinge from directions on the cranial supraspinatus muscle and tendon and are responsible for the symptoms of impingement syndrome (Fig. 9.37). This is true in only a few patients. In most cases the cause of the impingement is located at a more anterior and lateral location near the edge

of the acromion. Although frequently stressed in textbooks, the degenerated acromioclavicular joint is more likely to be a result of impingement and not the cause.

9.5.6
Greater Tuberosity

Degenerative changes in the greater tuberosity on radiographs, such as cortical flattening, sclerosis, eburnation, irregularity, bone proliferation, and cyst formation have been linked to impingement

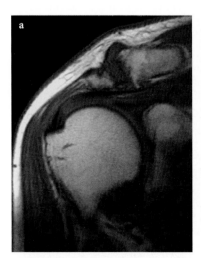
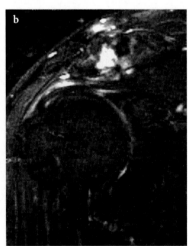
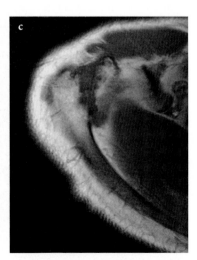

Fig. 9.36a–c. Acromioclavicular joint degeneration in a patient suffering from impingement syndrome. Oblique coronal T1-weighted (a) and STIR image (b), axial T1-wieghted image (c). Erosions and irregularities in the acromioclavicular joint in combination with bone marrow edema adjacent to the joint space are present. Fluid in the subacromial–subdeltoid bursa and subacromial bone appositions are also identified

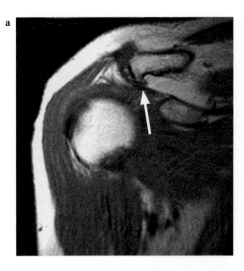

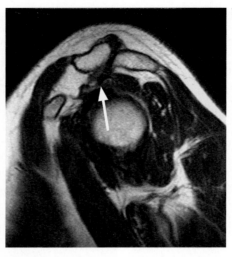

Fig. 9.37a, b. Acromioclavicular joint degeneration. The caudal orientated spurs are in contact with the rotator cuff (*arrows*) (**a, b**)

syndrome and rotator cuff tears (Harrison 1949; Cotton and Rideout 1964; Cone et al. 1984; Hardy et al. 1986; Bernageau 1990). These studies were uncontrolled and were biased toward more severe disease. Huang et al. (1999) correlated radiographic findings of cortical thickening, subcortical sclerosis, and cyst-like lesions with MR evidence of rotator cuff tears and tendinopathy. Interobserver agreement for the three radiographic findings was poor to fair. Cortical thickening of the greater tuberosity and subcortical sclerosis are not associated with rotator cuff disease. For some observers, identifying cyst-like lesions is associated with rotator cuff disease, but the clinical usefulness of this observation is limited by a high interobserver variability and poor positive predictive value (Fig. 9.38).

Bone marrow edema in the greater tuberosity can be occasionally seen in patients with chronic or acute shoulder problems undergoing MRI. It is seen in 1.3% of these patients (McCauley et al. 2000). A total of 82% of these patients also had partial or full thickness rotator cuff tears indicating a relationship between rotator cuff disease and bone marrow edema of the greater tuberosity (Fig. 9.39). It was argued that trauma with avulsion forces at the greater tuberosity may be responsible for these bone marrow edema areas (Mason et al. 1999; Zanetti et al. 1999). Since the mean anteroposterior measurement of the edema was 2.1 cm (1.5–3.2 cm) and in the transverse dimension 2.2 cm (1.0–3.6 cm), it is more likely that chronic compression rather avulsion caused the edema.

Sano et al. (1998) looked for cystic changes of the humeral head on MR images. They observed cystic changes in 35% of their patients in the bare bone area of the anatomical neck and at the attachment of the supraspinatus tendon. Cystic changes in the bare

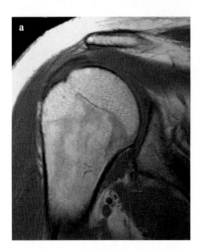

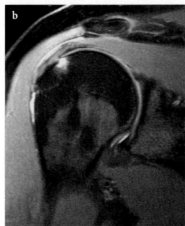

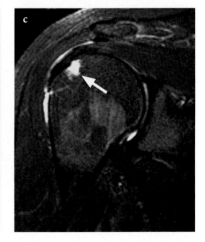

Fig. 9.38a–c. Patient with impingement syndrome. A cyst had developed in the greater tuberosity origination from the fibroosseous junction of the supraspinatus tendon (*arrow*). There is also bursal effusion and a thickened coracoacromial ligament

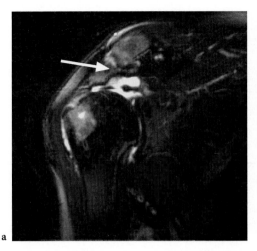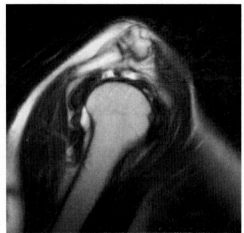

a   b

Fig. 9.39a, b. Full-thickness rotator cuff tear with bone marrow edema in the greater tuberosity. At the undersurface of the acromion, marked bone appositions had developed, causing a lateral down sloping of the acromion (*arrow*)

bone area were observed equally often in shoulders with or without rotator cuff tears (27% and 18%, respectively) and were more frequently observed in the elderly. Cystic changes at the attachment of the supraspinatus and subscapularis tendons were specific to rotator cuff tears: they were observed in 28% of rotator cuff tears, but in none of those with an intact cuff. They concluded that there are two distinct types of cystic changes: one at the attachment of the supraspinatus and subscapularis tendons, which is closely related to tears of these tendons, and the other in the bare bone area of the anatomical neck, which is related to aging.

9.6
Impingement Syndrome and Calcifying Tendinitis

The coincidence of the presence of calcified deposits within the rotator cuff tendons and chronic or acute shoulder pain and dysfunction are designated as calcifying tendinitis (UHTHOFF and SARKAR 1978). The clinical relevance of these calcified deposits to shoulder pain and dysfunction is still under discussion. Calcified deposits within the rotator cuff tendons have been regarded as one possible trigger of shoulder pain and dysfunction, but they may also be incidental radiographic findings in healthy, asymptomatic volunteers (BOSWORTH 1941). Approximately 30% of patients continue to have pain and shoulder dysfunction after curettage of the calcified material (MCKENDRY et al. 1982). At least in these patients, the calcified deposits cannot be the only explanation for shoulder pain and dysfunction.

The calcifications are mainly located in the supraspinatus tendon and only rarely in the infraspinatus or subscapularis tendons (BOSWORTH 1941). Single deposits are most common (68%), of which the highest proportion are in the supraspinatus (49%), 13% in the infraspinatus, 5% in the teres minor tendon, and 1% in the subscapularis tendon. Of the multiple deposits (32%) 17% involve the supraspinatus and infraspinatus, 7% the infraspinatus and teres minor, 4% supraspinatus, and subscapularis, 3% supraspinatus, infraspinatus and teres minor, and 1% all four tendons (Fig. 9.40) (LIPPMANN 1961).

Calcified deposits within the rotator cuff tendons are best detected using GRE sequences that are sensitive to susceptibility effects induced by such calcified deposits (i.e., field inhomogenities) (LOREDO et al. 1995). Deposits not detected on MRI images are mainly classified as type II according to DEPALMA and KRUPER (1961). When evaluating MRI morphologic criteria no statistically significant differences exist between type I and type II calcified deposits within the rotator cuff tendons according to DEPALMA and KRUPER (1961).

High rates of acromial spurs, cysts within the greater tuberosity, and increased signal intensity of the subdeltoid–subacromial bursa, are acknowledged signs of chronic impingement syndrome and are found in patients with calcified tendinitis. It has been shown that in calcific tendinitis neither inflammatory infiltrates nor degenerative scarring is present. The affected tendon is transformed into fibrocartilage and concomitant proliferation of vascular chan-

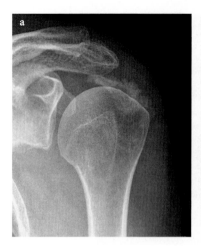 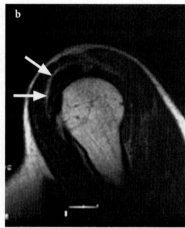 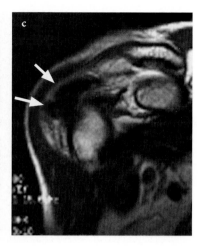

Fig. 9.40a–c. Calcifying tendonitis. The calcified deposits are of low signal intensity (*arrows*)

nels are found (UHTHOFF et al. 1976). MRI shows no substantial differences between patients with or without calcified deposits within the rotator cuff tendons, but does show distinct differences between such patients and healthy, asymptomatic volunteers (MAIER et al. 2001).

When evaluating the supraspinatus tendon in patients with calcified deposits, only a small number of patients was found to have normal-graded supraspinatus tendons (CARRINO et al. 1997). Most patients demonstrated an increased signal intensity of the supraspinatus tendon, which had to be classified as tendinosis according to CARRINO et al. (1997). Calcified deposits within the rotator cuff tendons are most probably an epiphenomenon of complex morphological alterations within the shoulder of patients with shoulder pain and dysfunction.

Although LOEW et al. (1996) did not find a clear correlation between calcifying tendinitis and subacromial impingement, MRI disclosed distinct morphological alterations in shoulders affected by calcified deposits, which may also be found in the shoulders of patients with similar shoulder pain and dysfunction but no signs of calcified deposits within the rotator cuff tendons (MAIER et al. 2001; LOEW et al. 1996). For patients with shoulder pain, shoulder dysfunction, and calcified deposits within the rotator cuff tendons, these calcified deposits are most probably not the main cause for the clinical symptoms (MAIER et al. 2001).

References

Allmann KH, Schafer O, Hauer M, Winterer J, Laubenberger J, Reichelt A, Uhl M (1999) Indirect MR arthrography of the unexercised glenohumeral joint in patients with rotator cuff tears. Invest Radiol 34:435–440

Aoki M, Ishii S, Usui M (1986) The slope of the acromion and rotator cuff impingement. Orthop Trans 10:228–235

Bachmann GF, Melzer C, Heinrichs CM, Mohring B, Rominger MB (1997) Diagnosis of rotator cuff lesions: comparison of US and MRI on 38 joint specimens. Eur Radiol 7:192–197

Balich SM, Sheley RC, Brown TR, Sauser DD, Quinn SF (1997) MR imaging of the rotator cuff tendon: interobserver agreement and analysis of interpretive errors. Radiology 204:191–194

Banas MP, Miller RJ, Totterman S (1995) Relationship between the lateral acromion angle and rotator cuff disease. J Shoulder Elbow Surg 4:454–461

Bennett WF (2001) Subscapularis, medial, and lateral head coracohumeral ligament insertion anatomy. Arthroscopic appearance and incidence of "hidden" rotator interval lesions. Arthroscopy 17:173–180

Bergman AG, Fredericson M (1998) Shoulder MRI after impingement test injection. Skeletal Radiol 27:365–368

Bernageau J (1990) Roentgenographic assessment of the rotator cuff. Clin Orthop 254:87–91

Bigliani LU, Levine WN (1997) Subacromial impingement syndrome. J Bone Joint Surg Am 79:1854–1868

Bigliani LU, Morrison D, April EW (1986) The morphology of the acromion and its relationship to rotator cuff tears. Orthop Trans 10:228

Bigliani LU, Ticker JB, Flatow EL, Soslowsky LJ, Mow VC (1991) The relationship of acromial architecture to rotator cuff disease. Clin Sports Med 10:823–838

Binkert CA, Zanetti M, Gerber C, Hodler J (2001a) MR arthrography of the glenohumeral joint: two concentrations of gadoteridol versus Ringer solution as the intraarticular contrast material. Radiology 220:219–224

Binkert CA, Zanetti M, Hodler J (2001b) Patient's assessment of discomfort during MR arthrography of the shoulder. Radiology 221:775–778

Bjorkenheim JM (1989) Structure and function of the rabbit's supraspinatus muscle after resection of its tendon. Acta Orthop Scand 60:461–463

Blanchard TK, Bearcroft PW, Dixon AK, Lomas DJ, Teale A, Constant CR, Hazleman BL (1997) Magnetic resonance imaging or arthrography of the shoulder: which do patients prefer? Br J Radiol 70:786–790

Blanchard TK, Constant CR, Bearcroft PW, Marshall TJ, Dixon AK (1998) Imaging of the rotator cuff: an arthrographic pitfall. Eur Radiol 8:817–819

Bosworth BM (1941) Calcium deposits in the shoulder and subacromial bursitis: a survey of 12,122 shoulders. JAMA 116:2477–2482

Brandt TD, Cardone BW, Grant TH, Post M, Weiss CA (1989) Rotator cuff sonography: a reassessment. Radiology 173: 323–327

Brenner ML, Morrison WB, Carrino JA, Nusser CA, Sanders TG, Howard RF, Meier P (2000) Direct MR arthrography of the shoulder: is exercise prior to imaging beneficial or detrimental? Radiology 215:491–496

Bretzke CA, Crass JR, Craig EV, Feinberg SB (1985) Ultrasonography of the rotator cuff. Normal and pathologic anatomy. Invest Radiol 20:311–315

Bright AS, Torpey B, Magid D, Codd T, McFarland EG (1997) Reliability of radiographic evaluation for acromial morphology. Skeletal Radiol 26:718–721

Brossmann J, Preidler KW, Pedowitz RA, White LM, Trudell D, Resnick D (1996) Shoulder impingement syndrome: influence of shoulder position on rotator cuff impingement–an anatomic study. AJR 167:1511–1515

Bureau NJ, Dussault RG, Keats TE (1996) Imaging of bursae around the shoulder joint. Skeletal Radiol. 25:513–517

Burk DL Jr, Karasick D, Kurtz AB, Mitchell DG, Rifkin MD, Miller CL, Levy DW, Fenlin JM, Bartolozzi AR (1989) Rotator cuff tears: prospective comparison of MR imaging with arthrography, sonography, and surgery. AJR 153:87–92

Burns WC, Whipple TL (1993) Anatomic relationships in the shoulder impingement syndrome. Clin Orthop 294:96–102

Carrino JA, McCauley TR, Katz LD, Smith RC, Lange RC (1997) Rotator cuff: evaluation with far spin-echo versus con-ventional spin-echo MR imaging. Radiology 202:533–539

Cervilla V, Schweitzer ME, Ho C, Motta A, Kerr R, Resnick D (1991) Medial dislocation of the biceps brachii tendon: appearance at MR imaging. Radiology 180:523–526

Chan TW, Dalinka MK, Kneeland JB, Chervrot A (1991) Biceps tendon dislocation: evaluation with MR imaging. Radiology 179:649–652

Chung CB, Dwek JR, Cho GJ, Lektrakul N, Trudell D, Resnick D (2000) Rotator cuff interval: evaluation with MR imaging and MR arthrography of the shoulder in 32 cadavers. J Comput Assist Tomogr 24:738–743

Codman EA, Akerson ID (1931) The pathology associated with rupture of the supraspinatus tendon. Ann Surg 93: 348–371

Cole BJ, Rodeo SA, O'Brien SJ, Altchek D, Lee D, DiCarlo EF, Potter H (2001) The anatomy and histology of the rotator interval capsule of the shoulder. Clin Orthop 390:129–137

Cone RO III, Resnick D, Danzig L (1984) Shoulder impingement syndrome: radiographic evaluation. Radiology 150: 29–33

Cotton RE, Rideout DF (1964) Tears of the humeral rotator cuff: a radiological and pathological necropsy survey. J Bone Joint Surg (Br) 46:314–328

Craig EV (1986) The acromioclavicular joint cyst. An unusual presentation of a rotator cuff tear. Clin Orthop 202: 189–192

Crass JR, Craig EV (1988) Noninvasive imaging of the rotator cuff. Orthopaedics 11:57–64

Davis SJ, Teresi LM, Bradley WG, Ressler JA, Eto RT (1991) Effect of arm rotation on MR imaging of the rotator cuff. Radiology 181:265–268

DePalma AF, Kruper JS (1961) Long-term study of shoulder joints afflicted with and treated for calcific tendinitis. Clin Orthop 20:61–72

Dines DM, Warren RF, Inglis AE, Pavlov H (1990) The coracoid impingement syndrome. J Bone Joint Surg Br 72:314–316

Edelson JG, Taitz C (1992) Anatomy of the coraco-acromial arch. Relation to degeneration of the acromion. J Bone Joint Surg Br 74:589–594

Edelson JG, Zuckerman J, Hershkovitz I (1993) Os acromiale: anatomy and surgical implications. J Bone Joint Surg (Br) 75:551–555

Edelson JG (1995) The 'hooked' acromion revisited. J Bone Joint Surg (Br) 77:284–287

Ellman H (1990) Diagnosis and treatment of incomplete rotator cuff tears. Clin Orthop 254:64–74

Emig EW, Schweitzer ME, Karasick D, Lubowitz J (1995) Adhesive capsulitis of the shoulder: MR diagnosis. AJR 164:1457–1459

Epstein RE, Schweitzer ME, Frieman BG, Fenlin JM Jr, Mitchell DG (1993) Hooked acromion: prevalence on MR images of painful shoulders. Radiology 187:479–481

Erickson SJ, Cox IH, Hyde JS, Carrera GF, Strandt JA, Estkowski LD (1991) Effect of tendon orientation on MR imaging signal intensity: a manifestation of the "magic angle" phenomenon. Radiology 181:389–392

Erickson SJ, Prost RW, Timins ME (1993) The "magic angle" effect: background physics and clinical relevance. Radiology 188:23–25

Evancho AM, Stiles RG, Fajman WA, Flower SP, Macha T, Brunner MC, Fleming L (1988) MR imaging diagnosis of rotator cuff tears. AJR 151:751–754

Farley TE, Neumann CH, Steinbach LS, Jahnke AJ, Petersen SS (1992) Full-thickness tears of the rotator cuff of the shoulder: diagnosis with MR imaging. AJR 158:347–351

Farley TE, Neumann CH, Steinbach LS, Petersen SA (1994) The coracoacromial arch: MR evaluation and correlation with rotator cuff pathology. Skeletal Radiol 23:641–645

Fiorella D, Helms CA, Speer KP (2000) Increased T2 signal intensity in the distal clavicle: incidence and clinical implications. Skeletal Radiol 29:697–702

Flannigan B, Kursunoglu-Brahme S, Snyder S, Karzel R, Del Pizzo W, Resnick D (1990) MR arthrography of the shoulder: comparison with conventional MR imaging. AJR 155: 829–832

Frost P, Andersen JH, Lundorf E (1999) Is supraspinatus pathology as defined by magnetic resonance imaging associated with clinical sign of shoulder impingement? J Shoulder Elbow Surg 8:565–568

Fuchs B, Weishaupt D, Zanetti M, Hodler J, Gerber C (1999) Fatty degeneration of the muscles of the rotator cuff: assessment by computed tomography versus magnetic resonance imaging. J Shoulder Elbow Surg 8:599–605

Fukuda H, Hamada K, Yamanaka K (1990) Pathology and pathogenesis of bursal-side rotator cuff tears viewed from en bloc histologic sections. Clin Orthop 254:75–80

Fukuda H, Hamada K, Nakajima T, Tomonaga A (1994) Pathology and pathogenesis of the intratendinous tearing of the rotator cuff viewed from en bloc histologic sections. Clin Orthop 304:60–67

Fukuda H, Hamada K, Nakajima T, Yamada N, Tomonaga A, Goto M (1996) Partial-thickness tears of the rotator cuff. A clinicopathological review based on 66 surgically verified cases. Int Orthop 20:257–265

Gagey N, Ravaud E, Lassau JP (1993) Anatomy of the acromial arch: correlation of anatomy and magnetic resonance imaging. Surg Radiol Anat 15:63–70

Gallino M, Battiston B, Annaratone G, Terragnoli F (1995) Coracoacromial ligament: a comparative arthroscopic and anatomic study. Arthroscopy 11:564–567

Gerber C, Krushell RJ (1991) Isolated rupture of the tendon of the subscapularis muscle. Clinical features in 16 cases. J Bone Joint Surg (Br) 73:389–394

Gerber C, Terrier F, Ganz R (1985) The role of the coracoid process in the chronic impingement syndrome. J Bone Joint Surg (Br) 67:703–708

Gerber C, Hersche O, Farron A (1996) Isolated rupture of the subscapularis tendon. J Bone Joint Surg (Am) 78:1015–1023

Getz JD, Recht MP, Piraino DW, Schils JP, Latimer BM, Jellema LM, Obuchowski NA (1996) Acromial morphology: relation to sex, age, symmetry, and subacromial enthesophytes. Radiology 199:737–742

Gold RH, Seeger LL, Yao L (1993) Imaging shoulder impingement. Skeletal Radiol 22:555–561

Goldberg BA, Nowinski RJ, Matsen FA III (2001) Outcome of nonoperative management of full-thickness rotator cuff tears. Clin Orthop 382:99–107

Goutallier D, Postel JM, Bernageau J, Lavau L, Voisin MC (1994) Fatty muscle degeneration in cuff ruptures. Pre- and postoperative evaluation by CT scan. Clin Orthop 304:78–83

Grainger AJ, Tirman PF, Elliott JM, Kingzett-Taylor A, Steinbach LS, Genant HK (2000) MR anatomy of the subcoracoid bursa and the association of subcoracoid effusion with tears of the anterior rotator cuff and the rotator-interval. AJR 174:1377–1380

Hamada K, Fukuda H, Mikasa M, Kobayashi Y (1990) Roentgenographic findings in massive rotator cuff tears. A long-term observation. Clin Orthop 254:92–96

Hardy DC, Vogler JB III, White RH (1986) The shoulder impingement syndrome: prevalence of radiographic findings and correlation with response to therapy. AJR 147:557–561

Harrison SH (1949) The painful shoulder: significance of radiographic changes in the upper end of the humerus. J Bone Joint Surg (Br) 31:418–422

Haygood TM, Langlotz CP, Kneeland JB, Iannotti JP, Williams GR Jr, Dalinka MK (1994) Categorization of acromial shape: interobserver variability with MR imaging and conventional radiography. AJR 162:1377–1382

Hijioka A, Suzuki K, Nakamura T, Hojo T (1993) Degenerative change and rotator cuff tears. An anatomical study in 160 shoulders of 80 cadavers. Arch Orthop Trauma Surg 112:61–64

Hodler J, Kursunoglu-Brahme S, Snyder SJ, Cervilla V, Karzel RP, Schweitzer ME, Flannigan BD, Resnick D (1992) Rotator cuff disease: assessment with MR arthrography versus standard MR imaging in 36 patients with arthroscopic confirmation. Radiology 182:431–436

Holt RG, Helms CA, Steinbach L, Neumann C, Munk PL, Genant HK (1990) Magnetic resonance imaging of the shoulder: rationale and current applications. Skeletal Radiol 19:5–14

Huang LF, Rubin DA, Britton CA (1999) Greater tuberosity changes as revealed by radiography: lack of clinical usefulness in patients with rotator cuff disease. AJR 172:1381–1388

Iannotti JP, Zlatkin MB, Esterhai JL, Kressel HY, Dalinka MK, Spindler KP (1991) Magnetic resonance imaging of the shoulder. Sensitivity, specificity, and predictive value. J Bone Joint Surg (Am) 73:1729

Jost B, Koch PP, Gerber C (2000) Anatomy and functional aspects of the rotator interval. J Shoulder Elbow Surg 9:336–341

Kaneko K, DeMouy EH, Brunet ME (1994) MR evaluation of rotator cuff impingement: correlation with confirmed full-thickness rotator cuff tears. J Comput Assist Tomogr 18:225–228

Kaplan PA, Bryans KC, Davick JP, Otte M, Stinson WW, Dussault RG (1992) MR imaging of the normal shoulder: variants and pitfalls. Radiology 184:519–524

Kessel L, Watson M (1977) The painful arc syndrome: clinical classification as a guide to management. J Bone Joint Surg (Br) 59:166–172

Kieft GJ, Bloem JL, Rozing PM, Obermann WR (1988) Rotator cuff impingement syndrome: MR imaging. Radiology 166:211–214

Kilcoyne RF, Reddy PK, Lyons F, Rockwood CA Jr (1989) Optimal plain film imaging of the shoulder impingement syndrome. AJR Am J Roentgenol 153:795–797

Kitchel SH, Butters KA, Rockwood CA (1984) The shoulder impingement syndrome. Orthop Trans 8:510–518

Kjellin I, Ho CP, Cervilla V, Haghighi P, Kerr R, Vangness CT, Friedman RJ, Trudell D, Resnick D (1991) Alterations in the supraspinatus tendon at MR imaging: correlation with histopathologic findings in cadavers. Radiology 181:837–841

Kneeland JB, Middleton WD, Carrera GF, Zeuge RC, Jesmanowicz A, Froncisz W, Hyde JS (1987) MR imaging of the shoulder: diagnosis of rotator cuff tears. AJR 149:333–337

Kolts I, Busch LC, Tomusk H, Raudheiding A, Eller A, Merila M, Russlies M, Paasuke M, Leibecke T, Kuhnel W (2002) Macroscopical anatomy of the so-called "rotator interval". A cadaver study on 19 shoulder joints. Ann Anat. 184:9–14

Kopka L, Funke M, Fischer U, Keating D, Oestmann J, Grabbe E (1994) MR arthrography of the shoulder with gadopentetate dimeglumine: influence of concentration, iodinated contrast material, and time on signal intensity. AJR 163:621–623

Kwak SM, Brown RR, Trudell D, Resnick D (1998) Glenohumeral joint: comparison of shoulder positions at MR arthrography. Radiology 208:375–380

Li XX, Schweitzer ME, Bifano JA, Lerman J, Manton GL, El-Noueam KI (1999) MR evaluation of subscapularis tears. J Comput Assist Tomogr 23:713–717

Liberson F (1937) Os acromiale: a contested anomaly. J Bone Joint Surg 19:683–689

Liou JT, Wilson AJ, Totty WG, Brown JJ (1993) The normal shoulder: common variations that simulate pathologic conditions at MR imaging. Radiology 186:435–441

Lippmann RK (1961) Observations concerning the calcific cuff deposits. Clin Orthop 20:49–60

Loew M, Sabo D, Wehrle M, Mau H (1996) Relationship between calcifying tendinitis and subacromial impingement: a prospective radiography and magnetic resonance imaging study. J Shoulder Elbow Surg 5:314–319

Lohr JF, Uhthoff HK (1987) The pathogenesis of degenerative rotator cuff tears. Orthop Trans 11:237–244

Loredo R, Longo C, Salonen D, Yu J, Haghighi P, Trudell D, Clopton P, Resnick D (1995) Glenoid labrum: MR imaging with histologic correlation. Radiology 196:33–41

MacGillivray JD, Fealy S, Potter HG, O'Brien SJ (1998) Multiplanar analysis of acromion morphology. Am J Sports Med 26:836–840

Maier M, Stäbler A, Schmitz C, Lienemann A, Kohler S, Durr HR, Pfahler M, Refior HJ (2001) On the impact of calcified deposits within the rotator cuff tendons in shoulders of patients with shoulder pain and dysfunction. Arch Orthop Trauma Surg 121:371–378

Mason BJ, Kier R, Bindleglass DF (1999) Occult fractures of the greater tuberosity of the humerus: radiographic and MR imaging findings. AJR 172:469–473

Matsen FA (1990) Subacromial impingement. In: Rockwood CA, Matsen FA (ed) The shoulder. Saunders, Philadelphia, pp 623–646

McCauley TR, Disler DG, Tam MK (2000) Bone marrow edema in the greater tuberosity of the humerus at MR imaging: association with rotator cuff tears and traumatic injury. Magn Reson Imaging 18:979–984

McKendry RJ, Uhthoff HK, Sarkar K, Hyslop PS (1982) Calcifying tendinitis of the shoulder: prognostic value of clinical, histologic, and radiologic features in 57 surgically treated cases. J Rheumatol 9:75–80

Mellado JM, Salvado E, Camins A, Ramos A, Merino X, Calmet J, Sauri A (2002) Fluid collections and juxta-articular cystic lesions of the shoulder: spectrum of MRI findings. Eur Radiol 12:650–659

Mink JH, Harris E, Rappaport M (1985) Rotator cuff tears: evaluation using double-contrast shoulder arthrography. Radiology 157:621–623

Mirowitz SA (1991) Normal rotator cuff: MR imaging with conventional and fat-suppression techniques. Radiology 180:735–740

Mitchell MJ, Causey G, Berthoty DP, Sartoris DJ, Resnick D (1988) Peribursal fat plane of the shoulder: anatomic study and clinical experience. Radiology 168:699–704

Mudge MK, Wood VE, Frykman GK (1984) Rotator cuff tears associated with os acromiale. J Bone Joint Surg (Am) 66:427–429

Nakagaki K, Ozaki J, Tomita Y, Tamai S (1994) Alterations in the supraspinatus muscle belly with rotator cuff tearing: evaluation with magnetic resonance imaging. J Shoulder Elbow Surg 3:88–93

Nakagaki K, Ozaki J, Tomita Y, Tamai S (1995) Function of supraspinatus muscle with torn cuff evaluated by magnetic resonance imaging. Clin Orthop 318:144–151

Nakagaki K, Ozaki J, Tomita Y, Tamai S (1996) Fatty degeneration in the supraspinatus muscle after rotator cuff tear. J Shoulder Elbow Surg 5:194–200

Needell SD, Zlatkin MB, Sher JS, Murphy BJ, Uribe JW (1996) MR imaging of the rotator cuff: peritendinous and bone abnormalities in an asymptomatic population. AJR 166:863–867

Needell SD, Zlatkin MB (1997) Comparison of fat-saturation fast spin echo versus conventional spin-echo MRI in the detection of rotator cuff pathology. J Magn Reson Imaging 7:674–677

Neer CS Jr (1972) Anterior acromioplasty for the chronic impingement syndrome in the shoulder: a preliminary report. J Bone Joint Surg (Am) 54:41–50

Neer CS Jr (1983) Impingement lesions. Clin Orthop 173:70–77

Neer CS Jr (1995) The components of our global exchange on surgery of the shoulder. J Shoulder Elbow Surg 4:477–480

Neer CS Jr, Welsh RP (1977) The shoulder in sports. Orthop Clin North Am 8:583–591

Nelson MC, Leather GP, Nirschl RP, Pettrone FA, Freedman MT (1991) Evaluation of the painful shoulder. A prospective comparison of magnetic resonance imaging, computerized tomographic arthrography, ultrasonography, and operative findings. J Bone Joint Surg (Am) 73:707–716

Neumann CH, Holt RG, Steinbach LS, Jahnke AH, Petersen SA (1992) MR imaging of the shoulder: appearance of the supraspinatus tendon in asymptomatic volunteers. AJR 158:1281–1287

Neviaser J (1945) Adhesive capsulitis of the shoulder: study of pathologic findings in periarthritis of the shoulder. J Bone Joint Surg 27:211–222

Neviaser R, Neviaser T (1987) The frozen shoulder diagnosis and management. Clin Orthop 223:59–64

Neviaser RJ, Neviaser TJ (1990) Observations on impingement. Clin Orthop 254:60–63

Nicholson GP, Goodman DA, Flatow EL, Bigliani LU (1996) The acromion: morphologic condition and age-related changes. A study of 420 scapulas. J Shoulder Elbow Surg 5:1–11

Nobuhara K, Ikeda H (1987) Rotator interval lesion. Clin Orthop 223:44–50

Ogata S, Uhthoff HK (1990) Acromial enthesopathy and rotator cuff tear. A radiologic and histologic postmortem investigation of the coracoacromial arch. Clin Orthop 254:39–48

Ozaki J, Fujimoto S, Nakagawa Y, Masuhara K, Tamai S (1988) Tears of the rotator cuff of the shoulder associated with pathological changes in the acromion. A study in cadavera. J Bone Joint Surg (Am) 70:1224–1230

Ozaki J, Nakagawa Y, Sakurai G, Tamai S (1989) Recalcitrant chronic adhesive capsulitis of the shoulder. J Bone Joint Surg (Am) 71:115–120

Palmer WE, Brown JH, Rosenthal DI (1993) Rotator cuff: evaluation with fat-suppressed MR arthrography. Radiology 188:683–687

Panni AS, Milano G, Luciana L, Fabbriciani C, Logroscino CA (1996) Histological analysis of the coracoacromial arch: correlation between age-related changes and rotator cuff tears. Arthroscopy 12:531–540

Park JG, Lee JK, Phelps CT (1994) Os acromiale associated with rotator cuff impingement: MR imaging of the shoulder. Radiology 193:255–257

Parsa M, Tuite M, Norris M, Orwin J (1997) MR imaging of rotator cuff tendon tears: comparison of T2*-weighted gradient-echo and conventional dual-echo sequences. AJR 168:1519–1524

Patte D (1990a) The subcoracoid impingement. Clin Orthop 254:55–59

Patte D (1990b) Classification of rotator cuff lesions. Clin Orthop 254:81–86

Patten RM (1994) Tears of the anterior portion of the rotator cuff (the subscapularis tendon): MR imaging findings. AJR 162:351–354

Paulson MM, Watnik NF, Dines DM (2001) Coracoid impingement syndrome, rotator interval reconstruction, and biceps
tenodesis in the overhead athlete. Orthop Clin North Am
32:485–493

Peh WC, Farmer TH, Totty WG (1995) Acromial arch shape:
assessment with MR imaging. Radiology 195:501–505

Petersilge CA, Lewin JS, Duerk JL, Hatem SF (1997) MR
arthrography of the shoulder: rethinking traditional imaging procedures to meet the technical requirements of MR
imaging guidance. AJR 169:1453–1457

Petersson CJ (1986) Spontaneous medial dislocation of the
tendon of the long biceps brachii. An anatomic study of
prevalence and pathomechanics. Clin Orthop 211:224–227

Petersson CJ, Redlund-Johnell I (1984) The subacromial space
in normal shoulder radiographs. Acta Orthop Scand 55:
57–58

Pfirrmann CW, Zanetti M, Weishaupt D, Gerber C, Hodler J
(1999) Subscapularis tendon tears: detection and grading
at MR arthrography. Radiology 213:709–714

Postacchini F, Perugia D, Gumina S (1993) Acromioclavicular
joint cyst associated with rotator cuff tear. A report of three
cases. Clin Orthop 294:111–113

Quinn SF, Sheley RC, Demlow TA, Szumowski J (1995) Rotator cuff tendon tears: evaluation with fat-suppressed MR
imaging with arthroscopic correlation in 100 patients.
Radiology 195:497–500

Rafii M, Firooznia H, Sherman O, Minkoff J, Weinreb J,
Golimbu C, Gidumal R, Schinella R, Zaslav K (1990) Rotator cuff lesions: signal patterns at MR imaging. Radiology
177:817–823

Reeder JD, Andelman S (1987) The rotator cuff tear: MR evaluation. Magn Reson Imaging 5:331–338

Reinus WR, Shady KL, Mirowitz SA, Totty WG (1995) MR diagnosis of rotator cuff tears of the shoulder: value of using
T2-weighted fat-saturated images. AJR 164:1451–1455

Resendes M, Helms CA, Eddy R, Knox K (1991) Double-echo
MPGR imaging of the rotator cuff. J Comput Assist Tomogr
15:1077–1079

Robertson PL, Schweitzer ME, Mitchell DG, Schlesinger F,
Epstein RE, Frieman BG, Fenlin JM (1995) Rotator cuff
disorders: interobserver and intraobserver variation in
diagnosis with MR imaging. Radiology 194:831–835

Rockwood CA Jr, Lyons FR (1993) Shoulder impingement
syndrome: diagnosis, radiographic evaluation and treatment with a modified Neer acromioplasty. J Bone Joint
Surg (Am) 75:409–424

Roger B, Skaf A, Hooper AW, Lektrakul N, Yeh L, Resnick
D (1999) Imaging findings in the dominant shoulder of
throwing athletes: comparison of radiography, arthrography, CT arthrography, and MR arthrography with
arthroscopic correlation. AJR 172:1371–1380

Sakurai G, Ozaki J, Tomita Y, Kondo T, Tamai S (1998) Incomplete tears of the subscapularis tendon associated with
tears of the supraspinatus tendon: cadaveric and clinical
studies. J Shoulder Elbow Surg 7:510–515

Sanders TG, Tirman PF, Feller JF, Genant HK (2000) Association of intramuscular cysts of the rotator cuff with tears of
the rotator cuff: magnetic resonance imaging findings and
clinical significance. Arthroscopy 16:230–235

Sano A, Itoi E, Konno N, Kido T, Urayama M, Sato K (1998)
Cystic changes of the humeral head on MR imaging. Relation to age and cuff-tears. Acta Orthop Scand 69:397400

Sarkar K, Taine W, Uhthoff HK (1990) The ultrastructure of the
coracoacromial ligament in patients with chronic impingement syndrome. Clin Orthop 254:49–54

Schippinger G, Bailey D, McNally EG, Kiss J, Carr AJ (1997)
Anatomy of the normal acromion investigated using MRI.
Langenbecks Arch Chir 382:141–144

Schraner AB, Major NM (1999) MR imaging of the subcoracoid bursa. AJR 172:1567–1571

Schweitzer ME, Magbalon MJ, Frieman BG, Ehrlich S, Epstein RE
(1994) Acromioclavicular joint fluid: determination of clinical
significance with MR imaging. Radiology 192:205–207

Seeger LL (1989) Magnetic resonance imaging of the shoulder.
Clin Orthop 244:48–59

Seeger LL, Gold RH, Bassett LW, Ellman H (1988) Shoulder
impingement syndrome: MR findings in 53 shoulders. AJR
150:343–347

Seibold CJ, Mallisee TA, Erickson SJ, Boynton MD, Raasch WG,
Timins ME (1999) Rotator cuff: evaluation with US and MR
imaging. Radiographics 19:685–705

Sher JS, Uribe JW, Posada A, Murphy BJ, Zlatkin MB (1995)
Abnormal findings on magnetic resonance images of
asymptomatic shoulders. J Bone Joint Surg (Am) 77:10–15

Singson RD, Hoang T, Dan S, Friedman M (1996) MR evaluation of rotator cuff pathology using T2-weighted fast spin-
echo technique with and without fat suppression. AJR 166:
1061–1065

Soble MG, Kaye AD, Guay RC (1989) Rotator cuff tear: clinical experience with sonographic detection. Radiology 173:
319–321

Sonin AH, Peduto AJ, Fitzgerald SW, Callahan CM, Bresler
ME (1996) MR imaging of the rotator cuff mechanism:
comparison of spin-echo and turbo spin-echo sequences.
AJR 167:333–338

Stiles RG, Resnick D, Sartoris DJ, Andre MP (1988) Rotator cuff
disruption: diagnosis with digital arthrography. Radiology
168:705–707

Stoller DW (1997) MR arthrography of the glenohumeral joint.
Radiol Clin North Am 35:97–116

Swen WA, Jacobs JW, Algra PR, Manoliu RA, Rijkmans J, Willems WJ, Bijlsma JW (1999) Sonography and magnetic resonance imaging equivalent for the assessment of full-thickness rotator cuff tears. Arthritis Rheum 42:2231–2238

Tasu JP, Miquel A, Rocher L, Molina V, Gagey O, Blery M (2001)
MR evaluation of factors predicting the development of
rotator cuff tears. J Comput Assist Tomogr 25:159–163

Thomazeau H, Rolland Y, Lucas C, Duval JM, Langlais F (1996)
Atrophy of the supraspinatus belly. Assessment by MRI in
55 patients with rotator cuff pathology. Acta Orthop Scand
67:264–268

Timins ME, Erickson SJ, Estkowski LD, Carrera GF,
Komorowski RA (1995) Increased signal in the normal
supraspinatus tendon on MR imaging: diagnostic pitfall
caused by the magic-angle effect. AJR 165:109–114

Tirman PF, Bost FW, Steinbach LS, Mall JC, Peterfy CG, Samp-
son TG, Sheehan WE, Forbes JR, Genant HK (1994) MR
arthrographic depiction of tears of the rotator cuff: benefit
of abduction and external rotation of the arm. Radiology
192:851–856

Trattnig S, Breitenseher M, Pretterklieber M, Kontaxis G, Rand
T, Helbich T, Imhof H (1997) MR-guided joint puncture and
real-time MR-assisted contrast media application. Acta
Radiol 38:1047–1049

Tuite MJ, Yandow DR, DeSmet AA, Orwin JF, Quintana FA
(1994) Diagnosis of partial and complete rotator cuff tears

using combined gradient echo and spin echo imaging. Skeletal Radiol 23:541–545

Tuite MJ, Turnbull JR, Orwin JF (1998) Anterior versus posterior, and rim-rent rotator cuff tears: prevalence and MR sensitivity. Skeletal Radiol 27:237–243

Uhthoff HK, Sarkar K (1978) Calcifying tendinitis. Its pathogenetic mechanism and a rationale for its treatment. Int Orthop 2:187–193

Uhthoff HK, Sarkar K, Maynard JA (1976) Calcifying tendinitis – a new concept of its pathogenesis. Clin Orthop Relat Res 118:164–168

Uhthoff HK, Hammond DI, Sakar K, Hooper GJ, Papoff WJ (1998) The role of the coracoacromial ligament in the impingement syndrome: a clinical, bursographic and histologic study. Int Orthop 12:97–103

Uri DS (1997) MR imaging of shoulder impingement and rotator cuff disease. Radiol Clin North Am 35:77–96

Uri DS, Kneeland JB, Herzog R (1997) Os acromiale: evaluation of markers for identification on sagittal and coronal oblique MR images. Skeletal Radiol 26:31–34

Uthoff HK, Hammond DI, Sakar K, Hooper GJ, Papof WJ (1988) The role of the coracoacromial ligament in the impingement syndrome: a clinical bursographic and histologic study. Int Orthop 12:97

Vahlensieck M (2000) MRI of the shoulder. Eur Radiol 10:242–249

Vahlensieck M, Pollack M, Lang P, Grampp S, Genant HK (1993) Two segments of the supraspinous muscle: cause of high signal intensity at MR imaging? Radiology 186:449–454

Walch G, Nove-Josserand L, Levigne C, Renaud E (1994) Tears of the supraspinatus tendon associated with "hidden" lesions of the rotator interval. J Shoulder Elbow Surg 3:353–360

Warner JJ, Higgins L, Parsons IM 4th, Dowdy P (2001) Diagnosis and treatment of anterosuperior rotator cuff tears. J Shoulder Elbow Surg 10:37–46

Watson M (1985) Major ruptures of the rotator cuff. The results of surgical repair in 89 patients. J Bone Joint Surg (Br) 67:618–624

Watson M (1989) Rotator cuff function in the impingement syndrome. J Bone Joint Surg (Br) 71:361–366

Winalski CS, Aliabadi P, Wright RJ, Shortkroff S, Sledge CB, Weissman BN (1993) Enhancement of joint fluid with intravenously administered gadopentetate dimeglumine: technique, rationale, and implications. Radiology 187:179–185

Wright RW, Fritts HM, Tierney GS, Buss DD (1998) MR imaging of the shoulder after an impingement test: how long to wait. AJR 171:769–773

Zanetti M, Gerber C, Hodler J (1998a) Quantitative assessment of the muscles of the rotator cuff with magnetic resonance imaging. Invest Radiol 33:163–170

Zanetti M, Weishaupt D, Gerber C, Hodler J (1998b) Tendinopathy and rupture of the tendon of the long head of the biceps brachii muscle: evaluation with MR arthrography. AJR Am J Roentgenol 170:1557–1561

Zanetti M, Weishaupt D, Jost B, Gerber C, Hodler J (1999) MR imaging for traumatic tears of the rotator cuff: high prevalence of greater tuberosity fractures and subscapularis tendon tears. AJR 172:463–467

Zlatkin MB, Iannotti JP, Roberts MC (1989) Rotator cuff tears: diagnostic performance on MR imaging. Radiology 172:223–229

10 Instability

A. Blum, Y. Carrillon, J.-J. Railhac, B. Roger, T. Tavernier

CONTENTS

A. Blum, MD
Professor of Radiology, Service d'Imagerie Guilloz, Hopital Central, CHU Nancy, 54035 Nancy Cedex, France
Y. Carrillon, MD
Clinique Saint Jean, 30 rue Bataille, 69008 Lyon, France
J.-J. Railhac, MD
Professor of Radiology, Service Central de Radiologie et d'Imagerie Médicale, Hôpital Purpan, 31059 Toulouse Cédex, France
B. Roger, MD
Service de Radiologie ostéo-articulaire, Hôpital Pitié Salpêtrière, Bd de l'Hôpital, 75013 Paris Cedex, France
T. Tavernier, MD
Clinique de la Sauvegarde, Avenue Ben Gourion, 69261 Lyon, France

10.1 Introduction

Glenohumeral instabilities are less and less perceived as simple recurrent dislocations responding to a single surgical treatment. Subtle forms are outlined, especially in high-level sports competition. Among athletes, the role of an underlying hyperlaxity should not be underestimated. Therapeutic practices have become much wider, particularly through arthroscopic procedures. However, the diagnosis and treatment of these instabilities remain difficult (Patte et al. 1980; Rowe 1987; Molé and Walch 1993).

According to clinical results, all cases require a specific X-ray evaluation, which is often sufficient to determine the severity of the lesions and indicate treatment, such as in acute or recurrent anterior glenohumeral dislocations. With the exception of the two latter conditions, a definite diagnosis can only be established through additional imaging methods, i.e., computed tomography (CT) arthrography, magnetic resonance imaging (MRI) or magnetic resonance (MR) arthrography) (Blum et al. 1997; Sanders et al. 2000; Zlatkin 1999). Glenohumeral instability is typically found in young athletes complaining of undefined shoulder pain. Indeed, these patients can be suffering from subtle forms of instability but also from rotator cuff pathologies or SLAP lesions (Rowe 1987; Blum et al. 2000a; Nizard 1997; Roger et al. 1999).

After a brief overview of shoulder anatomy and imaging techniques depicting shoulder instability, the several forms and various findings simulating instability will be reviewed.

10.2 Shoulder Anatomy

As a multi-axial joint, the stability of the glenohumeral joint is mainly due to capsulolabral structures, ligaments and to the rotator cuff.

10.2.1
Passive Mechanisms of Glenohumeral Joint Stability

The glenohumeral joint is formed by the humeral head and the glenoid surface of the scapula. Approximately 75% of the scapula displays a retroverted glenoid surface averaging 7°. In 25% cases, the glenoid surface has a 2–10° anteversion which could alter joint stability. In less common situations, joint stability may also be affected by hyper retroversion of the glenoid surface (Fig. 10.1). A posterior glenoid rim deficiency with a craniocaudal length of more than 12 mm could also affect the posterior glenohumeral stability (WEISHAUPT et al. 2000). Nevertheless, joint stability cannot be achieved through anatomical bone structures alone as the large spherical head of the humerus rotates against and not within a small shallow glenoid fossa.

The main stabilizing mechanisms of the glenohumeral joint are composed of capsulolabral structures and ligaments. The *glenoid labrum*, involved in passive stability of the joint, disperses the strains and pressure. As the glenoid articular surface is relatively flat compared to the humeral head, the presence of labrum increases the depth of the glenoid fossa from 2.5 to 5 mm (MOSELEY and OVERGAARD 1962). Schematically, its section is triangular and three-sided with a peripheral aspect connected to the capsule and the biceps tendon at the top, an internal aspect related to the peripheral glenoid surface and an external aspect gliding on the humeral head. Its shape, insertion and histological structures vary greatly according to individuals and its specific location on the glenoid rim (Fig. 10.2). Many different

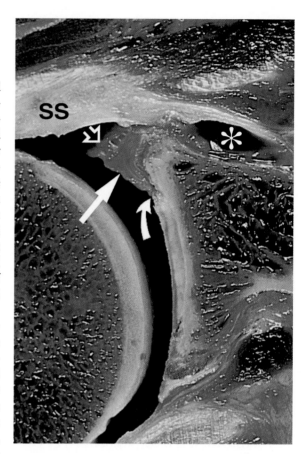

Fig. 10.2. Anatomic axial slice showing the anterior portion of the labrum *(straight arrow)*, coated with synovium *(hollow arrow)* and labrum-articular cartilage junction *(curved arrow)*. *SS*, subscapularis tendon; *asterisk*, anterior recess. (Courtesy of D Resnick MD, V.A. Medical center, San Diego)

types of labral classifications have been proposed. Generally, the glenoid surface is considered as a clock divided in twelve sections. The inferior labrum extends from a 4 o'clock to 8 o'clock position, the posterior from 8 to 11 o'clock, the superior from 11 to 1 o'clock and the anterior labrum from a 1 to 4 o'clock position (Fig. 10.3).

Its inferior portion is often large and attached to the glenoid, whereas its posterior portion can be partially free or attached to the glenoid. Its superior portion is usually shaped as a meniscus due to the presence of a sub-labral recess between the labrum and the glenoid rim (Fig. 10.4, 10.5) (MAFFET et al. 1995; TUITE and ORWIN 1996). Its appearance is more variable in its anterior portion. The labrum may be hypoplastic or missing. It may be shaped as a meniscus or be inserted at the articular cartilage periphery. In 13%–20% cases, the labrum is free in its anterosuperior portion (BRESLER et al. 1998;

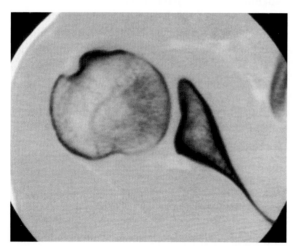

Fig. 10.1. CT scan showing hyper-retroversion of the glenoid surface

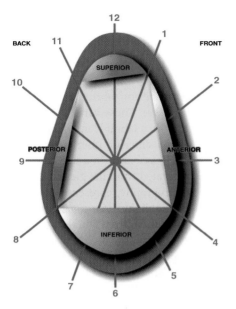

Fig. 10.3. Clock-like distribution of the glenoid rim and its four sectors: inferior, posterior, anterior and superior

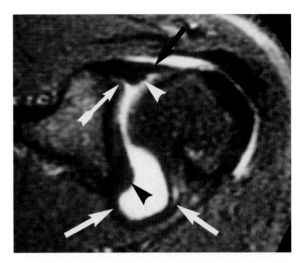

Fig. 10.5. Coronal slice with magnetic resonance arthrography pointing out the inferior glenohumeral complex comprised of the inferior glenohumeral ligament *(white arrows)* and the inferior labrum *(black arrowhead)*, the superior labrum *(white arrowhead)* and the sublabral recess *(finned white arrow)*

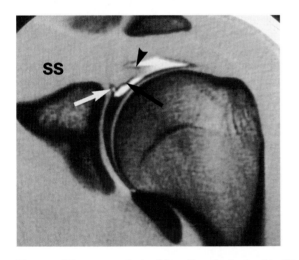

Fig. 10.4. Direct coronal shoulder slice obtained with CT arthrography highlighting the long biceps tendon *(arrowhead)* and its insertion at the supraglenoid tubercle, the superior labrum *(black arrow)*, the sublabral recess *(white arrow)* and the biceps tendon *(black arrow)*

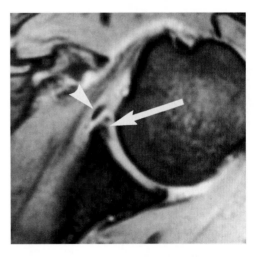

Fig. 10.6. Gradient echo axial slice showing a pseudo-cleft of the anterior portion of the labrum *(arrow)* and the middle glenohumeral ligament *(arrowhead)*

KREITNER et al. 1998). Finally, the labrum which is mainly a fibrous structure may display histological changes accounting for the signal intensity variations observed with MRI (specifically on gradient-echo sequences) (Fig. 10.6) (DETRISAC and JOHNSON 1988; COOPER et al. 1992; GARNEAU et al. 1991; KWACK et al. 1998a). Awareness of these normal variations is necessary in order to avoid excessive labral tear diagnoses.

The ligaments, and specifically the inferior glenohumeral ligament (IGHL), which reinforce the joint capsule are the most important stabilizing features of the glenohumeral joint. The middle glenohumeral ligament (MGHL) and the superior glenohumeral ligament (SGHL) have a lesser stabilizing effect on shoulder stability.

The *IGHL* is a complex structure strengthening the inferior capsule. It originates from the glenoid neck, adhering to the peripheral aspect of the labrum and inserts into the anatomical neck of the humerus. It is composed of anterior and posterior bands, and a hammock-shaped axillary pouch lying in between (Figs. 10.5, 10.7) (O'BRIEN et al. 1990; McMAHON at al. 1999).

The *MGHL* is inserted into the anterosuperior aspect of the labrum. Its attachment can be localized at 1 o'clock or much lower near the 4 o'clock position. Obliquely oriented towards the humerus just medial to the lesser tuberosity, it passes under the subscapularis tendon to which it adheres. In fact, this ligament can vary greatly in size or even be absent altogether. It may be very thin, in which case the anterior band of the IGHL is often quite thick. In 20% of cases, the MGHL takes a cord-like aspect. It appears thick and relatively rounded on axial slices and frequently

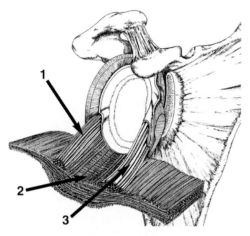

Fig. 10.7. Diagram of the inferior glenohumeral ligament. *1*, posterior band; *2*, axillary pouch; *3*, anterior band. (Adapted from O'BRIEN et al. 1990)

inserted on a large detached anterosuperior labrum (Fig. 10.8).

The "*Buford complex*" defines a normal variant in 1%–2% cases and is characterized by a cord-like MGHL, an insertion of the MGHL to the biceps tendon and no anterosuperior labrum (WILLIAMS et al. 1994) (Figs. 10.8, 10.9). These various patterns must not be confused with a labral tear. A labral tear is usually located in its anterior inferior portion, whereas in a cord-like ligament or in a Buford complex, the MGHL is separated from the glenoid on its entire surface. MR arthrography represents the most efficient technique to highlight these normal variations and to differentiate them from labral tear. Axial and sagittal slices clearly show the MGHL inserted in front of the large biceps and presenting a downward and external direction (TIRMAN et al. 1996; STOLLER 1997). When the MGHL is thick, it can act as an important secondary restraint to anterior translation if the anterior portion or the inferior glenohumeral ligament is damaged.

The *SGHL* which is the smallest of the glenohumeral ligaments is inserted at the superior portion of the glenoid rim and is attached to the biceps tendon, the labrum and the MGHL. It is part of the biceps tendon stabilizing process and of the so-called pulley system. Horizontally directed, it inserts itself at the top of the bicipital groove after joining the coracohumeral ligament. The SGHL is an anterior and inferior stabilizer in the hanging arm position. The coracohumeral ligament contributes to posterior stability.

Other passive mechanisms have a stabilizing effect on the glenohumeral joint. Negative pressure present within the joint together with a highly viscous articular liquid help to maintain an articular surface

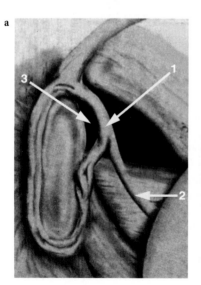

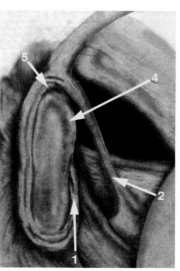

Fig. 10.8a, b. Normal variants of the labrum (*1*) and of the middle glenohumeral ligament (*2*) (adapted from WILLIAMS et al. 1994) **a** Cord-like middle glenohumeral ligament (MGHL) and loose anterosuperior labrum (*3*). **b** Buford complex characterized by a cord-like MGHL without anterosuperior labrum (*4*). *5*, Superior portion of the labrum and long head of the biceps tendon insertion

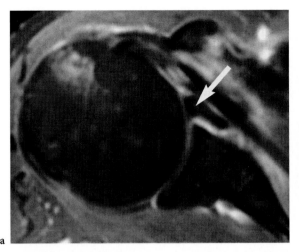 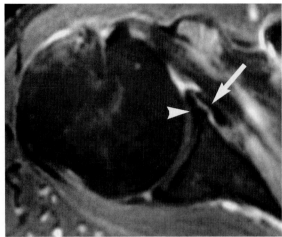

a

b

Fig. 10.9a, b. Buford complex. **a** Axial slice cutting through the superior portion of the glenohumeral joint showing a thick middle glenohumeral ligament *(arrow)* without anterosuperior labrum. **b** Axial slice cutting through the inferior portion of the glenohumeral joint depicting the anterior labrum *(arrowhead)*

cohesion and adhesion while preserving its mobility (MATSEN et al. 1990; HURSCHLER et al. 2000). Finally, a contrast is noticed between the strong anterior capsuloligamentar structures and the looser posterior capsule where no ligament is present. This pattern probably accounts for the scarcity of posterior glenoid fractures.

10.2.2
Active Mechanisms of Glenohumeral Joint Stability: The Rotator Cuff

Active mechanisms of glenohumeral joint stability are linked to the rotator cuff. These muscles play an essential role in dynamic and functional shoulder stability. They contribute to what BONNEL (1988) described as a dynamic three-dimensional recentering. Recent studies confirmed that the substantial anterior dynamic stability to the glenohumeral joint in the end-range as well as in the mid-range of motion is provided by the rotator cuff (LEE et al. 2000).

Supraspinatus and subscapularis tendons are separated by a space referred to as the rotator interval. This space is outlined by the coracohumeral ligament and the SGHL. The coracohumeral ligament originates from the external coracoid process and fuses with the capsule before dividing into a medial and a lateral portion. The medial portion blends with the SGHL before ending on the internal ridge of the bicipital groove, joining the superficial aspect of the

subscapularis tendon. In merging, the coracohumeral ligament and SGHL encircle and stabilize the biceps tendon at the top of the bicipital groove (Fig. 10.10).

The lateral portion ends at the lateral ridge of the bicipital groove. Finally, the transverse ligament which is inserted on the two bicipital groove ridges amalgamates with the two coracohumeral ligament portions. This ligament may also contain some subscapularis tendon fibers.

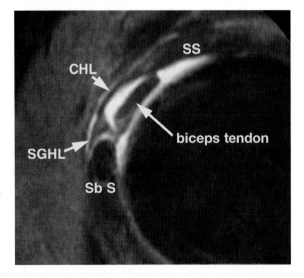

Fig. 10.10. Magnetic resonance arthrography in sagittal plane pointing out the rotator interval separating the supraspinatus tendon (*SS*) from the subscapularis tendon (*Sb S*). This space is outlined by the coracohumeral ligament (*CHL*) and the superior glenohumeral ligament (*SGHL*) which encircle the biceps tendon

10.3
Clinical Classification of Instabilities

Medical history and clinical evaluation help to classify shoulder instability according to the degree, direction, chronology, etiology, context and associated lesions, if any (NEER 1990; SILLIMAN and HAWKINS 1993).

10.3.1
Degree of Instability

Dislocation of the glenohumeral joint is the complete separation of the articular surfaces. In this case, if immediate, spontaneous relocation does not occur, it has to be reduced.

Contrary to the above-mentioned description, glenohumeral *subluxation* is characterized by a spontaneous relocation of the humeral head regardless of the severity of its displacement. As in some cases this displacement is fleeting so proof of instability is difficult to assess.

Clinical diagnosis will be inferred by getting to the source of the accident, and by identifying previous episodes of dislocation. It can also be suspected when a sharp fleeting pain occurs in abduction and external rotation of the arm associated with dysesthesia of the entire superior limb. There are no associated neurological signs and the symptoms disappear within a few hours. These manifestations known as the *dead-arm syndrome*, as described by ROWE (1987), are related to an anterior glenohumeral subluxation.

In subtle or *occult glenohumeral subluxation*, the separation of the articular surfaces is not perceived and pain is the only complaint of the patient. Therefore, this affection is classified in the sole painful shoulder syndrome. Athletes are often affected by this syndrome, complaining of pain at cocking phase in sports such as base-ball or tennis but also when the arm is in elevation and abduction (alpinism). Occult glenohumeral subluxation and above all its anterior or posterior direction, remains difficult to identify as the accompanying pains are not characteristic (GARTH et al. 1987; PAPPAS et al. 1983; LIU et al. 1996). According to ROCKWOOD, pain occurring in the early cocking phase is due to anterior instability whereas symptoms occurring during the late cocking or acceleration phases tend to be related to posterior instability (ROCKWOOD 1984). According to JOBE and coworkers (1991), the sole painful athlete's shoulder may be due to subacromial impingement syndrome related to an acquired ligament distension result-

ing in excess mobility of the shoulder head. Finally, according to WALCH, pain occurring at the cocking phase can be attributed to an impingement between the humeral head and the posterosuperior portion of the glenoid rim (WALCH et al. 1991; WALCH 1996).

10.3.2
Directions of Instability

Instabilities are most often anterior, rarely posterior, and exceptionally multidirectional. In glenohumeral dislocation, clinical history and radiography are sufficient to determine the direction of instability. Anterior dislocations represent 95% of all glenohumeral dislocations. In acute dislocation, the range of displacement determines the severity of the capsuloligamentous damage and the risk of vascular or neurological complications. According to the position of the humeral head, anterior glenohumeral dislocation are classified into subcoracoid (the most frequent), subglenoid, subclavicular, or intrathoracic dislocations.

In contrast, in subtle or occult forms of instability triggered or due to sports activities, the direction of instability is usually difficult to pinpoint. In such cases, symptoms are not specific and X-rays are often normal. The diagnosis can only be reached by using additional techniques, able to identify soft tissue alteration such as labral tears (CT arthrography, MRI or arthrography).

10.3.3
Chronology of Instability

A glenohumeral dislocation is acute if observed within the first day. After this delay, and within 3 weeks, it becomes chronic. After 3 weeks, reduction is difficult and the dislocation is considered as fixed or locked. Recurrent instability consists of repeated glenohumeral dislocations and/or subluxations.

10.3.4
Etiology and Context of Instability

Instability may be traumatic and in such cases involuntary, or atraumatic and generally voluntary (Fig. 10.11). The latter is often associated with hyperlaxity or hypermobility of the shoulder.

Instability and hyperlaxity must be clearly differentiated. Instability is a functional pathology associ-

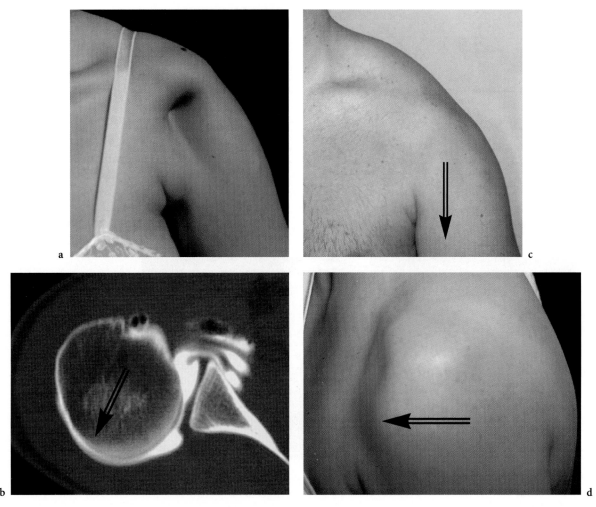

Fig. 10.11a–d. Some examples of atraumatic voluntary subluxations of the glenohumeral joint. **a** Left posterior subluxation in a young female patient. **b** CT arthrography showing a right voluntary posterior subluxation in a young female patient ruling out any other glenohumeral abnormalities. **c** Left inferior subluxation in a young male patient with hypermobility syndrome. **d** Left anterior subluxation in a young female patient with hypermobility syndrome

ated with discomfort, pain or apprehension and is most often unilateral but rarely multidirectional. In contrast, hyperlaxity is a physical characteristic, not pathological in itself, but which may induce instability (McFarland et al. 1996).

Hyperlaxity may be acquired when doing intensive sports activities stressing the IGHL, therefore only affecting the involved shoulder. For the most part, hyperlaxity is congenital, and found in women more often than men (Brown et al. 2000). It appears bilateral and may be part of a hyperlaxity syndrome. Beighton's score is used to establish clinical diagnosis of hypermobility syndrome, according to one's ability to perform the following nine maneuvers (Figs. 10.12, 10.13) (Beighton et al. 1973):

1: Passive dorsiflexion of the fifth MCP to 90° (scoring one point on each side)

2: Apposition of the thumb to the flexor aspect of the forearm

3: Hyperextension of the elbow beyond 90°

4: Hyperextension of the knee beyond 90°

5: Forward trunk flexion placing hands flat on floor with knees extended (score one point)

The diagnosis of hypermobility syndrome is only valid when scoring at least 4 or 5 points out of 9.

Shoulder hyperlaxity is always multidirectional. It is often highlighted by an anterior or posterior drawer test and especially by the sulcus test where the patient sits with his arm relaxed at his side and the examiner pulls the arm downward. The test is positive when a sulcus appears inferior to the acromion (Fig. 10.14). To conclude, instability and hyperlaxity are two different entities. The former is always pathological and most often unidirectional.

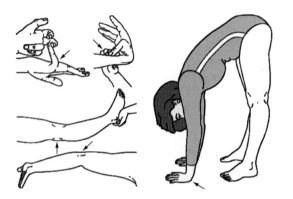

Fig. 10.12. Standard maneuvers depicting hypermobility syndrome. (Adapted from BEIGHTON et al. 1973)

The latter is a physical characteristic with multidirectional patterns. However, American authors often omit to differentiate these two conditions resulting in confusing terminology.

10.3.5
Associated Lesions

Instabilities may be associated with rotator cuff tears (generally after the age of 40), superior labral tears, neurological lesions or bone fractures.

Overall, glenohumeral instabilities occur in a wide range of forms. Since NEER's studies, *TUBS* are

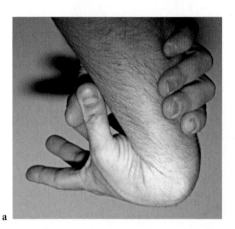
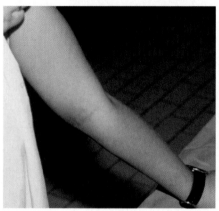

a   b

Fig. 10.13a, b. Examples of generalized hypermobility syndrome according to BEIGHTON et al. (1973). **a** Apposition of the thumb alongside the flexor aspect of the forearm. **b** Hyperextension of the elbow beyond 90°

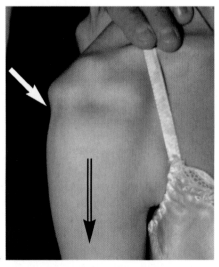
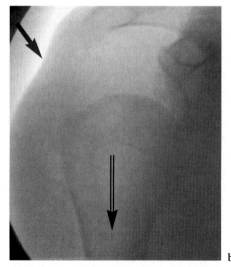

a   b

Fig. 10.14a, b. Demonstration of the sulcus sign. **a** Right upper arm downward traction (*hollow arrow*) highlights a sulcus under the acromion (*white arrow*). **b** Radiograph obtained with downward traction of the arm (*hollow arrow*) underlines the sulcus (*black arrow*) associated with the inferior subluxation of the humeral head

opposed to *AMBRI* and are classified at opposite ends of the clinical spectrum. TUBS refers to patients with a *traumatic* shoulder instability, usually *unilateral* with a *Bankart* lesion and requiring *surgery*. AMBRI corresponds to patients with an *atraumatic* initial injury, *multidirectional* hyperlaxity with a *bilateral* instability and who usually respond to a *rehabilitation* program. However, if surgery is needed, the surgeon must pay particular attention to performing an *inferior* capsular shift, a surgical procedure described by Neer (Matsen et al. 1990; Neer 1990). In all cases, it is important to differentiate instability from hyperlaxity in order to avoid surgical mistakes:

- Unnecessary surgery consists in treating patients with hyperlaxity as patients with shoulder instability. This surgery is detrimental to the patient and could lead to future shoulder pain and stiffness.
- Inadequate treatment of patients presenting true instability favoured by hyperlaxity. If treated solely for instability, surgical procedure may be ineffective.

10.4
Shoulder Imaging Techniques

Several imaging techniques may be used to explore the unstable shoulder such as standard X-Rays, CT, CT arthrography, MRI and MR arthrography.

10.4.1
X-Ray Evaluation

X-ray evaluation is always recommended even though clinical diagnosis has been reached. This exploration may be sufficient to determine the severity of the lesion and to specify therapeutic options such as in acute or recurrent anterior dislocation (Fig. 10.13). When X-rays are negative, more precise exploratory methods such as CT arthrography, MRI or MR arthrography are usually indicated (Blum et al. 1996; Nizard 1997; Rockwood et al. 1990; Engebretsen and Craig 1993).

10.4.2
CT and CT Arthrography

CT may be indicated to highlight bony glenoid or humeral head lesions but is ineffective to evaluate

the labrum or the capsuloligamentous structures. However, its efficiency seems to be improved by such technical refinements as helical acquisition which enables high quality multiplanar and three-dimensional (3D) reconstructions to be obtained (Fig. 10.15) (Godefroy and Chevrot 1996).

CT arthrography is a minimally invasive method enhanced by helical acquisition and multislice CT acquisition. Arthrography may be done as single or double contrast. The CT procedure gives the most valuable information but its efficacy is in direct relation to the quality of the arthrographic examination (Blum et al. 1995, 2000a; Dosch et al. 1996). Double contrast CT arthrography requires less contrast media diminishing the morbidity of this procedure and improving the quality of the images obtained with soft tissue windowing.

CT arthrography (and CT scan) must be performed with thin slices (thickness ≤2 mm), particularly to improve the viewing of the supraspinatus tendon (obliquely directed in a downward direction), the long head of the biceps tendon as it enters the bicipital groove, the high portion of the subscapularis tendon, the superior and inferior labrum and finally the inferior and superior glenoid rim. Acquisition with internal or external rotating position of the arm may be needed to detect a labral tear. Acquisition with internal rotation of the arm is associated with a more complete filling of the anterior recess and usually allows a better delineation of the anterior lesions. In external rotation posterior alterations of the labrum are usually better underlined (Soulez et al. 1991).

However, this usually well codified and tolerated technique may not be without risk due to intra-articular injection of contrast media. Shoulder pain or discomfort may occur hours after the procedure. This late occurrence explains why such complaints are frequently overlooked by radiologists. They usually respond to regular pain killers but the patient should be warned of possible undesirable effects. The frequency of symptoms are related to the amount, osmolality and concentration of the injected media (Hall et al. 1981; Blum et al. 2000b).

10.4.3
MRI

Published results about the value of MRI in shoulder disorders are rapidly outdated due to the constant improvement of equipment and pulse sequences.

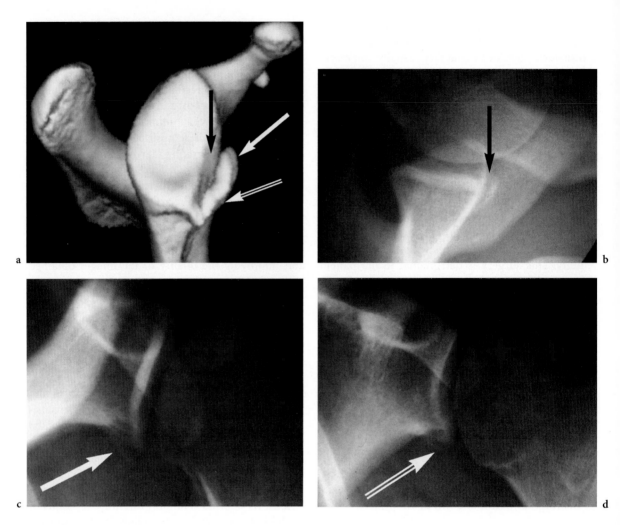

Fig. 10.15a–d. Various radiographic data necessary for the evaluation of the anteroinferior aspect of the glenoid rim. **a** Three-dimensional surface shaded image of the scapula showing a large anteroinferior fracture of the glenoid rim (*arrows* indicating the direction of the X-ray beam, *black arrow* for glenoidal profile, *white arrow* for apical oblique view and *hollow arrow* for the AP view). **b** Glenoidal profile showing the anterior portion of the fractured glenoid fragment (*black arrow*). **c** Apical oblique view highlighting the middle portion of the fracture (*white arrow*). **d** AP view of the glenohumeral joint (with a 30° caudal tilt of the X-ray beam) demonstrating the inferior portion of the fracture (*hollow arrow*). These combined radiographs are required to detect the small localized fracture of the anteroinferior glenoid rim

The aspect of the different anatomical structures of the shoulder vary according to the different pulse sequences used. This aspect has to be taken into consideration when analysing images on unfamiliar machines. Moreover, some sequences which seem identical may yield quite different results depending upon the machine or even from one version to the next on the same machine. Therefore, each machine requires a specific protocol suited to the clinical situation and the machine performance.

The best results are usually obtained with the fast spin-echo moderately T2-weighted sequence associated with a fat suppression signal (Fat Sat). The echo train length must not be set too high in order to limit blurring artifacts. Besides, intravenous gadolinium injection with T1-weighted images seems to effectively outline labral or capsular lesions.

10.4.4
MR Arthrography

Debatable MRI performances have led some authors to propose the injection of contrast media within the glenohumeral joint prior to performing MR examination. This technique labelled MR arthrography improves the analysis of the labrum, ligaments and capsular structures as it increases intra-articular contrast and distends the capsule.

Two different techniques have been adopted (ZANETTI and HODLER 1997). Firstly, T1-weighted sequences are obtained after intra-articular gadolinium injection, diluted either with physiological serum or iodinated contrast media. This technique is widely used and its excellent ability to detect articular abnormalities has been reported in many studies. It is probably the best available method on low field machines (LOEW et al. 2000). However, in most countries, intra-articular injection of gadolinium is not approved by administrative authorities and informed consent of the patient has to be obtained.

In the second procedure, iodinated contrast media (or physiological serum) is injected solely and fast spin-echo T2-weighted sequences are obtained. The second method offers substantial advantages as it combines two widely used methods (arthrography and MRI) and does not require any complex manipulation of contrast media. It does not involve intra-articular gadolinium injection. Moreover, examinations are of high quality and images are rapidly available. Finally, T2-weighted sequences which are used in this technique constitute the basis of shoulder exploration (TUITE and ORWIN 1996; WILLEMSEN et al. 1996; BLUM et al. 2000a).

Some studies report that high volume intra-articular injection of solution (15–40 ml) in distending the capsule of patients with capacious joint cavities improves the accuracy of this technique (WILLEMSEN et al. 1998). However, 40 ml is an enormous quantity of fluid that might rupture the extra-capsular synovial recesses and generally 10–15 ml is sufficient.

To put stress on the anteroinferior labrocapsular structures and therefore to obtain a higher definition of their lesions, acquisition with abduction and external rotation of the arm (ABER) or in the apprehension test position can be performed (WINTZELL et al 1999a; CVITANIC et al. 1997; KWAK et al. 1998b). ABER positioning is also recommended for exploring the painful athlete's shoulder (ROGER et al. 1999).

Finally, indirect MR arthrography with intravenous injection of gadolinium has been recommended by some authors for the exploration of anterior shoulder instability (WINTZELL et al. 1998a,b; VAHLENSIECK et al. 1998). Although special positioning of the shoulder such as the ABER position or apprehension test position improves the value of this technique, it is not well-suited for the detection of capsular or labroligamentous lesions since indirect injection of gadolinium does not increase joint fluid and, therefore, joint structure distension is limited.

10.5
Anterior Instability

Imaging is fundamental in exploring instabilities; however, subsequent explorations vary according to clinical findings. On the one hand, in the most common types of instabilities such as recurrent dislocation, surgery is indicated and the procedure is essentially dependent upon the importance of glenoid rim lesions. In this case, a standard X-ray evaluation is usually sufficient. The three anteroposterior views of the glenohumeral joint (external, neutral and internal rotation), apical oblique view described by GARTH and the glenoid profile described by BERNAGEAU et al. (1976) are standard procedures (BLUM et al. 1998; GARTH et al. 1984). In order to identify bony lesions, CT-scan may eventually be used. CT arthrography or MRI give more specific details as to the severity of the lesions, particularly soft tissue alterations; however, these data do not alter standard therapeutic protocol.

On the other hand, in subtle forms of instability, diagnosis or instability direction are not clearly assessed clinically and standard X-ray evaluation is usually normal. In this case, further imaging with CT arthrography, MRI or MR arthrography are recommended to confirm the diagnosis of instability and to evaluate its direction. The technique of choice is undoubtedly MR arthrography; however, the imaging technique used depends mostly on several factors, principally quality, performance and access to the machines.

10.5.1
Diagnosis of Bony Lesions Associated with Instability

Bony lesions associated with anterior instability are mainly represented by a posterolateral osteochondral compression fracture of the humeral head and by a lesion appearing on the anteroinferior portion of the glenoid rim.

Outlining these lesions enables one to establish the instability but also points out its direction (anterior). However, glenoid alterations only determine therapeutic procedures. Both lesions are usually highlighted using standard X-rays.

10.5.1.1
Humeral Head Defect

Humeral head defect (Malgaigne or Hill-Sachs lesion) is due to a compression fracture of the superoposterolateral aspect of the humeral head displaced anteriorly and impacted at the anteroinferior portion of the glenoid rim. In fact, depending upon the direction of the displacement, the impaction may be observed higher or lower on the humeral head. In acute dislocations, the incidence of the defect ranges between 30% and 100% in various series. This discrepancy can be partially explained by the different exploratory methods used: standard radiographs frequently overlooked small lesions and more specifically pure cartilage lesions, whereas arthroscopy is the more sensitive technique. In recurrent dislocations, defects are larger and are identified by standard X-rays in more than 80% of cases. These defects, variable in size, do not influence therapeutic procedure although according to some authors, patients with larger lesions are more prone to recurrent dislocations (MOLÉ and WALCH 1993; ROCKWOOD 1984; WALCH 1996; CALANDRA et al. 1989).

Humeral head defect is usually outlined by the anteroposterior (AP) view of the shoulder with the arm in internal rotation or by the apical oblique view described by GARTH (Fig. 10.16) (GARTH et al. 1984). Other less applied methods have been described such as the "Stryker notch view" or the "20/20 incidence" discussed by JOHNER et al. (1982) (ROCKWOOD et al. 1990; ENGEBRETSEN and CRAIG 1993).

CT scan or CT arthrography are more efficient than the above-mentioned methods to diagnose these abnormalities as they are more efficient in detecting small bony defects and sometimes underline a pure cartilaginous defect or reveal sclerosis of the humeral

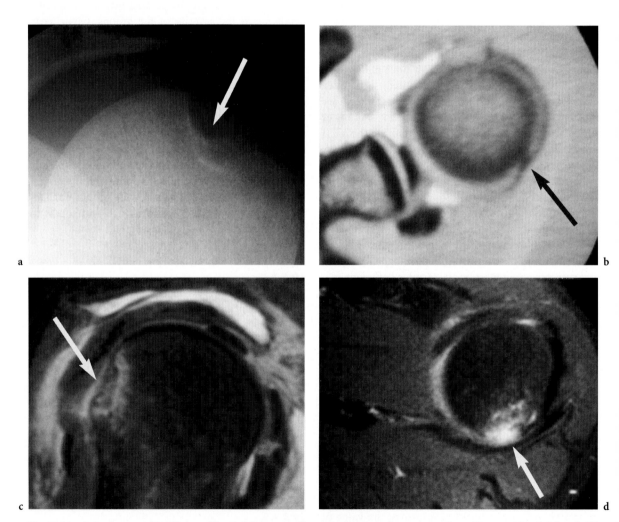

Fig. 10.16a–d. Some examples of humeral head defects. **a** Radiograph showing a large posterolateral humeral head defect. **b** CT arthrography of the left shoulder pointing out a pure chondral defect of the posterolateral aspect of the humeral head (*arrow*). **c** Fast spin-echo (FSE) T2-weighted image with fat saturation obtained in the sagittal plane showing a large posterolateral defect of the humeral head underlined by bone marrow edema. **d** FSE T2-weighted with fat saturation obtained in the axial plane showing a posterolateral defect of the humeral head with underlying bone marrow edema

head due to impaction (Fig. 14) (DELGOFFE et al. 1984). Finally, MRI is a valuable method to detect humeral head fractures, especially if performed shortly after the accident. These cases show bone marrow edema as well as the bony compression fracture at the posterolateral aspect of the humeral head (Fig. 10.15). However, when bone marrow edema is no longer visible, small defects are less detectable with MRI than with CT scan.

10.5.1.2
Anteroinferior Lesions of the Glenoid Rim

Bony lesions appearing on the anteroinferior portion of the glenoid rim are not always present but can be highlighted by specific standard exploration in more than 90% of cases using an AP view of the glenohumeral joint added to an apical oblique view (GARTH) and glenoid profile (BERNAGEAU) (Fig. 13) (GARTH et al. 1984; BERNAGEAU et al. 1976). However, the latter may be difficult to perform in patients unable to fully abduct their arm. In all cases, best results are obtained using fluoroscopy. Finally, the comparative glenoid profile of the other shoulder may be useful. The "West Point method" is also advised by some Anglo-Saxon authors (ROCK-WOOD et al. 1990). When in doubt, CT scan or CT arthrography are the best techniques to highlight and define bony lesions.

This evaluation permits one to point out fractures, non-union or a partial wear and tear of the glenoid rim (Figs. 10.17, 10.18). It can also reveal a periosteal

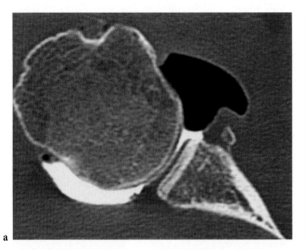
a

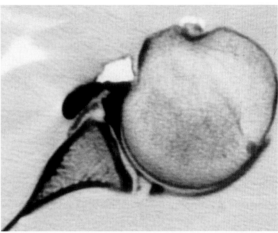
b

Fig. 10.17. a CT arthrography showing a glenoid rim fracture with a medially displaced fragment. b CT arthrography showing a small glenoid rim fracture and a periosteal reaction

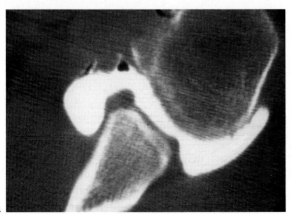
a

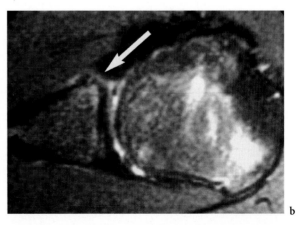
b

Fig. 10.18. Comparison of CT arthrography and MRI in the evaluation of capsulolabral lesions. a CT arthrography showing a partial wear and tear of the anteroinferior glenoid rim indicating anterior recurrent instability; paradoxically, the labrum appears intact. b MRI with IV gadolinium injection reveals fibrous scar tissue mimicking a labrum with enhancement at the bone base (*white arrow*)

reaction at the anterior aspect of the neck of the scapula indicating a capsuloperiosteal avulsion.

Fracture is linked to either IGHL avulsion occurring when the patient is in external rotation or sectioning of the glenoid rim caused by direct impact of the humeral head. Fractures can heal completely, sometimes showing a callus or evolve as a non-union. The wear and tear is present in more than 40% of recurrent dislocation. It is caused by repetitive rubbing of the humeral head against the glenoid rim. Its aspect varies from a softening of the bone to a complete corner cut off.

10.5.1.3
Associated Lesions

Some bone fractures can be related to a former dislocation: greater tuberosity fracture and coracoid process fracture. The latter normally occurs in older patients with severe rotator cuff tears. An osteochondral defect of the glenoid fossa, although uncommon, has a high association with instability and also with labral tear and intraarticular bodies (Fig. 10.19) (Yu et al. 1998).

10.5.2
Soft Tissue Lesions

The demonstration of labrocapsuloligamentous lesions is essential to establish the diagnosis of anterior instability when no bony lesions are identified. This evaluation is based on CT arthrography, MRI or arthro-MRI, but before proceeding any further, we must eliminate the possibility of a hyperlaxity.

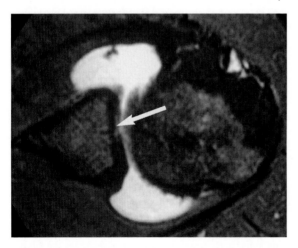

Fig. 10.19. MR arthrography showing a chondral lesion at the inferior portion of the glenoid surface (*arrow*)

Thanks to a good spatial resolution in the different available planes, an excellent intra-articular contrast and a distension of the IGHL, an extensive analysis of capsuloligamentous structures can only be obtained with MR arthrography. However, this method remains less accurate than arthroscopy which yields a precise classification of the lesions.

10.5.2.1
Determination of a Hyperlaxity

Hyperlaxity is mostly defined by clinical evaluation but it can also be determined by a stress view with inferior traction of the arm showing the inferior exclusion of the humeral head associated to the sulcus sign (JALOVAARA et al. 1992). Quantification of hyperlaxity would be helpful; however, no study has been performed to validate the usefulness of these radiographs. If arthrography or MR arthrography are performed, a large axillary pouch is apparent (Fig. 10.20).

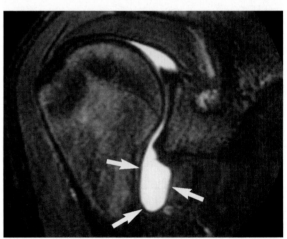

Fig. 10.20. MR arthrography showing a large axillary pouch and a thinning of the inferior glenohumeral ligament (*arrows*) associated with shoulder hyperlaxity

10.5.2.2
Capsulolabral Detachments

Capsulolabral detachments are referred to as the Bankart lesion. These lesions are in fact variable depending on the direction of the humeral head displacement, the strength of the different anatomical components and the frequency of recurrence of dislocation. The labrum is usually detached at its anteroinferior portion (Fig. 10.21), but it may remain intact. On the contrary, the tear can extend to its

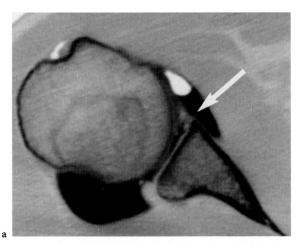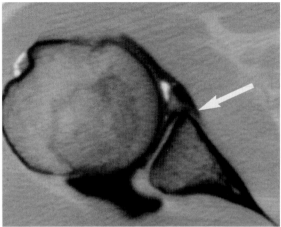

a   b

Fig. 10.21a, b. CT arthrography detecting a labral tear (*white arrow*) which is better observed in external rotation than in neutral rotation. **a** Neutral rotation. **b** External rotation

anterosuperior and superior portion. The tearing of the capsule and of the IGHL usually extends inward as far as the periosteum at the anterior neck of the scapula. It may also extend upward with a tearing of the MGHL. The healing process results in a more or less weak fibrous scar. When healing does not occur, a large pouch as described by BROCA and HARTMANN is noticed (BROCA and HARTMANN 1890).

The ALPSA (anterior labroligamentous periosteal sleeve avulsion) lesion is an avulsion of the antero-inferior glenoid labrum with an intact scapular periosteum. The ALPSA lesion differs from the Bankart lesion in that the ALPSA lesion has an intact anterior scapular periosteum allowing the labroligamentous structures to displace medially and rotate inferiorly on the scapular neck. In the Bankart lesion, the anterior scapular periosteum rupture results in displacement of the labrum and attached ligaments anterior to the glenoid rim. In the ALPSA lesion, the anterior labrum with stripped periosteum are displaced medially and rotated inferiorly (BELTRAN et al. 1997; LEE et al. 2000).

CT arthrography, MRI or MR arthrography can show different pathological patterns whose relationship with arthroscopic data can be difficult to estab-

lish. For example, a fibrous scar may mimic an intact labrum on CT arthrography and a wear and tear of the anteroinferior glenoid rim can be observed with a pseudo intact labrum. In this case, MRI with intravenous gadolinium injection can show a tissue enhancement at the base of the pseudo-labrum indicating the presence of fibrous tissues (see Fig. 10.18). The most characteristic patterns are described in Table 10.1.

An irregular or severed anteroinferior recess is due to a fibrous scar and is usually well defined when the joint is filled with contrast media (Fig. 10.22). Therefore, it can be demonstrated with CT arthrography or MR arthrography but is barely visible with MRI. As previously mentioned, a slight periosteal reaction is due to an extension of the tearing of the capsule at its insertion together with a periosteal tearing. This process is better observed with CT or CT arthrography (Fig. 10.22).

The value of the different imaging methods in the diagnosis of labral tears remains controversial. In a prospective study involving 30 patients aged 19–39 and presenting shoulder instability or unexplained painful shoulder syndrome, CHANDNANI et al. (1993) demonstrated that CT arthrography, MRI and MR

Table 10.1. Most characteristic patterns of anterior instabilities observed with CT arthrography, MRI or MR arthrography

Patterns	CT arthrography	MRI	MR arthrography
Irregular or severed anteroinferior recess	++	0	++
Slight periosteal reaction at the anterior aspect of the neck of the scapula	++	0	0
Detached anteroinferior labral tear	++	++	+++
Uneven aspect, thickening or detachment of the inferior glenohumeral ligament	0	0	+++

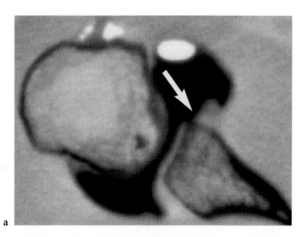
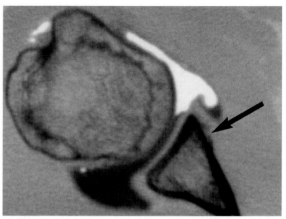

Fig. 10.22a, b. Different CT arthrography examples of capsulolabral lesions. **a** Severed anteroinferior recess (*white arrow*) due to scar tissue at the anterior aspect of the glenoid neck. **b** Slight periosteal reaction at the anterior aspect of the glenoid neck

arthrography sensitivities in the diagnosis of labral tears were respectively 73%, 93% and 96%. However, other studies indicate that MRI sensitivity varies between 19%–95% and specificity from 78%–93% (JAHNKE et al. 1992; BALICH et al. 1996).

Therefore, it is difficult to assess whether standard MRI is more efficient than CT arthrography, when their sensitivity and specificity vary respectively from 73% to 93% and from 73% to 80% (CALLAGHAN et al. 1988; JAHNKE et al. 1992). Taking into account these large variations in accuracy, many authors advocate the use of MR arthrography as the most reliable method with a 90% accuracy to evaluate labrocapsular structures and to detect labral tears (Fig. 10.23).

IGHL tearing can occur at three different locations. It appears most often at its attachment on the glenoid neck and is generally associated with a labral tear. Less commonly, the ligament is detached and torn at its humeral neck insertion. The avulsion of the anterior band of the inferior glenohumeral ligament complex from the humerus is called HAGL (humeral avulsion of the glenohumeral ligament). Finally, the axillary pouch or the anterior or posterior band of the ligament may be distended or severed. These alterations may occur separately or together. MR arthrography or arthrography (less accurate) are the only imaging techniques able to detect these abnormalities. Arthrography may depict a leak at the IGHL insertions or a large and irregular axillary pouch indicating a stretching of the axillary pouch fibers. (In order to obtain an easier diagnosis, it is advised to inject the contrast media at the upper portion of the glenohumeral joint in the event of contrast media reflux which could be misinterpreted as a leaky tear). In addition, MR arthrography can depict the actual tearing of the ligament (Figs. 10.24, 10.25).

10.5.2.3
Other Soft Tissue Lesions

Complete rotator cuff tears associated with glenohumeral instability are unusual before the age of 40. However, through arthroscopy, partial tears can be identified in up to 20% of acute luxation and highlighted in 5% of recurrent luxation cases. In the specific case of anterior luxations in elderly patients, large rotator cuff tears are almost always present (LEVY et al. 1999).

In 1% of cases, a cartilage lesion at the anteroinferior portion of the glenoid surface can be associated with a labral tear (Fig. 10.26). This association, called GLAD (glenoid labral articular disruption), results from a forced adduction injury occurring from the position of abduction and external rotation of the arm (NEVIASER 1993; SANDERS et al. 1999).

10.5.3
Therapeutic Aspects of Anterior Instability

10.5.3.1
Treatment and Prognosis
of Acute Anterior Dislocation

The most frequently recommended treatment of acute dislocation is an orthopedic method (closed reduction, immobilization, reeducation). A stabilising procedure may sometimes be indicated for young athletes or certain manual workers who seem to be prone to recurrent dislocations. Imaging plays a major role in determining the severity of the lesions, suggesting the eventual possibility of recurrence and guiding towards appropriate surgical options.

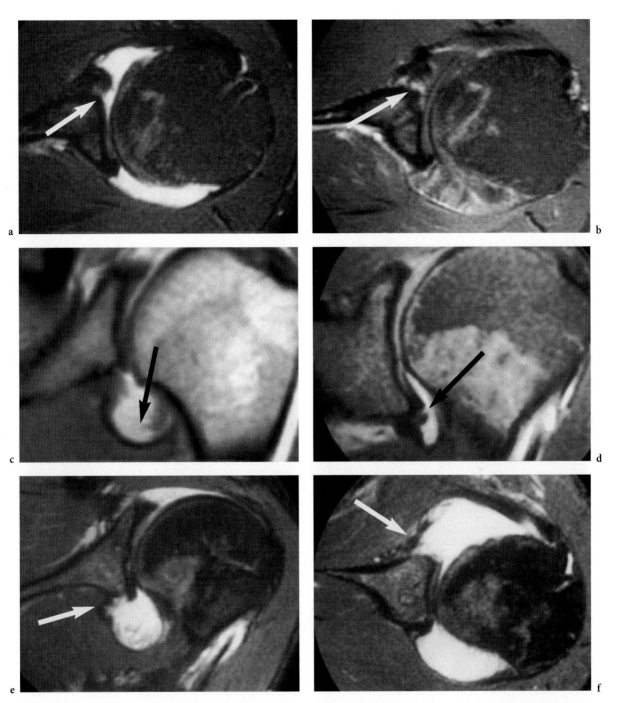

Fig. 10.23. MR arthrography examples of capsulolabral lesions obtained with iodinated contrast media (without intraarticular gadolinium injection). **a** Fast spin-echo (FSE) T2-weighted image with fat saturation. **b** Spin-echo (SE) T1-weighted image with fat saturation after IV gadolinium (Dotarem) injection in the axial plane showing a capsulolabral tear (*white arrow*) better visible with second acquisition. **c** SE T2-weighted coronal image showing a tearing of the inferior glenohumeral ligament (*arrow*). **d.** FSE T2-weighted coronal image showing a Bankart lesion. Coronal (**e**) and axial (**f**) SE T2-weighted image showing a recurrent capsuloligamentous tear following a Bankart procedure, with a thickened and irregular aspect below and in front of the scapular neck (*white arrow*)

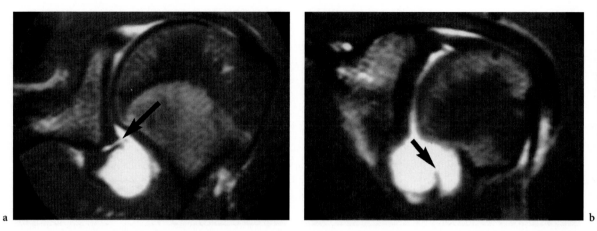

Fig. 10.24a, b. MR arthrography showing a Bankart lesion (*arrow*) (**a**) associated with an avulsion of the anterior band of the inferior glenohumeral ligament (*arrow*) (**b**)

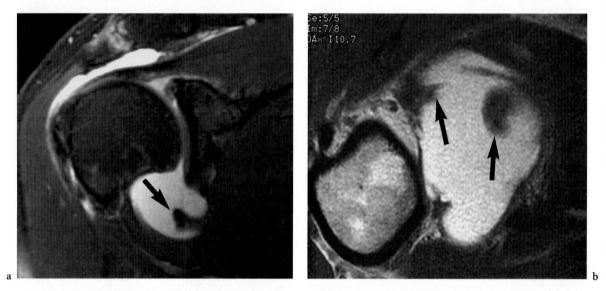

Fig. 10.25a, b. MR arthrography showing a tearing of the anterior band of the inferior glenohumeral ligament (*arrows*)

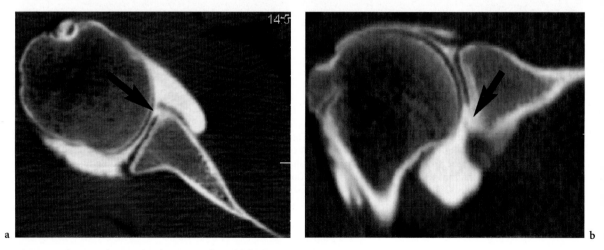

Fig. 10.26a, b. CT arthrography showing a glenoid labral articular disruption lesion (*arrow*). Axial view (**a**) and coronal multi-planar reformation (**b**) highlighting an anteroinferior articular lesion (*arrow*)

According to specific studies, acute anterior gleno-humeral dislocation will evolve in 40%–92% of cases towards recurrent dislocation (MATSEN et al. 1990; VERMEIREN et al. 1993). HOVELIUS (1987) showed that after more than 5 years, patients under 30 who originally underwent 3 weeks of immobilization had a 58% rate of recurrent dislocation.

The younger the patient, the greater the risk of recurrent dislocation. This finding may seem paradoxical as the healing potential tends to diminish with age. Certain lesions are probably more prone to reoccur and arise more specifically in young patients, but no poor prognostic factor has ever been identified beyond a type 2 SLAP lesion (MOLÉ et al. 1996). On the other hand, the low intensity of the initial trauma and intense sports activities are classically recognized as factors leading to poor prognosis.

Treatment quality is not negligible. The immobilization period does not seem to be the main factor but a specific rehabilitation program leads to a 25% decrease in recurrence rate. Finally, articular flushing seems to improve the healing process of labrocapsular and ligamentous lesions (WINTZELL et al. 1999b,c). In a study involving 30 patients under 30 who underwent arthroscopic procedure including articular flushing following initial trauma, the rate of recurrence was only 20% over a 24-month period (MOLÉ et al. 1996).

10.5.3.2
Treatment of Recurrent Dislocation

All recurrent instabilities must be treated surgically. However, in occult or subtle cases, surgery may only be considered when the diagnosis has been confirmed through arthroscopy or other imaging methods. Four major types of surgical procedures are identified: surgical capsular repairs, coracoid transfers, arthroscopic repairs and capsular shift and repair (MATSEN et al. 1990; ROCKWOOD 1984; WALCH 1996).

Surgical capsular repairs consist in stretching the capsule and the IGHL and reinserting them into the anterior glenoid rim. This procedure is inspired by the Bankart procedure and staples are commonly used to secure the capsule to the bone. The main advantages of this method reside in its similarity to normal anatomical structures and its good clinical results. However, the strength of the treated joint is not always satisfactory and the risk of recurrence is approximately 3%–8%.

The most common coracoid transfer method is derived from the Latarjet procedure. The coracoid process along with the biceps and the coracobrachialis tendons is transferred to the anteroinferior aspect of the neck of the scapula. Stability is the result of abutment of the humeral head against the coracoid process and of the short head of the biceps which belts the weak anteroinferior point when the arm is in abduction/external rotation. The main advantage of this method is its great mechanical performance. Recurrences are uncommon. However, this technique is seen by some authors as being too far removed from natural anatomy. The risk of osteoarthritis is significant, particularly if the coracoid process protrudes from the articular surface.

Arthroscopic repairs are the most recent techniques to restore anterior stability (NELSON and ARCIERO 2000). Metallic anchors are used to reattach the capsule to the neck of the capsula. This neat and elegant technique is free of ugly scarring or subsequent infections. Early procedures were plagued by a high rate of recurrence in the absence of fibrous tissue scarring; however, due to technical refinements such as artificial exacerbation of fibrous tissue, a scar-like effect is created improving the stability of the joint.

Capsular shifts are defined as capsular incisions performed in order to reduce the capsule redundancy. This technique first applied by NEER (1990) (inferior capsular shift) is indicated when capsule distension is present. There are several other less commonly used surgical methods.

The choice of the surgical procedure depends on a number of factors such as the degree of instability, the severity of the lesions and the presence of hyperlaxity. In major forms of instability (recurrent dislocations), coracoid transfers are usually preferred because of their mechanical reliability. In minor or occult forms of instability, arthroscopic or surgical capsular repairs may be favoured. Isolated and recent capsulolabral tears are easily sutured. Chronic tearing of the capsule and fibrous scarring of the IGHL may need complementary capsular repair. Fracture or non-union of the anteroinferior portion of the glenoid rim requires a coracoid transfer. In the case of underlying hyperlaxity with capsule redundancy, a capsular shift is additionally performed.

10.6
Posterior Instabilities

Posterior instabilities essentially include acute and traumatic posterior dislocations which evolve towards fixed dislocations when misdiagnosed, voluntary and atraumatic subluxations associated with acquired or constitutional shoulder hyperlaxity and occult or minor instabilities essentially found in athletes (BLUM et al. 2000a; GERBER 1991).

10.6.1
Acute Traumatic Posterior Dislocations

Acute dislocations are misdiagnosed in about 50% of cases. This can be partially explained when considering this particular population (alcoholics, epileptics, polytraumatized patients) who don't always receive proper medical care, and considering the radiographic data which are sometimes incomplete or difficult to assess. Diagnosis can be suggested on the AP view of the glenohumeral joint when the humeral head seems to be fixed in internal rotation with a pseudo-widening of the articular space. On the contrary, posterior dislocation is suggested when the articular space cannot be visualized without bony overlapping (Fig. 10.27). A fracture–impaction of the humeral head, visible as a vertical and dense line on the medial portion of the head, is also significant. Finally, a rising of the humeral head is characteristic but non specific (BERNAGEAU and PATTE 1980).

At this phase, the true scapulolateral X-ray (the Y view) described by LAMY or the scapular outlet view discussed by NEER (1990) are the most useful views (Fig. 10.27). The diagnosis of posterior dislocation is confirmed when the humeral head sits posterior to the glenoid articular surface. The axillary lateral radiograph is recommended by some authors; however, it may be difficult to obtain in the trauma situation (PETERSON 2000). CT scan is usually performed when associated fractures are suspected or with polytraumatized patients. This technique clearly shows the position of the humeral head and the anteromedial defect of the humeral head due to its impaction on the posterior glenoid rim. It may reveal a fracture of the posterior glenoid rim; however, this lesion is uncommon.

Acute posterior dislocations require emergency closed reduction. Surgery is only recommended in cases such as major displacement of an associated lesser tuberosity fragment, major fragment of the posterior glenoid rim, irreducible dislocation, open dislocation or unstable reduction. Recurrence of common forms of posterior dislocation are exceptional.

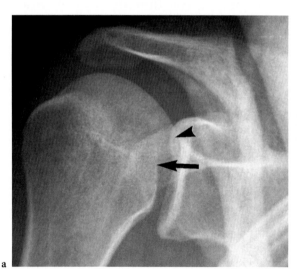

a

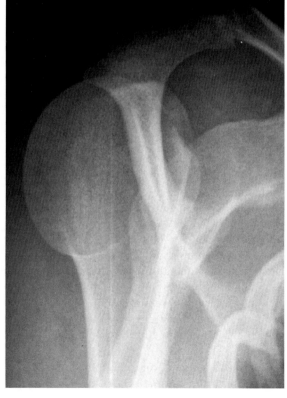

b

Fig. 10.27a, b. Posterior dislocation. **a** Front view aspect of posterior dislocation characterised by an elevation of the humeral head, the lack of visibility of the glenohumeral space (*arrowhead*) and an anterior impaction fracture (*arrow*). **b** Neer profile view confirming the posterior displacement of the humeral head

10.6.2
Fixed Posterior Dislocations

If not treated within 3 weeks, dislocations become fixed. The gravity of these lesions can be explained by four major complications:
- The occurrence of fibrosis and soft tissue retraction which precludes the performance of a closed reduction in more than 60%.
- The anteromedial defect of the humeral head which progressively becomes larger increasing the risk of recurrence after reduction. This defect will require surgical filling.
- The lesions of anterior circumflex artery branches which may lead to an avascular necrosis of the humeral head.
- Osteoarthritis which is the final course of this lesion despite joint mobility and activity reduction.

The size of the humeral head defect and the delay between the onset of the trauma and the diagnosis are the main factors determining surgical procedures. CT scan represents the most pertinent technique to evaluate the size of the humeral head defect classified according to the percentage of destroyed articular surface or according to RANDELLI's classification (Figs. 10.28, 10.29, 10.30) (RANDELLI 1988; DUPARC et al. 1996).

When the diagnosis can be reached within 6 months and the defect covers less than 50% of the humeral head, conservative surgical treatment is indicated. The surgical procedure includes an anterior deltopectoral approach, disinsertion of the sub-scapularis tendon or of the lesser tuberosity, resection of the fibrous scar tissue and reduction of the humeral head. The defect is then filled with the lesser tuberosity (Hawkins-Neer procedure) or with the subscapularis tendon (McLaughlin procedure).

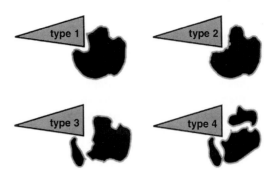

Fig. 10.29. Posterior dislocation classification (RANDELLI 1988)

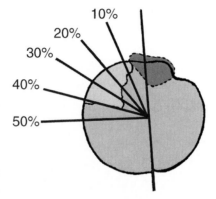

Fig. 10.30. Posterior dislocation classification according to the size of the humeral head defect and the percentage of damaged articular surface

10.6.3
Atraumatic Voluntary Subluxations

Atraumatic voluntary subluxations are usually associated with hyperlaxity of the shoulder and sometimes with a hypermobility syndrome (see Fig. 10.11). They usually affect young patients and especially female teenagers (BROWN et al. 2000). Subluxations are painless. Imaging techniques are not usually prescribed as they do not reveal any lesion. X-rays possibly combined with video recording, CT or MRI can be performed to confirm the subluxation direction. In most cases, voluntary subluxations are only posterior, but they can also be compounded with anterior or inferior voluntary subluxations. If performed, arthrography, CT arthrography or MR arthrography outline a capacious axillary pouch but no specific treatment is necessary. However, a rehabilitation program may be advised. Rarely is a posteroinferior capsular shift required (FUCHS at al. 2000; TILLANDER et al. 1998). However, when painful or involuntary episodes of subluxation occur subsequently, CT arthrography, MRI or MR arthrography are indicated as they may reveal capsulolabral alterations.

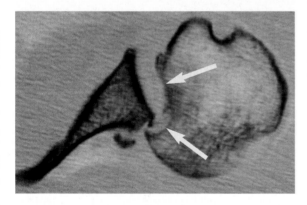

Fig. 10.28. CT scan demonstrating a fixed posterior instability with a large humeral head defect (*arrows*)

10.6.4
Occult Forms of Instability

Minor forms of instability are difficult to assess clinically as they are not always accompanied by trauma. Moreover, episodes of subluxations are often misinterpreted by the patient (Fig. 10.31). This specific type of instability is essentially found in athletes with possible acquired hyperlaxity of the glenohumeral joint.

Since bony lesions (such as a fracture of the posterior glenoid rim) are uncommon, X-rays are usually not contributive to the diagnosis. CT arthrography, MRI or MR arthrography are indicated to identify a posterior labral tear (Fig. 10.32). This tear may be

associated with the development of a labral or a retrolabral cyst. If the cyst becomes larger and extends towards the spinoglenoidal region, it may compress the suprascapular nerve resulting in infraspinatus muscle edema and amyotrophy (Figs. 10.33, 10.34).

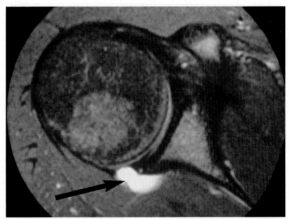

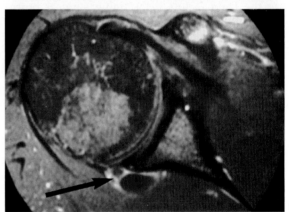

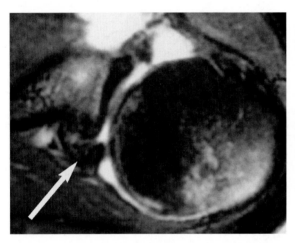

Fig. 10.31. Axial fast spin-echo T2-weighted image with fat sat showing a fracture of the posterior glenoid rim (*white arrow*) in a patient with undetected recurrent posterior subluxations

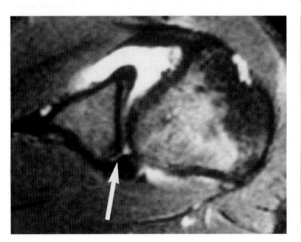

Fig. 10.32. Axial fast spin-echo T2-weighted image with fat saturation showing a posterior labral tear (*white arrow*) in a young female athlete with shoulder pain at the end of the cocking phase

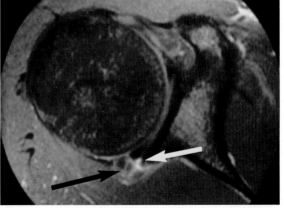

Fig. 10.33a–c. MRI showing a posterior labral tear (*white arrow*) associated with a labral cyst (*black arrow*) in a rugby player with an occult form of posterior instability. **a** Axial fast spin-echo T2-weighted image with fat saturation. **b, c** Axial spin-echo T1-weighted image with fat saturation

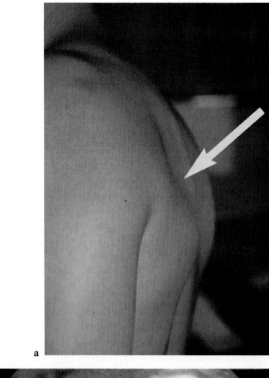

Fig. 10.34a–d. Young male athlete with left shoulder pain and infraspinatus muscle atrophy. **a** Posterolateral view showing an isolated infraspinatus muscle atrophy. **b** CT arthrography poorly delineating a spinoglenoidal cyst (*arrow*) and missing a posterior labral tear. **c** Axial fast spin-echo T2-weighted image with fat saturation showing a spinoglenoidal cyst (*black arrow*) communicating with the glenohumeral joint through a posterior labral tear (*black arrow*) and revealing infraspinatus muscle edema. **d** Sagittal spin-echo T2-weighted image showing the cyst and highlighting the isolated amyotrophy and edema of the infraspinatus muscle. *SS*, supraspinatus muscle; *SbS*, subscapularis muscle; *IS*, infraspinatus muscle; *D*, deltoid muscle; *TM*, teres minor muscle

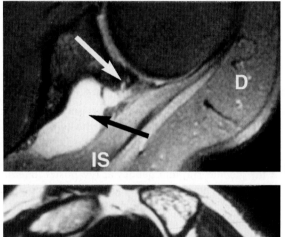

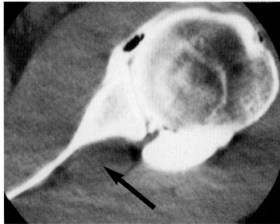

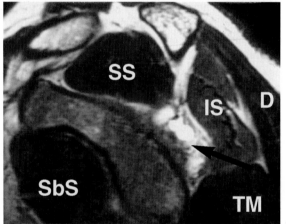

Surgical treatment of such instabilities is hazardous. This is due to the scarcity of anatomical lesions, psychological factors (voluntary instability) and the frequent presence of an associated glenohumeral hyperlaxity. When a hyper-retroversion of the glenoid surface (>10°) is present, it is considered a contributing factor in posterior instability and therefore some authors suggest correcting it using a posterior glenoid neck osteotomy (HAWKINS 1996). In other cases, surgery is suggested with some reserve. Surgery may include capsular shift and repair and infraspinatus shortening or iliac or acromial transfer fixed

at the posterior aspect of the scapular neck (ESSADKI et al. 2000; TILLANDER et al. 1998).

10.7
Simulated Forms of Instability

Most forms of instability are easily identified with clinical data and standard imaging procedures. However, in certain cases, particularly in minor forms of instability, other aetiologies of the painful shoulder syndrome must be ruled out in order to establish a clear cut diagnosis (ROGER et al. 1999).

10.7.1
Rotator Cuff Alterations

When confronted with a painful shoulder syndrome, specially in athletes, tendinopathy or partial tear of the rotator cuff tendons must be ruled out (PATTE et al. 1980; JOBE et al. 1991; ELLMANN 1990). The latter can be identified with ultrasound, CT arthrography, MRI or more precisely using MR arthrography.

However, a posterosuperior impingement syndrome as described by WALCH et al. (1991) which is responsible for shoulder pain at the cocking phase is sometimes difficult to differentiate from a minor form of instability. This syndrome is due to repetitive impingement of the posterior portion of the supraspinatus tendon against the posterosuperior rim. Lesions include a partial rotator cuff tear, alterations of the posterosuperior portion of the labrum or of the glenoid rim and geodes at the posterolateral aspect of the humeral head (Fig. 10.35). A hypo-retrotorsion of the humerus (of less than 10°) is considered a contributing factor in this syndrome (WALCH et al. 1991; BOILEAU et al. 1993).

Differentiation of instability from posterosuperior impingement syndrome might be difficult when the partial tear is not identified. Posterosuperior alterations of the labrum or of the glenoid rim may simulate posterior instability alterations and humeral head lesions may mimic Hill-Sachs defects. However, these conditions identified together do not fit the description of instability. Moreover, humeral head lesions are usually quite large in posterosuperior impingement syndrome, whereas they appear minimal in subtle forms of instability (Fig. 10.36). Finally, MRI with ABER positioning may help in the diagnosis by outlining the impingement of the posterior portion of the supraspinatus tendon against the posterosuperior portion of the glenoid rim.

10.7.2
Superior Labral Lesions

Superior labral lesions, also named SLAP lesions (superior labral anterior to posterior lesion) can lead to symptomatic and painful shoulder syndrome. Several types of lesions have been identified and have been classified by SNYDER into four types (SNYDER et al. 1990) (Fig. 10.37). The type 1 lesion, which is today considered as a common degenerative alteration requiring no particular treatment, consists in fraying of the free edge of the superior labrum with an intact biceps tendon. Type 2 lesions consist in an avulsion of the labral-biceps anchor from the

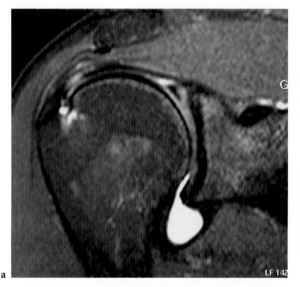
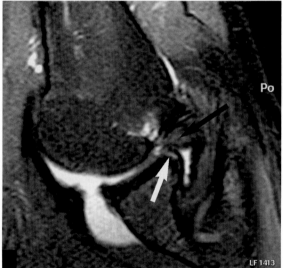

a   b

Fig. 10.35a, b. MR arthrography with fast spin-echo T2-weighted image with fat saturation demonstrating a posterosuperior impingement syndrome (arthrography is normal). **a** Coronal view obtained in standard position showing a posterior humeral head alteration with a mid-substance partial tear of the posterior portion of the supraspinatus tendon. **b** ABER positioning demonstrating the posterosuperior impingement of the supraspinatus tendon (*black arrow*) impacted between the humeral head and the posterosuperior glenoid rim. The labral tear (*white arrow*), alteration of the humeral head and the impacted supraspinatus tendon can be observed on the same slice

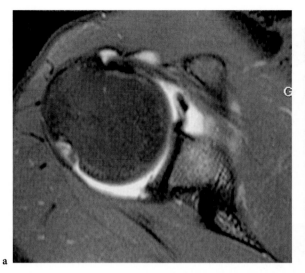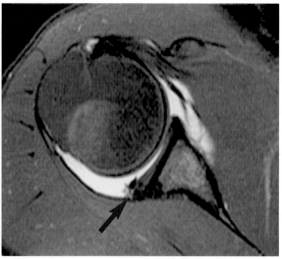

a   b

Fig. 10.36a, b. MR arthrography with fast spin-echo T2-weighted images and fat saturation demonstrating a posterosuperior impingement syndrome (arthrography is normal). **a** Axial view showing a large notch at the posterolateral aspect of the humeral head mimicking a Hill-Sach lesion. **b** Lower section demonstrating a posterior labral tear (*arrow*). These two lesions do not correspond to instability, however, they agree with the specifications of a posterosuperior impingement syndrome

glenoid (Fig. 10.38). They may be difficult to differentiate from a large sublabral recess. According to BENCARDINO et al. , a sublabral recess is medially oriented while SLAP 2 lesions are distally oriented; however, these findings are controversial (BENCARDINO et al. 2000; JEE 2001). Type 3 lesions are represented by a bucket-handle tear of the superior labrum below the biceps tendon which remains intact. Type 4 lesions are defined as a bucket handle tear of the superior labrum extending into the long head biceps tendon.

SLAP lesions are primarily encountered among athletic males in their thirties involved in throwing sports or sports with blocked cocking phase (baseball, handball, volley-ball, tennis, combat sports, etc.) or in gymnastics, rowing, etc. SLAP lesions can be isolated or associated with a rotator cuff tear or with shoulder instability. In the latter, type 2 SLAP lesions seem to be more common but ultimately, they must be differentiated from an upper extension of the anterior labral tear (Fig. 10.39). As clinical and standard imaging data are not specific, arthroscopy is often required to reach a clear cut diagnosis, in order to determine the severity of the lesions and at the same time to apply the proper therapeutic procedure.

MR arthrography is the most reliable imaging technique to outline superior labral lesions with a 90% accuracy rate (PARK et al. 2000). MRI is not dependable enough due to insufficient intraarticular contrast; moreover, the value of CT arthrography

even with spiral CT remains debatable (BRESLER et al. 1998; DOSCH et al. 1996; HUNTER et al. 1992; SMITH et al. 1996; DE MAESENEER et al. 2000). In certain cases, especially when using CT arthrography or MRI, type 2 SLAP lesions are sometimes difficult to differentiate from minor forms of posterior instability when only the posterior extension of the tear is visible. Therefore, we advocate the primary use of MR arthrography in cases of aspecific painful shoulder syndrome in athletes.

10.7.3
Suprascapular Nerve Entrapment

Suprascapular nerve entrapment occurs most often at the suprascapular notch area in the general population. In the athlete, however, the nerve is often entrapped distally as it passes around the base of the acromion to innervate the infraspinatus (Figs. 10.40, 10.41). Nerve compression may be due to a large and posterior synovial cyst or labral cyst (LEVY et al. 1997). In the latter case, the cyst is usually associated with a labral tear indicating a minor form of posterior instability. Suprascapular nerve entrapment as an identification of posterior instability is a recent finding (BLUM et al. 1998).

When compression occurs at the suprascapular notch area, both the supraspinatus and the infraspinatus muscles are denervated. When occurring

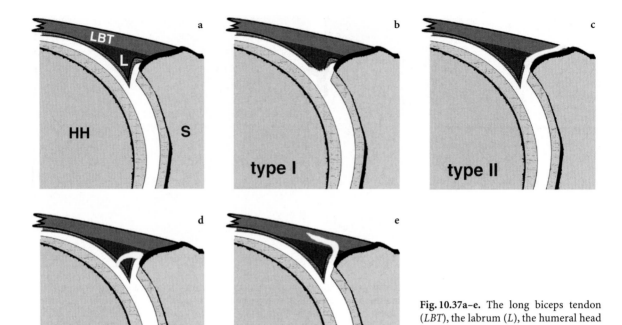

Fig. 10.37a–e. The long biceps tendon (*LBT*), the labrum (*L*), the humeral head (*HH*) and the scapula (*S*) in an oblique coronal plane. **a** Normal aspect; **b** SLAP lesion type I; **c** SLAP lesion type II; **d** SLAP lesion type III; **e** SLAP lesion type IV

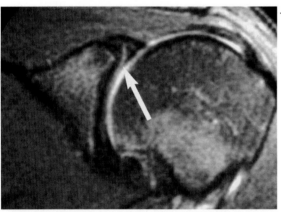

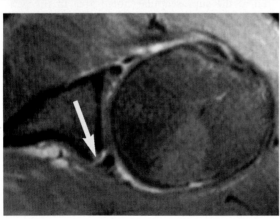

◁ **Fig. 10.38a, b.** SLAP lesion type 2. **a** Coronal fast spin-echo (FSE) T2-weighted image with fat saturation showing the tear of the superior portion of the labrum (*arrow*). **b** Axial FSE T2-weighted image with fat saturation showing the tear of the posterosuperior portion of the labrum (*arrow*)

Fig. 10.39. CT arthrography showing the upward extension of a Bankart lesion with great mobility of the superior portion of the labrum (*arrow*)

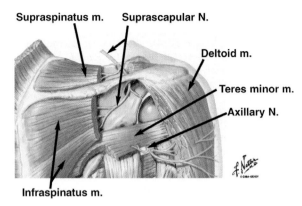

Fig. 10.40. Posterior shoulder view (adapted from NETTER 1987)

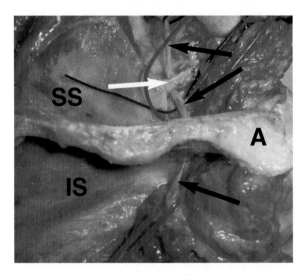

Fig. 10.41. Dissection (posterosuperior view of the left shoulder) showing the staggered trajectory of the suprascapular nerve (*black arrows*). The suprascapular nerve enters the supraspinatus fossa through the suprascapular notch closed by a ligament (*white arrow*) and winds around the lateral border of the spine of the scapula to reach the infraspinatus fossa. *SS*, supraspinatus muscle; *IS*, infraspinatus muscle; *A*, acromion

at the base of the acromion, only the infraspinatus is denervated and the supraspinatus is spared. Clinical examination reveals muscle amyotrophy involving both the supraspinatus and the infraspinatus muscles, or only the infraspinatus muscle depending on the site of entrapment. Pain is variable and often misdiagnosed as tendinitis. Electromyography is essential to confirm muscle denervation.

Standard X-rays are usually normal and diagnosis may be incomplete with CT arthrography as the cyst or the labral tear may be overlooked. MRI is the best technique to identify the cysts and the muscle dener-

vation which is characterized by early muscle edema and later by amyotrophy and fatty muscle degeneration (Figs. 10.26, 10.27). The identification of a posterior labral tear indicates that posterior instability is the primum movens of this pattern and therapeutic procedures must take this fact into account.

10.7.4
Snapping Scapula

Snapping scapula, or scapulothoracic crepitus, is of uncertain origin that should seldom be considered as pathologic. Snapping must not be confused with voluntary subluxations of the glenohumeral joint. Snapping is both audible and palpable posteriorly. Pain is usually minimal or absent. Imaging methods usually cannot identify any characteristic abnormality. At times, there may be an asymmetry of the scapula with hypertrophy of the Luschka tubercle or hypertrophy of the subscapularis or anterior serratus muscles (SANS et al. 1999). Exceptionally, a scapula or a rib exostosis are discovered.

10.8
Conclusion

To summarize, shoulder instabilities appear in various and unexpected forms. Depending upon the clinical data, we would like to propose the following practical approach:

1. In recurrent anterior instability, an established standard X-ray protocol is often sufficient.

2. In fixed posterior dislocations, the best results are obtained with simple CT scan.

3. In case of suspicion of a minor form of instability, CT arthrography, MRI or MR arthrography are indicated; however, we recommend the use of MR arthrography.

4. In voluntary, atraumatic and painless subluxations, exploratory methods should be avoided.

Acknowledgements
We would like to thank Jacqueline Zevnick for her help in reviewing the manuscript.

References

Balich SM, Sheley RC, Brown TR, Sausor D, Quinn SF (1996) MR Imaging evaluation of the glenoid labrum. Radiology 201:430

Beighton P, Solomon L, Soskolne CL (1973) Articular mobility in an African population. Ann Rheum Dis 32:413–418

Beltran J, Rosenberg ZS, Chandnani VP,Cuomo F, Beltran S, Rokito A (1997) Glenohumeral instability: evaluation with MR Arthrography. RadioGraphics 17:657–673

Bencardino JT, Beltran J, Rosenberg ZS, Rokito A, Schmahmann S, Mota J, Mellado JM, Zuckerman J, Cuomo F, Rose D (2000) Superior labrum anterior-posterior lesions: diagnosis with MR arthrography of the shoulder. Radiology 214:267–271

Bernageau J, Patte D (1980) Les luxations postérieures de l'épaule. J Radiol 61:511–519

Bernageau J, Patte D, Debeyre J, Feranne J (1976) Intérêt du profil glénoïdien dans les luxations récidivantes de l'épaule. Rev Chir Orthop [Suppl II] 62:142–147

Blum A, Molé D, Bresler F, Grignon B, Deneuville M, Delfau F, Régent D (1995) Baert AL, Grenier P, Willi UV (Eds) CT-arthrography of the shoulder. In: Syllabus musculoskeletal. ECR'95, Vienna, pp 25–31

Blum A, Molé D, Bresler F, Grignon B, Deneuville M, Delfau F, Régent D (1996) Imagerie des instabilités gléno-humérales. In: Railhac (ed) Imagerie et pathologie sportive. Sauramps, Montpellier pp 269–362

Blum A, Quirin-Cosmidis I, Henrot P, Roland J (1997) Les instabilités de l'épaule. Société Française de Radiologie. Cours de perfectionnement post-universitaire SFR Paris

Blum A, Bourrel V, Henrot P, Payafar A, Walter F, Bresler F, Coudane H, Molé D (1998) L'exploration de l'épaule et de la ceinture scapulaire. In: Blum A (ed) Imagerie en traumatologie du sport. Masson, Paris, pp 113–164

Blum A, Coudane H, Molé D (2000a) Gleno-humeral instabilities. Eur Radiol 10:63–82

Blum A, Simon JM, Cotten A, Quirin-Cosmidis I, Boyer B, Boutry N, Antonini JP (2000b) Comparison of double-contrast CT arthrography image quality with nonionic contrast agents. Invest Radiol 35:604–310

Boileau P, Walch G, Mazzoleni N, Urien JP (1993) In vitro study of humeral retrotorsion. J Shoulder Elbow Surg 2: 12–18

Bonnel F (1988) L'épaule: articulation à recentrage rotatoire tridimensionnel. L'épaule douloureuse chirurgicale. Cahiers d'Enseignement de la SOFCOT, vol 33. Expansion Scientifique Française, Paris, pp 1–12

Bresler F, Blum A, Braun M, Simon JM, Cossin M, Régent D, Molé D (1998) Assessment of the superior labrum of the shoulder joint with CT-arthrography and MR-arthrography: correlation with anatomical dissection. Surg Radiol Anat 19:57–62

Broca A, Hartmann H (1890) Contribution à l'étude des luxations de l'épaule. Bull Soc Anat Paris 4:312–336

Brown GA, Tan JL, Kirkley A (2000) The lax shoulder in females. Issues, answers, but many more questions. Clin Orthop 372:110–122

Calandra JJ, Baker CL, Uribe J (1989) The incidence of Hill-Sachs lesions in initial anterior shoulder dislocations. Arthroscopy 5:254–257

Callaghan JJ, McNiesh LM, De HJ, Savory CG, Polly DJ (1988) A prospective comparison study of double contrast computed tomography (CT) arthrography and arthroscopy of the shoulder. Am J Sports Med 16:13–20

Chandnani VP, Yeager TD, De Berardino T, Christensen K, Gagliardi JA, Heitz DR, Baird DE, Hansen MF (1993) Glenoid labral tears: prospective evaluation with MR imaging, MR arthrography and CT arthrography. AJR 161: 1229–1235

Cooper DE, Arnoczky SP, O'Brien SJ, Warren RF, Di Carlo E, Allen AA (1992) Anatomy, histology and vascularity of the glenoid labrum. An anatomical study. J Bone Joint Surg [Am] 74:46–52

Cvitanic O, Tirman PF, Feller JF, Bost FW, Minter J, Carroll KW (1997) Using abduction and external rotation of the shoulder to increase the sensitivity of MR arthrography in revealing tears of the anterior glenoid labrum. AJR 169: 837–844

Delgoffe C, Fery A, Regent D, Kurdziel JC, Claudon M, Verdon J, Treheux (1984) Apport de la scanographie dans l'étude de l'instabilité antérieure de l'épaule. J Radiol 65:737–745

De Maeseneer M, van Roy F, Lenchik L, Shahabpour M, Jacobson J, Ryu KN, Hendelberg F, Osteaux M (2000) CT and MR arthrography of the normal and pathologic anterosuperior labrum and labral-bicipital complex. RadioGraphics 20: S67–S81

Detrisac DA, Johnson LL (1988) Arthroscopic shoulder anatomy: pathologic and surgical implications. Slack, Thorofare NJ

Dosch JC, Kempf JF, Nerisson D, Dupuis MG (1996) Les "SLAP lesions" de l'épaule. In: La coiffe des rotateurs et son environnement. Laredo JD, Bard H (Eds). Sauramps Médical, Montpellier, pp 263–270

Duparc F, Postel JM, Levigne C, Gazielly DF, Goutallier D (1996) Report of the 2nd meeting of the Study Group of shoulder and elbow. Paris, 6 Nov 1995. Traumatic posterior dislocations of the shoulder. Rev Chir Orthop 82:767–771

Ellmann H (1990) Diagnosis and treatment of incomplete rotator cuff tears. Clin Orthop 254:64–74

Engebretsen L, Craig EV (1993) Radiologic features of shoulder instability. Clin Orthop Relat Res 29:29–44

Essadki B, Dumontier C, Sautet A, Apoil A (2000) Posterior shoulder instability in athletes: surgical treatment with posterior bone block. Rev Chir Orthop 86:765–772

Fuchs B, Jost B, Gerber C (2000) Posterior-inferior capsular shift for the treatment of recurrent, voluntary posterior subluxation of the shoulder. J Bone Joint Surg [Am] 82: 16–25

Garneau RA, Renfrew DL, Moore TE, El-Khoury GY, Nepola JV, Lempke JH (1991) Glenoid labrum: evaluation with MR imaging. Radiology 179:519–522

Garth WJ, Allman FJ, Armstrong WS (1987) Occult anterior subluxations of the shoulder in non contact sports. Am J Sports Med 15:579–585

Garth WP, Slappey CE, Ochs CW (1984) Roentgenographic demonstration of instability of the shoulder: the apical oblique projection. J Bone Joint Surg [Am] 66: 1450–1453

Gerber C (1991) L'instabilité postérieure de l'épaule. Cahiers d'enseignement de la SOFCOT, 40:223–245

Godefroy D, Chevrot A (1996) Apport du scanner hélicoïdal dans l'étude de la coiffe. In: La coiffe des rotateurs et son environnement. Laredo JD, Bard H (Eds). Sauramps Médical, Montpellier, pp 147–155

Hall FM, Rosenthal DI, Goldberg RP (1981) Morbidity from

shoulder arthrography: etiology, incidence and prevention. AJR 136:59–62

Hawkins RH (1996) Glenoid osteotomy for recurrent posterior subluxation of the shoulder: assessment by computed axial tomography. J Shoulder Elbow Surg 5:393–400

Hovelius L (1987) Anterior dislocation of the shoulder in teenagers and young adults. Five year prognosis. J Bone Joint Surg [Am] 69:393–399

Hunter JC, Blatz DJ, Escobedo EM (1992) SLAP lesions of the glenoid labrum: CT arthrography and arthroscopic correlation. Radiology 184:513–518

Hurschler C, Wülker N, Mendila M (2000) The effect of negative intraarticular pressure and rotator cuff force on Glenohumeral translation during simulated active elevation. Clin Biomech 15:306–314

Jahnke AJ, Petersen SA, Neumann C, Steinbach L, Morgan FA (1992) A prospective comparison of computerized arthrotomography and magnetic resonance imaging of the glenohumeral joint. Am J Sports Med 20:695–700

Jalovaara P, Myllyla V, Paivansalo M (1992) Autotraction stress roentgenography for demonstration anterior and inferior instability of the shoulder joint. Clin Orthop 284:136–143

Jee WH, McCauley TR, Katz LD, Matheny JM, Ruwe PA, Daigneault JP (2001) Superior Labral Anterior Posterior (SLAP) Lesions of the glenoid labrum: reliability and accuracy of MR arthrography for diagnosis. Radiology 218:127–132

Jobe FW, Tibone JE, Jobe C, Kvitne RS, Glousmann RE (1991) Anterior capsulolabral reconstruction of the shoulder in athletes in overhead sports. Am J Sport Med 19:428–434

Johner RT, Joz-Roland P, Burch HB (1982) Luxation antérieure de l'épaule: nouveaux aspects diagnostiques et thérapeutiques. Rev Méd Suisse Romande 102:1143–1150

Kreitner KF, Botchen K, Rude J, Bittinger F, Krummenauer F, Thelen M (1998) Superior labrum and labral-bicipital complex: MR imaging with pathologic-anatomic and histologic correlation. AJR 170:599–605

Kwak SM, Brown RR, Resnick D, Trudell D, Applegate GR, Haghighi P (1998a) Anatomy, anatomic variations and pathology of the 11- to 3-o'clock position of the glenoid labrum: findings on MR-arthrography and anatomic sections. AJR 171:235–238

Kwak SM, Brown RR, Trudell D, Resnick D (1998b) Glenohumeral joint: comparison of shoulder positions at MR arthrography. Radiology 208:375–380

Lee SB, Kim KJ, O'Driscoll SW, Morrey BF, An KN (2000) Dynamic glenohumeral stability provided by the rotator cuff muscles in the mid-range and end-range of motion. A study in cadavera. J Bone Joint Surg (Am) 82:849–857

Lee SU, Lang P (2000) MR and MR arthrography to identify degenerative and posttraumatic diseases in the shoulder joint. Eur Radiol 35:126–135

Levy P, Roger B, Tardieu M, Ghebontni L, Thelen P, Richard O, Grenier P (1997) Compression kystique du nerf sus-scapulaire. Intérêt de l'imagerie. A propos de 6 cas et revue de la littérature. J Radiol 78:123–130

Levy O, Pritsch M, Rath E (1999) An operative technique for recurrent shoulder dislocations in older patients. J. Shoulder Elbow Surg. 8:452–457

Liu S, Henry M, Nuccion S, Shapiro M, Dorey F (1996) Diagnosis of glenoid labral tears. A comparison between magnetic resonance imaging and clinical examinations. Am J Sports Med 24:149–154

Loew R, Kreitner KF, Runkel M, Zoellner J, Thelen M (2000) MR arthrography of the shoulder: comparison of low-field (0.2 T) vs high-field (1.5 T) imaging. Eur Radiol 10:989–996

Maffet MW, Gartsman GM, Moseley B (1995) Superior labrum-biceps tendon complex lesions of the shoulder. Am J Sports Med 23:93–98

Matsen FA, Thomas SC, Rockwood CA (1990) Glenohumeral instability. In: Rockwood CA, Matsen FA (eds) The shoulder. Saunders, Philadelphia, pp 526–622

McFarland EG, Campbell G, McDowell J (1996) Posterior shoulder laxity in asymptomatic athletes. Am J Sports Med 24:468–471

McMahon PJ, Dettling J, Sandusky MD, Tibone JE, Lee TQ (1999) The anterior band of the inferior glenohumeral ligament. Assessment of its permanent deformation and the anatomy of its glenoid attachment. J Bone Joint Surg [Br] 81:406–413

Molé D, Walch G (1993) Traitement chirurgical des instabilités de l'épaule. Articulation Glénohumérale . Encycl Med Chir (Paris, France). Appareil locomoteur 44–265

Molé D, Coudane H, Rio B, Quievreux P, Benazet JP, Frank A, Kelberine F (1996) Place de l'arthroscopie lors du premier épisode de luxation antéro-interne de l'épaule. J Traumatol Sport 13:20–24

Moseley HF, Overgaard B (1962) The anterior capsular mechanism in recurrent dislocation of the shoulder. Morphological and clinical studies with special reference to the glenoid labrum and glenohumeral ligaments. J Bone Joint Surg (Br) 44:913–927

Neer CS (1990) Shoulder reconstruction. Saunders, Philadelphia

Nelson BJ, Arciero RA (2000) Arthroscopic management of glenohumeral instability. Am J Sports Med 28:602–614

Netter FH (1978) Netter collection of medical illustrations, vol 8, part I. Musculoskeletal system, anatomy, physiology and metabolic disorders. Ciba-Geigy Corporation, Summit New-Jersey

Neviaser TJ (1993) The GLAD lesion: another cause of anterior shoulder pain. Arthroscopy 9:22–23

Nizard R (1997) Quel type d'imagerie diagnostique et pré-thérapeutique (médicale ou chirurgicale) faut-il réaliser devant une épaule instable? Rev Rhum 64:59S–68S

O'Brien SJ, Neves MC, Arnoczky SP, Rozbruck SR, Dicarlo EF, Warren RF, Schwartz R, Wickiewicz TL (1990) The anatomy and histology of the inferior glenohumeral ligament complex of the shoulder. Am J Sports Med 1:449–456

Pappas AM, Goss TP, Kleinman PK (1983) Symptomatic shoulder instability due to lesions of the glenoid labrum. Am J Sports Med 11:279–288

Park YH, Lee JY, Moon SH, Mo JH, Yang BK, Hahn SH, Resnick D (2000) MR arthrography of the labral capsular ligamentous complex in the shoulder. AJR 175:667–672

Patte D, Bernageau J, Rodineau J, Gardes JC (1980) Epaules douloureuses et instables. Rev Chir Orthop 66:157–165

Randelli M (1988) La fracture-luxation postérieure de l'épaule: nouveaux éléments de classification et thérapeutiques. 2e congrès de la Société Européenne de Chirurgie de l'épaule et du coude, Berne

Rockwood CA (1984) Subluxations and dislocations about the shoulder. In: Rockwood CA, Green DP (eds) Fractures in adults, 2nd edn. Lippincott, Philadelphia, pp 722–950

Rockwood CA, Szalay EA, Curtis RJ, Young DC, Kay SP (1990) X-Ray evaluation of shoulder problems. In: Rockwood CA,

Matsen FA (eds) The shoulder. Saunders, Philadelphia, pp 178–207

Roger B, Skaf A, Hooper AW, Lektrakul N, Yeh L, Resnick D (1999) Imaging findings in the dominant shoulder of throwing athletes: comparison of radiography, arthrography, CT arthrography, and MR arthrography with arthroscopic correlation. AJR 172:1371–1380

Rowe CR (1987) Recurrent transient subluxation of the shoulder; the "Dead arm" syndrome. Clin Orthop 223:11–19

Sanders TG, Tirman PF, Linares R, Feller JF, Richardson R (1999) The glenolabral articular disruption lesion: MR arthrography with arthroscopic correlation. AJR 172: 171–175

Sanders TG, Morrison WB, Miller MD (2000) Imaging techniques for the evaluation of glenohumeral instability. Am J Sports Med 28:414–434

Sans N, Jarlaud T, Sarrouy P, Giobbini K, Bellumore Y, Railhac JJ (1999) Snapping scapula: the value of 3D imaging. J Radiol 80:379–381

Silliman JF, Hawkins RJ (1993) Classification and physical diagnosis of instability of the shoulder. Clin Orthop 291: 7–19

Smith DK, Chopp TM, Aufdemorte TB, Witkowski EG, Jones RC (1996) Sublabral recess of the superior glenoid labrum: study of cadavers with conventional nonenhanced MR imaging, MR arthrography, anatomic dissection, and limited histologic examination. Radiology 201:251–256

Snyder SJ, Karzel RP, Del Pizzo W, Ferkel RD, Friedman MJ (1990) SLAP lesions of the shoulder. Arthroscopy 6: 274–279

Soulez G, Vallee C, Chevrot A, Wybier M, Gires F, Pallardy G (1991) Etude du bourrelet glénoïdien en arthroscanner opaque, aspects normaux et pathologiques. Rev Im Med 3:389–396

Stoller DW (1997) Magnetic Resonance Imaging in orthopaedics and sports medecine, 2nd edn. Lippincott-Raven, Philadelphia

Tillander B, Lysholm M, Norlin R (1998) Multidirectional hyperlaxity of the shoulder: results of treatment. Scand J Med Sci Sports 8:421–425

Tirman PF, Feller JF, Palmer WE, Carroll KW, Steinbach LS, Cox I (1996) The Buford complex a variation of normal shoulder anatomy: MR arthrographic imaging features. AJR 166:869–873

Tuite MJ, Orwin JF (1996) Anterosuperior labral variants of the shoulder appearance on gradient-recalled-echo and fast spin-echo MR images. Radiology 199:537–540

Vahlensieck M, Sommer T, Textor J, Pauleit D, Lang P, Genant HK, Schild HH (1998) Indirect MR arthrography: techniques and applications. Eur Radiol 8:232–235

Vermeiren J, Handelberg F, Casteleyn P, Opdecam P (1993) The rate of reccurence of traumatic anterior dislocation of the shoulder. A study of 154 cases and a review of the literature. Int Orthop 17:337–341

Walch G (1996) Chronic anterior gleno-humeral instability. J Bone Joint Surg (Br) 78:670–677

Walch G, Liotard JP, Boileau P, Noel E (1991) Le conflit glénoïdien postéro-supérieur: un autre conflit de l'épaule. Rev Chir Orthop 77:571–574

Weishaupt D, Zanetti M, Nyffeler RW, Gerber C, Hodler J (2000) Posterior glenoid rim deficiency in recurrent (atraumatic) posterior shoulder instability. Skeletal Radiol 29:204–210

Willemsen UF, Wiedemann E, Brunner U, Pfluger T, Scheck RJ, Hahn K (1996) Evaluation of MR arthrography with intraarticular saline in patients with shoulder instability. Radiology 201:156

Willemsen UF, Wiedermann E, Brunner U, Scheck R, Pfluger T, Kueffer G, Hahn K (1998) Prospective evaluation of MR arthrography performed with high-volume intraarticular saline enhancement in patients with recurrent anterior dislocations of the shoulder. AJR 170:79–84

Williams MW, Snyder SJ, Buford D (1994) The Buford complex: the " cord-like " middle glenohumeral ligament and absent antero-superior labrum complex a normal anatomic capsulolabral variant. Arthroscopy 10:241–247

Wintzell G, Haglung-Akerlind Y, Larsson H, Zyto K, Larsson S (1998a) Joint fluid enhancement at MRI of the glenohumeral joint with intravenous injection of gadodiamide in standard and triple dose: a prospective comparative study of stable and unstable shoulders. Skeletal Radiol 27:87–91

Wintzell G, Larsson H, Larsson S (1998b) Indirect MR arthrography of anterior shoulder instability in the ABER and the apprehension test positions: a prospective comparative study of two different shoulder positions during MRI using intravenous gadodiamide contrast for enhancement of the joint fluid. Skeletal Radiol 27:488–494

Wintzell G, Haglund-Akerlind Y, Larsson H, Zyto K, Larsson S (1999a) Open MR imaging of the unstable shoulder in the apprehension test position: description and evaluation of an alternative MR examination position. Eur Radiol 9: 1789–1795

Wintzell G, Haglund-Akerlind Y, Ekelund A, Sandstrom B, Hovelius L, Larsson S (1999b) Arthroscopic lavage reduced the recurrence rate following primary anterior shoulder dislocation. A randomised multicentre study with 1-year follow-up. Knee Surg Sports Traumatol 7: 192–196

Wintzell G, Haglund-Akerlind Y, Nowak J, Larsson S (1999c) Arthroscopic lavage compared with nonoperative treatment for traumatic primary anterior shoulder dislocation: a 2-year follow-up of a prospective randomized study. J Shoulder Elbow Surg 8:399–402

Yu JS, Greenway G, Resnick D (1998) Osteochondral defect of the glenoid fossa: cross-sectional imaging features. Radiology 206:35–40

Zanetti M, Hodler J (1997) Contrast media in MR arthrography of the glenohumeral joint: intra- articular gadopentetate vs saline: preliminary results. Eur Radiol 7:498–502

Zlatkin MB (1999) Techniques for MR imaging of joints in sports medicine. Magn Reson Imaging Clin North Am 7:1–21

11 The Postoperative Shoulder 1: Soft Tissues

M. B. Zlatkin

CONTENTS

M. B. ZLATKIN, MD, FRCP (C)
President, National Musculoskeletal Imaging, 13798 NW 4th
St. Suite 305, Sunrise, Fl 33325, USA

Text and images are adapted from ZLATKIN (2002) with permission.

11.1 Introduction

11.1.1 General Features

Performing magnetic resonance imaging (MRI) in patients who have previously been operated upon presents difficulties in that the normal anatomic appearances are altered by the procedures that have been carried out. For this reason it is important to have some understanding of the more commonly performed surgical or arthroscopic procedures or both, and how they affect the appearance of the relevant anatomic structures. The pathology that is discovered in these situations may be a residual or recurrent problem that remains or develops despite the surgery, a complication of the surgery itself, or a new problem unrelated to the original problem or the surgery performed for it. This chapter will review the common surgical procedures performed for rotator cuff disease, as well as those for shoulder instability and other labral pathology including SLAP lesions. The expected MRI findings that are seen following these procedures will be discussed as well, as the residual and recurrent pathology that may be identified with the use of MRI and MR arthrography. General complications that may occur subsequent to these procedures as seen on MRI will also be reviewed. One persistent problem in our understanding of imaging of the postoperative shoulder is the lack of a large body of published data on this topic, with both conventional MRI (OWEN et al. 1993; HAYGOOD et al. 1993; GAENSLEN et al. 1996; MAGEE et al. 1997; GUSMER et al. 1997; LONGOBARDI et al. 1997; FELLER et al. 1998; ZANETTI et al. 1999; RAND et al. 1999a; SPEILMAN et al. 1999) and MR arthrography (RAND et al. 1996, 1999b).

11.1.2
Technical Considerations

One of the considerable problems associated with imaging patients who have undergone prior surgery is the presence of postoperative artifact. This includes ferromagnetic screws, or staples. Small metal shavings from the use of a burr, for example during an acromioplasty, may also yield considerable artifact. The use of weakly ferromagnetic material such as titanium or the use of plastics may help minimize this. The use of gradient echo sequences should also be minimized in this situation. This can impair visualization of important structures such as the rotator cuff, glenoid labrum and capsule (Fig. 11.1). In this regard turbo spin echo (TSE) or fast spin echo (FSE) imaging is useful as the multiple 180° pulses (echo train) help to minimize the degree of magnetic susceptibility artifact (Fig. 11.2), in conjunction with the use of large matrices. Additionally, fat saturation may be not be reliable, again due to the presence of magnetic susceptibility effects and ferromagnetic artifact related to the prior surgery. Fast spin echo inversion recovery sequences may prove useful in this situation. Postoperative scar formation may limit evaluation by distorting the anatomy and by making tissue planes difficult to differentiate. MR arthrography may then become a useful tool to help image postoperative patients more successfully (Fig. 11.2) (RAND et al. 1996, 1999b; ZLATKIN 2000).

11.2
Impingement and Rotator Cuff Disease

11.2.1
General Considerations

Traditional impingement involving the rotator cuff occurs when the latter is impacted against the undersurface of the anterior edge of the acromion, the coracoacromial ligament, or the acromioclavicular joint (primary extrinsic impingement) (NEER 1972, 1983; MATSEN et al. 1998; ROCKWOOD and LYONS 1993; FU et al. 1991). Different causes of this condition include overuse syndromes and altered acromion morphology (BIGLIANI et al. 1986). Inferiorly projecting subacromial spurs also have a high association with the clinical syndrome of impingement. Shoulder instability may cause secondary extrinsic impingement (KVITNE and JOBE 1993; ARROYO et al. 1997). A spectrum of changes may occur in the cuff progressing in these circumstances from edema, to tendinosis, eventually resulting in rotator cuff tears, partial and complete.

Conservative treatment for the symptoms associated with this condition includes modification of activities, physical therapy and anti-inflammatory medication (MATSEN et al. 1998; ARROYO and FLATOW 1999; BOKOR et al. 1993). Steroid injections may also be used. With failure of conservative treatment, surgery may be needed. This will usually

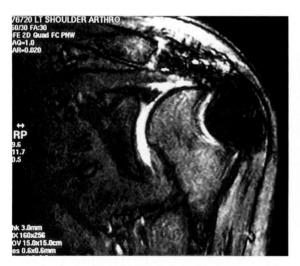

Fig. 11.1. Coronal oblique T2* gradient echo image. The image is significantly degraded by artifact from the prior rotator cuff repair. The tendon is obscured

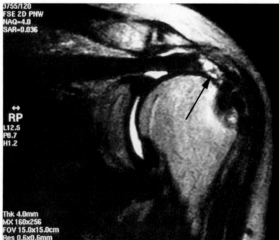

Fig. 11.2. Coronal oblique T2 weighted fast spin echo. Same patient as in Fig. 11.1. The patient is status post supraspinatus tendon repair and anterior acromioplasty. A recurrent defect in the anterior supraspinatus tendon is present (*arrow*). The post repair artifact from suture anchors in the bone trough is minimized by multiple 180° echoes

involve decompression of the coracoacromial arch, often with debridement of tendinosis or a partial tear, or repair of a torn rotator cuff (NEER 1972, 1983; MATSEN et al. 1998; ARROYO and FLATOW 1999; BURKHEAD et al. 1995; BURKHART 1994, 1996).

MRI and MR arthrographic evaluation of the rotator cuff disease and impingement in the postoperative patient may prove more difficult than the evaluation of patients not previously operated upon. A baseline postoperative study can be helpful, if available. Recent studies have described the MRI findings in asymptomatic patients after rotator cuff surgery (ZANETTI et al. 1999; SPEILMAN et al. 1999).

The most common causes of failure after shoulder surgery for rotator cuff disease are residual bony changes of impingement after subacromial decompression, advancing rotator cuff tendinosis, residual and recurrent rotator cuff tears both partial and complete, postoperative adhesions, and weakening of the deltoid muscle from detachment or denervation (OGILVIE-HARRIS et al. 1990; BIGLIANI et al. 1992; DeORIO and COFIELD 1984).

11.2.2
Subacromial Decompression Without Rotator Cuff Repair

11.2.2.1
Surgical Techniques

Assessment of the symptomatic postoperative rotator cuff can be divided into two categories. The first category of postoperative patients are those who have had a prior acromioplasty for impingement, with an intact rotator cuff and no rotator cuff repair. This procedure may be done as an open procedure, via an anterolateral deltoid splitting incision (NEER 1972, 1983; MATSEN et al. 1998; ROCKWOOD and LYONS 1993; ARROYO and FLATOW 1999), or via arthroscopy (ESCH 1993; GARTSMAN 1990; BEACH and CASPARI 1993; HURLEY et al. 1992; PAULOS and FRANKLIN 1990; PETERSON and ALTCHEK 1996) (Fig. 11.3). The anteroinferior acromion is removed, from the AC joint to the deltoid insertion, removing that portion anterior to the clavicle. Most often the subdeltoid bursa is also inflamed and is resected at the time of the acromioplasty. The insertion as well as a variable part of the coracoacromial ligament may be removed, although the coracoacromial ligament is often preserved in order to prevent superior migration of the humeral head (MATSEN et al.

1998). In young athletic patients, in which the CA ligament may just be thickened, debridement only may be performed (ARROYO and FLATOW 1999). The AC joint and the distal 2.5 cm of the clavicle may also be removed if the patient is symptomatic, or if there are large osteophytes (MUMFORD 1941; FLATOW et al. 1995).

Arthroscopic subacromial decompression requires various arthroscopic shavers and burrs to remove the subacromial bursa, subdeltoid fat pad, and anterior edge and inferior surface of the acromion (ESCH 1993; GARTSMAN 1990; BEACH and CASPARI 1993; HURLEY et al. 1992; PAULOS and FRANKLIN 1990; PETERSON and ALTCHEK 1996). A cautery is used to release the coracoacromial ligament. The distal clavicle can be resected using a burr. A combined open and arthroscopic approach (GARTSMAN 1990; BEACH and CASPARI 1993; PAULOS and FRANKLIN 1990; BLEVIS et al. 1996) may be used, especially if a full thickness tear is found. MRI may help in this decision by determining the status of the rotator cuff prior to surgery.

11.2.2.2
Results of Treatment

The incidence of failure (i.e. persistence or recurrence of pain) after subacromial decompression is reported to be between 3%–11% (NEER 1972; FU et al. 1991; OGILVIE-HARRIS et al. 1990; PAULOS and FRANKLIN 1990; HURLEY and ANDERSON 1990). The interpretation of these results is difficult because of the admixture of patients with intact cuffs, and those with cuff tears, partial and complete (MATSEN et al. 1998) in reported studies. Arthroscopic decompressions may carry a higher incidence of recurrence (GARTSMAN 1990; BEACH and CASPARI 1993; PAULOS and FRANKLIN 1990), where there may be insufficient excision of the acromion. Arthroscopic acromioplasty has the advantage of not needing a deltoid splitting incision, therefore not putting the deltoid at risk (MATSEN et al. 1998).

11.2.2.3
MRI Findings

MRI findings typically associated with acromioplasty (Fig. 11.3) include a flattened acromial undersurface, non-visualization of the anterior one third of the acromion, and decreased marrow signal in the remaining distal acromion, due to marrow fibrosis (OWEN et al. 1993). Low signal due to artifacts from small metal fragments are often present and related to burring of the acromion. These particles are typically too

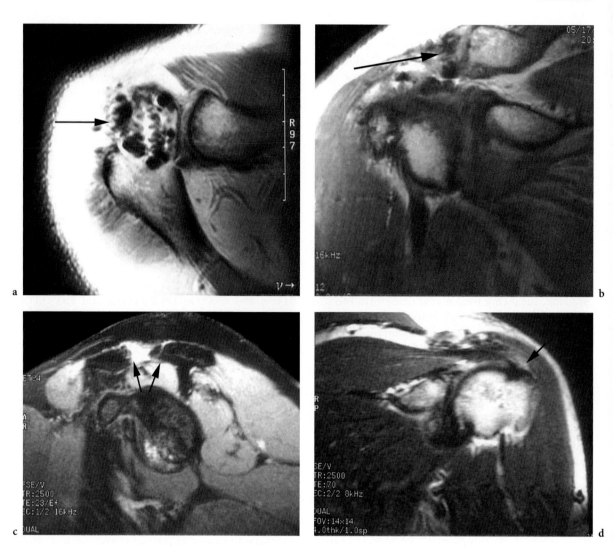

Fig. 11.3a–d. Anterior acromioplasty. **a** Axial proton density weighted image. Metal artifact outlines the site of the anterior acromioplasty (*arrow*). **b** Coronal oblique proton density weighted image. Same patient as in (**a**). Absence of the anterior portion of the acromion is evident (*arrow*). **c** Sagittal oblique proton density weighted image in another patient. The anterior acromion and AC joint have been excised. Sagittal oblique images may best show the extent of the decompression (*arrows*). **d** Coronal T2 weighted image. Same patient as in (**c**). Resection or debridement of the subdeltoid bursa (*arrow*) results in increased signal in this region

small to be seen on plain radiographs or computed tomographic images (HAYGOOD et al. 1993). The appearance the acromion is related to how much is removed at the time of decompression or whether the decompression is open or arthroscopic. Removal of the subacromial bursa and subdeltoid fat pad results in the absence of these structures on postoperative studies. These structures are often replaced by scar tissue of intermediate signal intensity (LONGOBARDI et al. 1997). After resection of the bursa there is often a small amount of fluid signal identified in this region on images with T2 contrast (ZANETTI et al. 1999; SPEILMAN et al. 1999) (Fig. 11.3). This renders fluid

in the subdeltoid bursa not useful as a secondary sign of cuff injury or of bursal inflammation.

The anatomy of the coracoacromial arch after decompression may be best viewed on sagittal oblique images (Figs. 11.3, 11.4). These are best obtained with a proton density and T2 weighted FSE sequence. Preservation or excision of the acromioclavicular joint may also be readily apparent. If the AC joint has also been excised (Fig. 11.3), scar tissue may be the most prominent finding. In the more recent postoperative period, increased signal intensity about the margins of the excised joint may persist for months (LONGOBARDI et al. 1997).

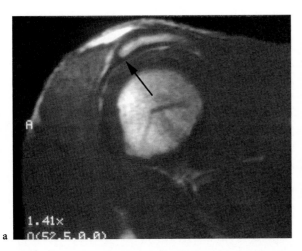
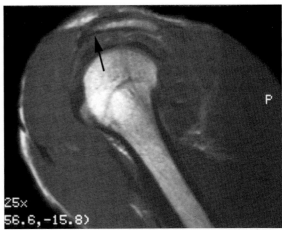

Fig. 11.4a, b. Sagittal oblique T1 weighted images before (**a**) and after (**b**) acromioplasty. Note the conversion from a type 2–3 acromion, to a type 1 acromion, after surgery (*arrows*)

After subacromial decompression, some improvement of the altered signal in the rotator cuff tendon and in the peritendinous tissues, that may be the result of inflammation, may be seen over time, but resolution of any signal or morphologic alterations that are related to rotator cuff tendinosis are less likely (OWEN et al. 1993; MAGEE et al. 1997; GUSMER et al. 1997; LONGOBARDI et al. 1997).

An additional cause of failed subacromial decompression is the failure to recognize secondary extrinsic impingement mediated by anterior shoulder instability, whereby performance of an acromioplasty without addressing the instability may in fact worsen the situation (KVITNE and JOBE 1993). Another cause of persistent postacromioplasty pain is related to osteoarthrosis of the acromioclavicular joint (Fig. 11.5) (OGILVIE-HARRIS et al. 1990). After acromioplasty, there may be progression of rotator cuff disease (Figs. 11.5, 11.6a), including the interval development of a rotator cuff tear, partial or complete. Unrecognized partial tears or small complete tears may extend. Progression may occur if the acromioplasty and decompression are inadequate, with persistent subacromial roughening (MATSEN et al. 1998; OGILVIE-HARRIS et al. 1990). The ability of MRI to detect residual bony impingement has been evaluated. One study showed a relative insensitivity to the determination of persistent bony changes of impingement (OWEN et al. 1993). The sensitivity was 64%, the specificity 82%, and the accuracy 74%. In another study by MAGEE et al. (1997) the performance of MRI was better, with a sensitivity of 84% and a specificity of 87%. Current MRI criteria for persistent impingement are extrapolations of those used with plain radiographic exam. Correlative plain radiographs are helpful. Sagittal oblique MR images best evaluate

the adequacy of the decompression and any persistent impingement due to insufficient acromion resection, or the persistence of a large subacromial spur. Additionally large osteophytes projecting from the acromioclavicular joint are best identified in the sagittal oblique plane. MRI may also be valuable in the determination of deltoid detachment. Excessive acromial resection and dense postoperative scarring between the cuff and the acromion may also lead to persistent or recurrent symptoms (MATSEN et al. 1998).

In the setting of interval development of a cuff tear or extension and/or progression of existing cuff

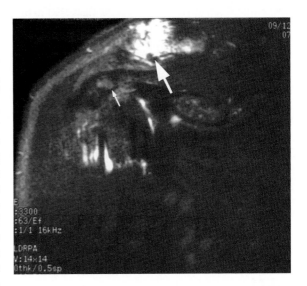

Fig. 11.5. Post acromioplasty pain. Coronal oblique T2 weighted fast spin echo sequence with fat saturation. There is persistent AC joint arthritis, with marginal edema and fluid in the AC joint (*large arrow*). A small undersurface partial tear is seen (*small arrow*)

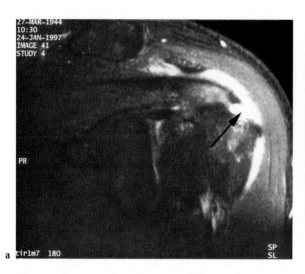
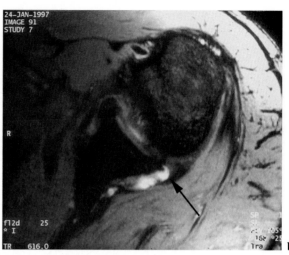

a

b

Fig. 11.6a, b. Progression of rotator cuff disease after acromioplasty. **a** Coronal oblique, turbo inversion recovery sequence. The patient has had an anterior acromioplasty. There has been interval development of a full thickness tear of the supraspinatus tendon, anterodistally (*arrow*). **b** Axial T2* gradient echo image, in the same patient. There is also a posterior labral tear noted with a paralabral cyst (*arrow*)

pathology such as tendinosis, or partial thickness tears, clinical findings are not considered to be specific (Fu et al. 1991). MRI is therefore indicated, in the setting of persistent postoperative symptoms. The integrity of the cuff is more difficult to determine in the postoperative situation due to the alterations related to the decompression described above, as well as persistent intermediate signal within the rotator cuff tendons that may be present on T2 weighted images post acromioplasty (Owen et al. 1993). Studies show that in this setting MRI remains sensitive, but less specific than MRI in the patient who has not had prior surgery. The usual criteria (Zlatkin et al. 1989; Iannotti et al. 1991; Needel and Zlatkin 1997) for a rotator cuff tear may still be applied. According to most studies, however, a tear can only be diagnosed confidently when a definite region of discontinuity in the cuff can be identified, accompanied by fluid signal within the defect on images with a long TR/TE acquisition (Owen et al. 1993), on STIR or T2* weighted gradient echo sequences, or when contrast extravasation is seen through the cuff defect at MR arthrography (Rand et al. 1996, 1999b; Zlatkin 2000).

11.2.3
Rotator Cuff Repair or Debridement

11.2.3.1
Surgical Techniques

The second category involves patients who have had a prior rotator cuff repair. In patients with partial thick-

ness tears treatment depends on the area, depth and severity of tendon involvement. The most common partial tears occur along the cuff undersurface, in the anterior aspect of the supraspinatus tendon, near its insertion into the greater tuberosity. Treatment may vary from debridement of frayed tissue, in more superficial partial tears, to completely excising the area of the partial defect and repairing the remaining healthy cuff tissue (Matsen et al. 1998; Arroyo and Flatow 1999; Burkhart 1994; Esch 1993; Blevins et al. 1996), as if it were a small full thickness defect. Simple debridement may more often be used in younger patients without prominent bony changes about the coracoacromial arch, or those who may have cuff injuries related to instability or internal impingement (Arroyo and Flatow 1999; Burkhead et al. 1995; Burkhart 1994; Budoff et al. 1988; Andres et al. 1985; Snyder et al. 1991). Simple debridement may be less satisfactory in older patients and in patients with deeper partial tears. Repairs are usually done in tears involving greater than 50% of the tendon thickness, with either a side-to-side or tendon-to-bone repair being done (Matsen et al. 1998; Arroyo and Flatow 1999; Burkhart 1994; Esch 1993; Blevins et al. 1996). Either of these treatments may be accompanied by decompression (Matsen et al. 1998; Arroyo and Flatow 1999; Burkhart 1994; Esch 1993; Blevins et al. 1996). Both of these methods are often done arthroscopically (Esch 1993; Peterson and Altchek 1996; Peterson et al. 1998), although the repairs and acromioplasty may be done open or with a combined approach.

Knowing the type of surgery performed and its extent is important when interpreting MR images of these patients. As such it is important to obtain the details of these surgical interventions, if possible from the surgical reports, or other patient records. The general principle of rotator cuff repairs is sub-acromial decompression, rotator cuff mobilization and repair of the tendon, if possible back to the tuberosity (ARROYO and FLATOW 1999). Most open repairs are done through an anterosuperior approach through a split or takedown of the proximal deltoid. Mini open repairs are those that employ only a split of the deltoid, without any takedown of the origin (BLEVINS et al. 1996). Arthroscopic approaches gen-erally involve three bursal portals, anterior, lateral and posterior (BEACH and CASPARI 1993; ELLMAN et al. 1993; BAKER and LIU 1995; GARTSMAN and HAMMERMAN 1997). Repair of small full thickness tears can usually be carried out with a side-to-side suturing technique, or if distal small tears, with a tendon-to-bone repair. Larger tears with retraction require reattaching the tendon to bone. Traditionally this was done into a trough-in-bone at the greater tuberosity (MCLAUGHLIN 1963). Currently this is less commonly done, with most surgeons now freshening the bone at the articular–tuberosity junction (ARROYO and FLATOW 1999). The repairs are done with nonab-sorbable suture material, tied to each other, or with suture anchors. Suture anchors are more commonly used with arthroscopic repairs. Suture anchors can be composed of various materials, including ferro-magnetic metal, nonferromagnetic metal (titanium), plastic and bioabsorbable polymers. Larger or mas-sive defects require mobilization of the remaining portions of the cuff (HAWKINS et al. 1985) or incor-poration of the long head of biceps or subscapularis, to achieve an effective repair. Other authors advocate the use of allograft material or synthetic material (NEVIASER et al. 1978; OZAKI et al. 1986). In mas-sive tears some have advocated debridement alone (MELILO et al. 1997). In the majority of rotator cuff repairs an acromioplasty is also performed; however, recently some surgeons have reserved acromioplasty for patients with definite subacromial spurs, rough-ening, or "abnormal acromial shapes" such as a type 3 anterior acromion (BUDOFF et al. 1988). Removal of the osteophytes and/or resection of the distal one third of the clavicle may be carried out in patients with advanced AC joint disease, or those that are tender or symptomatic. A bursal release is generally performed for exposure and to relieve the cuff of any bursal adhesions. If the biceps is torn or subluxed it is tenodesed or incorporated into the repair.

11.2.3.2
Results of Treatment

In general the results of rotator cuff repair are good. COFIELD (1985) reviewed many different series of rotator cuff repairs and found that pain relief occurred in 87%. Early results of mini open and arthroscopic repairs (GARTSMAN and HAMMERMAN 1997; WEBER 1997) have shown similar results. In those patients who do fail treatment, causes of recurrent pain or dimin-ished function following rotator cuff repair include failure of the repair. This can be due to fixation fail-ure, or tendon tissue failure. Inadequate subacromial decompression can lead to continued impingement, resulting in recurrent tendon failure. In addition, if the tendinous tissue is of poor quality due to atrophy or degenerated tissue a new tear may develop, perhaps due to continued impingement or excessive tension at the repair site, particularly in larger tears. Occasion-ally, iatrogenic cuff tears may occur due to portal placement (NORWOOD and FOWLER 1989). Aggressive debridement of the subacromial bursa can also lead to delamination and penetration of an intact region of the rotator cuff.

11.2.3.3
MRI Findings

Limited experience with MRI in patients after rotator cuff repairs (OWEN et al. 1993; HAYGOOD et al. 1993; GAENSLEN et al. 1996; MAGEE et al. 1997; GUSMER et al. 1997) shows that its accuracy is decreased, although the determination of an intact tendon or a recurrent complete tear remain good. MRI findings following cuff repair (Fig. 11.7) include distortion of the soft tissues adjacent to the cuff and non-visualiza-tion of the subdeltoid fat pad and bursa, as well as fluid in the region of the subdeltoid bursa (ZANETTI et al. 1999; SPEILMAN et al. 1999). Soft tissue metal or suture artifacts occur due to nonabsorbable sutures and suture anchors, especially if ferromagnetic suture anchors are used. These can create a large balloon artifact (OWEN et al. 1993; HAYGOOD et al. 1993; GAENSLEN et al. 1996; LONGOBARDI ET AL. 1997). Granulation tissue surrounding sutures may result in intermediate or high signal intensity on imaging sequences with T2 weighted contrast in the peritendinous tissues (OWEN et al. 1993; GAENSLEN et al. 1996). A surgical trough in the humeral head is present when tendon-to-bone repairs have been per-formed. Intermediate signal within the rotator cuff substance may be present on T1 and proton density weighted images, presumably due to granulation

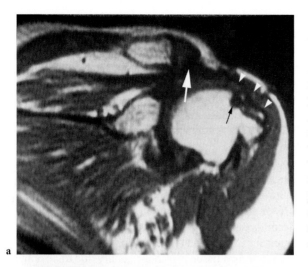

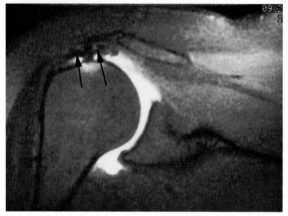

Fig. 11.7a, b. Intact rotator cuff, post repair. **a** Coronal oblique proton density weighted image. The patient has had an anterior acromioplasty and tendon-to-bone repair (*large arrow*). Note the distorted soft tissues overlying the cuff, the defect from the trough-in-bone (*small arrow*) and the intact low signal tendon (*arrowheads*). **b** MRI arthrogram. Coronal oblique T1 image with fat suppression. Note the artifact from the sutures in this tendon to tendon repair (*arrows*). Contrast outlines an intact tendon repair

tissue (OWEN et al. 1993) and the diagnosis of tendinosis or intrasubstance degeneration is difficult in the repaired tendon. Further distortion occurs with repair of large or massive tears if allograft is utilized, or if there is transfer of other tendons. Mild superior subluxation of the humeral head may occur, due to capsular tightening, scarring, cuff atrophy, or bursectomy (RAND et al. 1999a). Decreased acromiohumeral distance does not necessarily predict a retear of the rotator cuff, but may cause increased stress on the cuff by the humerus (RAND et al. 1999a).

Several findings associated with full thickness tears in the preoperative shoulder may be seen in an intact repaired shoulder. These include small to moderate joint effusions, fluid in the region of the subdeltoid bursa, and increased signal in the cuff on images with T2 weighted contrast. Increased signal in the tendon after rotator cuff repair can be due to postoperative hyperemic granulation tissue or disorganized granulation tissue at the repair site, which may contain or imbibe fluid. The increased signal in the tendon should not be equivalent to the signal of the fluid in a tendon defect. Mild bone marrow edema in the humeral head may also be seen (43% of subjects) (SPEILMAN et al. 1999), even up to 5 years after surgery. Fluid in the subdeltoid bursa, may be used as a secondary finding of a rotator cuff tear in the non-operated tendon (ZLATKIN et al. 1989; IANNOTTI et al. 1991; MITCHELL et al. 1988; RAFII et al. 1993; FARLEY et al. 1992), but can be seen after surgery due to bursal resection or leakage of fluid from the joint, into the subdeltoid bursal region (CALVERT et al. 1986; HARRYMAN et al. 1991) from a functional, but not watertight repair. In the postoperative setting this finding is not reliable as a secondary finding of a cuff defect (OWEN et al. 1993; LONGOBARDI et al. 1997; ZANETTI et al. 1999; SPEILMAN et al. 1999). A nonwatertight repair can be associated with patient satisfaction and pain relief, the presence of a cuff defect affects shoulder strength (HARRYMAN et al. 1991). Its size may be best quantified with MR arthrography.

Fluid signal on T2 weighted images seen within a recurrent rotator cuff tendon defect or non visualization of a portion of the cuff are the more reliable indicators of full thickness tears in the postoperative patient according to one study (OWEN et al. 1993), but the most specific finding of a recurrent tear is complete absence of the tendon (Fig. 11.8). In the postoperative situation there may be a higher incidence of low signal tears, due to chronic granulation tissue, which are more difficult to discern with conventional imaging sequences (see Fig. 11.12) (RAFII et al. 1993). Use of secondary signs such as muscle atrophy, and tendon retraction, may also be of value in these cases (RAFII et al. 1993). A baseline postoperative study (ZANETTI et al. 1999; SPEILMAN et al. 1999) is useful, and MR arthrography (Fig. 11.9) can document leakage of contrast through a cuff defect directly, and the cuff tissues and the tendon edges may be better delineated with this technique (Fig. 11.9).

Both conventional MRI (Fig. 11.8) and MR arthrography (Figs. 11.9, 11.10, 11.11) can outline severe muscle atrophy, tendon retraction, or fragmentation of the tendon edges in recurrent tears to help determine the feasibility of a second repair. Muscle retraction may be visible in larger defects,

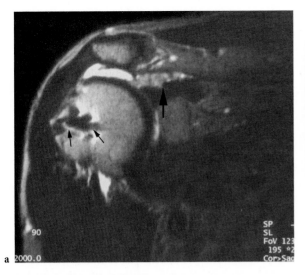
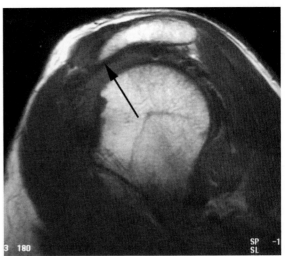

Fig. 11.8a, b. Recurrent rotator cuff tear. **a** Coronal oblique T2 weighted image. The supraspinatus tendon has retracted to the medial glenoid margin (*large arrow*). There is severe muscle atrophy. There is metal artifact in the humeral head from suture anchors (*small arrows*). **b** Sagittal oblique Turbo spin echo proton density weighted image. There is a persistent hook-like anterior acromion (*arrow*), post rotator cuff repair and decompression

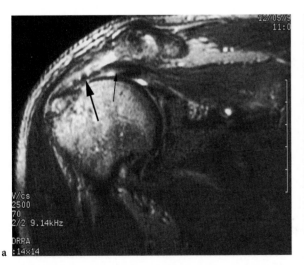
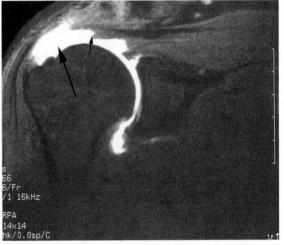

Fig. 11.9a, b. Recurrent rotator cuff tear. MR arthrography. **a, b** Coronal oblique T2 weighted image in (**a**), and MR arthrogram in (**b**). In (**a**) the artifact from surgery gives a false impression of an intact tendon (*large arrow*). MR arthrography in (**b**), better demonstrates the moderate size supraspinatus tendon defect (*large arrow*). Contrast imbibition in (**b**) better outlines the degenerated tendon edges [*small arrows* in (**a**) and (**b**)]

but the location of the musculotendinous junction is not a reliable secondary finding of a cuff tear after surgery, because its position may change if the cuff is mobilized during surgery (LONGOBARDI et al. 1997).

Recurrent partial tears may be difficult to detect. The criteria for a partial tear according to GAENSLEN et al. (1996) is fluid signal on images with T2 weighted contrast replacing a portion of the tendon. In this study, however, this fluid signal could not always be distinguished from edematous degeneration of the tendon as seen around sutures (GAENSLEN et al. 1996). In another earlier study (OWEN et al. 1993) it was noted that occasionally a small recurrent full thickness tear might be underestimated to be a partial tear. MR arthrography may help to resolve these difficulties (ZLATKIN 2000).

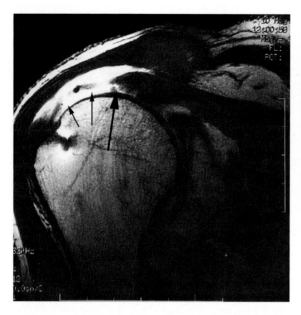

Fig. 11.10. Coronal oblique T1 weighted MR arthrogram. Moderately sized recurrent tear of the supraspinatus tendon is identified. Images were carried out with small field of view and larger matrix (512 384). Fat suppression was not applied in order to obtain better signal to noise. Note the excellent depiction of the tear size (*small arrows*) and status of the tendon edges (*large arrow*) with MR arthrography

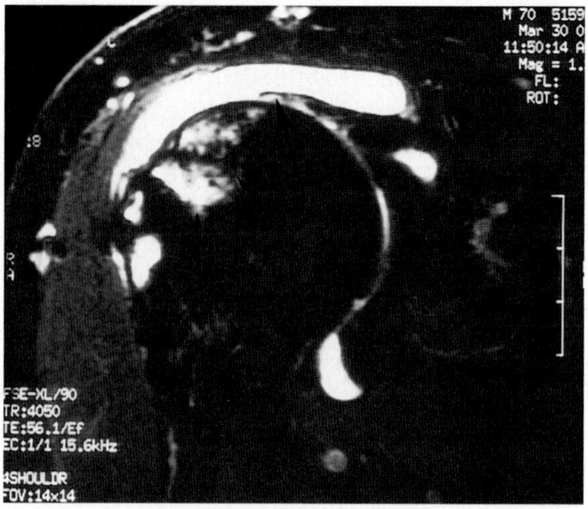

Fig. 11.11. Coronal oblique T2 weighted fast spin echo, MR arthrogram image. A recurrent tear in the posterior supraspinatus tendon is observed. The tear is well delineated (*arrow*). The multiple refocusing echoes used limit the metal artifact from the suture anchors in the greater tuberosity (*small arrow*)

11.2.3.4
MRI Results

In a recent study, SPIELMANN and coworkers (1999) evaluated MRI in 15 asymptomatic individuals after rotator cuff repair. They found that only 10% of patients after surgery had "normal" tendons. Mildly increased signal in the tendon was present in 53% of subjects, felt to be due to inflammation and or scarring and difficult to distinguish from tendinosis. More than one third of the patients had MRI findings similar to those seen in partial and complete tears, although these were not surgically confirmed. Other imaging findings in these patients included partial or complete loss of the peribursal fat in all, subacromial–subdeltoid bursal fluid in 67%, and small or moderate effusions in 93%. They found mild bone marrow edema in 40%, subchondral cysts in 60% and AC joint osteophytes in 70%. ZANETTI and coworkers (1999) studied 15 asymptomatic volunteers after rotator cuff repair. They found recurrent tears in 33% of patients. The retears were small with a mean diameter of 8 mm. A similar sized sample of patients studied with recurrent or residual pain had retears in 45%, but the mean size was 3.4 cm. Fluid in the subacromial–subdeltoid bursa was seen in nearly all

patients. Thus findings similar to those considered pathologic can be seen in asymptomatic individuals and therefore should be interpreted with caution in postoperative patients.

The sensitivity and specificity of MRI for rotator cuff tears in the postoperative shoulder has been evaluated. MAGEE et al. (1997) found the sensitivity and specificity for rotator cuff tears (partial and complete) was 100% and 87%, respectively. For partial thickness tears only, the sensitivity was 83% and the specificity 83%. In an earlier study (OWEN et al. 1993) of complete cuff tears the sensitivity was 86% and the specificity was 92%. Partial thickness tears were felt to be indistinguishable from repaired tendons in this earlier study. The lack of fat suppressed images may have contributed to this poorer sensitivity to partial tears.

11.2.3.5
MR Arthrography

MRI after intraarticular contrast injection may be useful in the postoperative rotator cuff (Figs. 11.7, 11.9–11.11). Conventional arthrography has been used in the past to try to diagnose recurrent rotator cuff tears (DEORIO and COFIELD 1984; CALVERT et al.

1986). Conventional arthrography has been considered unreliable because contrast material may leak through an incompletely healed but well repaired tendon, and conversely contrast material may fail to leak from the joint due to scar tissue, despite a tear. With the addition of MRI after contrast injection the size and nature of the defect leading to the leak can be directly visualized to determine its significance. If there is scar formation intraarticular contrast improves visualization of the cuff anatomy over conventional MRI and better outlines the morphologic alterations needed to diagnose tears obscured by scar. Intraarticular contrast can help confirm the presence of an intact cuff, in a situation where the cuff may have high signal on images with T2 weighted contrast, due to postoperative granulation tissue, edema, or fluid contained in residual nonabsorbable sutures, by revealing the absence of contrast extravasation through the cuff, into the bursa. As noted above, MR arthrography can be helpful in determining the size and location of a recurrent defect and better determine the integrity of the tendon edges for preoperative planning. MRI arthrography may potentially increase the sensitivity for recurrent partial tears of the cuff undersurface. A recent study has described the use of MR arthrography in evaluating the postoperative rotator cuff (RAND et al. 1996, 1999b).

11.2.3.6
Deltoid Detachment

Postoperative detachment of the deltoid from its insertion to the acromion may occur. With open repairs through an arthrotomy, the shoulder is accessed through a deltoid splitting incision. If the closure of the deltoid muscle is inadequate, or if it dehisces, deltoid detachment may occur. Another cause can be due to aggressive resection of the anterior portion of the acromion, which can result in inadvertent deltoid release from its acromial attachment. On MRI images (Fig. 11.12), the presence of deltoid detachment can be identified by retraction of the deltoid from the acromion, with fluid filling the defect (OXNER 1997). If the detachment is chronic, atrophy will be present. In the study by MAGEE et al. (1997), all five cases of deltoid muscle retraction found at surgery were correctly diagnosed by MRI.

11.2.3.7
Biceps Tendon

MRI is accurate in the diagnosis of biceps tendon rupture (MAGEE et al. 1997) in patients after sur-

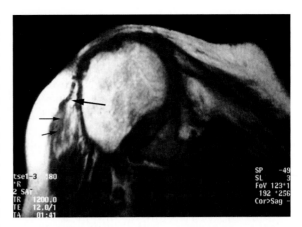

Fig. 11.12. Deltoid detachment. Coronal oblique proton density weighted turbo spin echo image. The deltoid muscle is retracted distally (*large arrow*) and shows atrophy (*small arrows*). The patient has a large rotator cuff tear after open rotator cuff surgery and subacromial decompression. There is no anatomic or functional depressor of the humeral head, which has migrated superiorly

gery. This is diagnosed by lack of visualization of the biceps tendon in the intertubercular groove. In the study by MAGEE et al. (1997), this was correctly identified in eight of ten shoulders found to have this complication after surgery. Biceps tendon dislocations with associated tears of the subscapularis tendon were found in eight of the 50 patients studied by MAGEE et al. (1997). This diagnosis is made by visualizing the empty intertubercular groove and medial displacement of the biceps tendon. The subscapularis, if torn, is retracted from its insertion into the lesser tuberosity.

11.3
Shoulder Instability

11.3.1
Clinical Features

Shoulder instability is most commonly unidirectional, and may be anterior, posterior, inferior or very rarely superior. Anterior instability is most common, and represents approximately 95% of cases (CAIN et al. 1987). Instability can be traumatic, either due to a single episode, or due to repetitive microtrauma as in athletics. It may be atraumatic as well, related to ligament and capsular laxity. Anterior instability is most commonly due to prior anterior dislocation associated with avulsion of the complex of the labrum, adjacent capsule, and glenohumeral ligaments (anterior inferior labroligamentous complex) from the bony glenoid (Bankart lesion and its variants).

The other more common clinical situation encountered is multidirectional instability, which is instability in more than one direction. This is often seen in patients with ligamentous laxity, in which case it may often be bilateral, or in throwing athletes with secondary stretching of the capsule. Patients with unidirectional instability most commonly are treated surgically. Patients with multidirectional instability will be treated conservatively with a vigorous rehabilitation regime, prior to any consideration of surgery.

11.3.2
Surgical Approach

The surgical treatment of patients with anterior instability has involved different approaches. Currently a direct repair of the labral and capsular lesions is done most commonly, usually a Bankart type repair (BANKART 1938), or less commonly the staple capsulorraphy described by DU TOIT and ROUX (1956). Other types of repair are those that tighten the capsule indirectly, usually through manipulation of the subscapularis, most commonly the Putti-Platt (OSMOND-CLARKE 1948) or Magnusson-Stack procedure (MAGNUSON and STACK 1943), and those that involve movement of the coracoid process, most commonly the Bristow (HELFET 1958) procedure.

11.3.2.1
Anatomic Repairs

Current techniques as noted are aimed at repairing the essential lesion of instability, as described by PERTHES (1906) and BANKART (1923, 1938). This is usually done via some modification of the repair originally described by BANKART in 1938 (Fig. 11.13). This was originally described as an open procedure via the deltopectoral interval to accomplish a reattachment of the torn capsulolabral complex to the bony glenoid rim. Drill holes are made in the glenoid, through which sutures may be passed to secure the labrum and capsule. In place of drill holes suture anchors may be used. These are usually placed at the 3, 4, and 5 0'clock positions. These suture anchors may have different compositions, and can be ferromagnetic (Fig. 11.13), especially in older repairs, but others may be made of nonferromagnetic substances, including plastic and bioabsorbable materials.

Arthroscopic capsulolabral repairs have become more common. Arthroscopic techniques minimize surgical dissection, damage to surrounding tissues and scarring (MATTHEWS and PAVLOVICH 1999). CASPARI (1991; CASPARI and SAVOIR 1990) described a technique in which the torn capsulolabral tissues are repaired via the passage of sutures from the capsulolabral tissue, through the glenoid neck and scapular body and secured over the fascia above the scapula. Newer techniques use suture anchors placed in the bony glenoid with arthroscopic graspers and

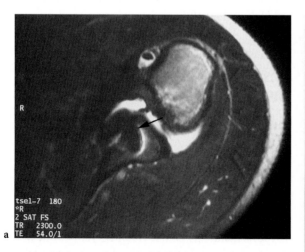
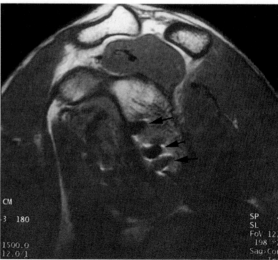

Fig. 11.13a, b. Post Bankart repair. **a** Axial turbo spin echo T2 weighted image. Note the postsurgical artifact from the suture anchor in the anterior inferior glenoid (*arrow*). **b** Sagittal oblique fast spin echo proton density weighted image in another patient. Artifact from the suture anchor outlines the site of placement for the anatomic repair (*arrows*)

knot pushers used to secure the labrum to the glenoid (WOLF et al. 1992). Another type of fixation used
in arthrosopic repairs is fixation with a stapling or
tacking device (LANE et al. 1993). Currently bioabsorbable tacks are used (SPEER et al. 1996).

In addition to repairing the torn labrum and capsule, many surgeons also perform a capsulorrhaphy
of redundant capsule. This can be done as part of
an open procedure or arthroscopically. When done
arthroscopically this may be done with absorbable
sutures, or with a holmium laser. The use of the laser
has been developed since arthroscopic techniques
are not that well suited to performing capsular shifts
(HAYASHI et al. 1996). The recurrence rate after open
Bankart repair is 5% or less (ROWE et al. 1978), but is
somewhat higher with arthroscopic repair (MORGAN
and BODENSTAB 1987; MORGAN 1991; HAWKINS 1989),
although CASPARI (1991; CASPARI and SAVOIR 1990)
reported results close to those with open techniques.

The staple capsulorrapy described by DUTOIT
and ROUX (1956) employs a staple to reattach the
anterior capsulolabral complex to the glenoid margin.
It is not commonly performed (LONGOBARDI et al.
1997), because of a high rate of failure (O'DRISCOLL
and EVANS 1993).

A glenoid fracture that involves more than 25%
of the glenoid fossa and is associated with shoulder
instability is an indication for surgery. This is usually done as an open reduction of the fragment with
screw fixation. CT can best determine fragment size
and displacement (MATTHEWS and PAVLOVICH 1999).
After surgery these patients are best imaged with MR
arthrography with FSE imaging or CT arthrography.

Pathology in the rotator interval may also contribute to shoulder instability (FRONEK et al. 1989) and
this may be identified on MRI. Closure of this interval
is often performed in conjunction with procedures
for shoulder instability (FIELD et al. 1995)

11.3.2.2
Indirect Repairs

The Putti-Platt (OSMOND-CLARKE 1948) and Magnuson-Stack procedures (MAGNUSON and STACK
1943), are not anatomic reconstructions and tighten
the capsule indirectly, through manipulations of
the subscapularis (Fig. 11.14). They do not directly
address the detached labrum and capsule. They prevent recurrent dislocations via restricting natural
motion. They are no longer commonly done. These
procedures have a higher rate of patient dissatisfac-
tion because of the decrease in motion, and have
higher rates of osteoarthritis. The subscapularis

tendon is split at its midpoint in the Putti-Platt procedure. Its lateral portion is attached to the glenoid,
and its medial portion is then imbricated over it. The
humerus must be rotated internally to a near neutral
position (OSMOND-CLARKE 1948). The recurrence
rate is between 2% and 10%. In the Magnuson-Stack
procedure (M-Stack) (MAGNUSON and STACK 1943)
the subscapularis is removed from its insertion into
the lesser tuberosity and transferred distal and lateral
to the greater tuberosity. The loss of external rotation
is usually less than with the Putti-Platt procedure.

11.3.2.3
Bristow Procedure

The Bristow procedure (HELFET 1958) involves
moving the coracoid process and using it as a bone
block to prevent recurrent anterior dislocation. The
bony tip of the coracoid process is transferred with
the conjoined tendon, and attached to the anterior
inferior glenoid rim through a split made in the
subscapularis. The conjoined tendon can then act as
a reinforcement of the capsule. The coracoid is fixed
with a cancellous screw. A high rate of subluxation
and hardware complications (YOUNG and ROCK-
WOOD 1991) has been reported with the modified
Bristow procedure. Failure of this procedure may
also be related to the fact that it does not address

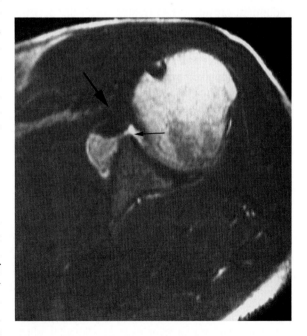

Fig. 11.14. Post Putti-Platt repair. Axial conventional spin echo
T2 weighted image. There is deformity in the subscapularis
tendon post repair (*large arrow*). The anterior labrum (*small
arrow*) is absent

the detached labrum and capsule (MATTHEWS and PAVLOVICH 1999). The Bristow procedure is no longer commonly performed.

Imaging of patients with Bristow procedures yield significant metal artifact arising from the cancellous screw, and is best done with MR arthrography with FSE imaging or CT arthrography. Assessing for failure of fixation, or for hardware complications may be best done with CT scanning.

11.3.2.4
Posterior Instability

The current approach in posterior instability is anatomic repair, through the infraspinatus muscle and tendon (FRONEK et al. 1989). Repair for posterior instability is generally modified from that done for anterior instability. Most commonly this is a repair of the reverse Bankart lesion, and if there is a redundant posterior capsule then a posterior capsular plication or shift is needed. If there is a bony deficiency it is treated with a posterior glenoid bone graft, or posterior opening wedge osteotomy (RAMSEY and KLIMKIEWICA 1999).

11.3.2.5
Multidirectional Instability

The pathology in these patients is generally a loose redundant capsule. When treated surgically patients are usually treated with an inferior capsular shift (NEER and FOSTER 1980; ALTCHECK et al. 1991; BIGLIANI et al. 1994). This procedure was devised for multidirectional anteroinferior instability. It reduces the volume of the glenohumeral joint anteriorly, inferiorly and posteriorly. This procedure may also be used for posteroinferior and other combinations of instability, with the region of capsular shift adjusted accordingly. The deltopectoral interval is used as the approach and the subscapularis traversed to expose the capsule. A "T" shaped incision is made in the capsule to allow the inferior capsule to be advanced in a superior direction, and the superior capsule to overlap it by advancing it inferiorly.

On MRI exam the most common finding is thickening of the anteroinferior capsule due to scar (LONGOBARDI et al. 1997). On coronal views in particular, the axillary pouch will be diminished in size. Low signal foci from suture material may be seen in the subscapularis and anterior capsule. Capsular plication may be best assessed with MRI arthrography, which determines any residual redundancy by distending the joint.

11.3.2.6
Isolated Labral Tears

Isolated labral tears such as SLAP lesions are often treated with debridement via an arthroscopic approach (ALTCHEK et al. 1992) (Fig. 11.15). In some situations, especially where there is an avulsion of the anterior superior labrum or avulsion of the biceps labral anchor complex, the lesions are debrided of loose tissue and a suture or staple repair back down to the bony glenoid bone may be carried out (MATTHEWS and PAVLOVICH 1999). Labral fraying or tearing may be present in regions other than SLAP lesions or anteroinferiorly (Bankart lesions). For example posterior labral fraying or detachment may occur in patients with internal impingement. In such patients the frayed portions can be debrided under arthroscopic visualization (PETERSON et al. 1998).

11.3.2.7
Normal Postoperative MRI Findings

The artifacts from surgery impair visualization, including metal and suture artifacts, especially screw fixation of the coracoid in the Bristow procedure, or the placement of suture anchors, staples or tacks with some of the other techniques described (Fig. 11.15). Scarring from the incisions as well as suture repair, may impair visualization resulting in disruption of normal tissue contrast, with areas of more prominent signal void arising. In Bankart repairs even nonferromagnetic suture anchors or other materials may be apparent within the glenoid neck (LONGOBARDI et al. 1997). If transglenoid sutures are placed, there will be channels seen traversing the glenoid neck and scapula. In addition, the suture knot placed posteriorly, that is tied over fascia, may show some surrounding intermediate or high signal on images with T2 type contrast, due to hyperemic granulation tissue. In patients with anatomic repairs such as the Bankart repair there should be an anatomic position and morphology of the labrum and capsule post repair (ROWE et al. 1978). In procedures that do not directly repair the labral and capsular lesions, as noted above, the abnormality from these lesions remains at imaging. HASHIUCHI and coworkers (2000) evaluated MR images following Putti-Platt procedure for recurrent anterior dislocation of the shoulder. After the Putti-Platt procedure the subscapularis tendon was thickened and increased signal on T2-weighted images were observed. The area of subscapularis tendons after operation was increased maximally 3.46-fold and the volume was increased on average 1.51-fold.

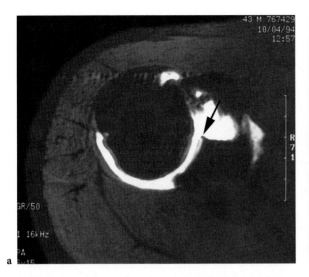 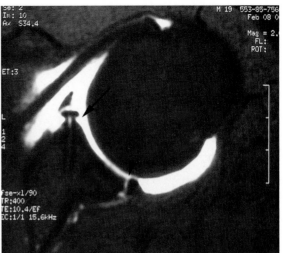

Fig. 11.15. **a** Labral debridement. MR arthrogram. Axial three-dimensional volume gradient echo image. A smooth, but attenuated anterior superior labrum is seen (*arrow*). **b** Labral repair with tack. MR arthrogram in a different patient than in (**a**). Axial T1 weighted image with fat suppression. A tack is seen in the anterior superior glenoid (*arrow*). Contrast outlines a detached posterior labrum (*arrowhead*)

The course of subscapularis muscle fibers before operation were described as a mild arc, but changed to a straight line after the procedure.

Owing to the difficulties in assessing the integrity of the repairs for instability after surgery has been performed, MR arthrography has been employed for this purpose. SUGIMOTO and colleagues (2002) studied the ability of MR arthrography in the assessment of anatomic reestablishment of the capsulolabral complex and correlated this with arthroscopic findings in 30 patients after suture-anchor Bankart repair. MR arthrographic findings of reattachment of the capsulolabral complex were in agreement with arthroscopic findings in 93 anchor points (accuracy, 93 of 98 anchor points; 95%). In 28 shoulders, oblique transverse images obtained with the shoulder in the abduction and external rotation position (ABER) showed that the anterior band of the inferior glenohumeral ligament (AIGHL) abutted the humeral head and that reattachment of the AIGHL to the glenoid rim was seamless. They concluded that MR arthrography can be reliably used for the postoperative assessment of suture-anchor Bankart repair.

11.3.2.8
Recurrent Lesions and MRI

The success rates for surgery for typical patterns of anterior glenohumeral instability are good. The recurrence rate for most instability procedures done in an open manner is 1%–10% (MATTHEWS and

PAVLOVICH 1999; ROWE et al. 1978, 1984; MATSEN et al. 1998; ROSENBERG et al. 1995). Procedures done arthroscopically have a rate of recurrence in the range of 15%–20% (CASPARI and SAVOIR 1990; CASPARI 1991; MORGAN and BODENSTAB 1987; MORGAN 1991; HAWKINS 1989; GUANCHE et al. 1996; PAGNANI et al. 1996; SNYDER and STAFFORD 1993). Recurrent problems after surgery may often be treated based on clinical grounds, or assessed via arthroscopy. The volume of cases referred for MRI for recurrent instability after surgical treatment is limited, and there is little in the literature on this topic. MRI may be helpful in diagnosing some of the abnormalities that may be present, although discerning true recurrent pathology from artifacts, scarring and residual untreated lesions is difficult. MRI arthrography may be helpful by improving tissue contrast (Fig. 11.16) (ZLATKIN 2000). WAGNER and colleagues (2002) studied 24 patients who underwent MRI after shoulder instability surgery and had recurrent instability requiring repeat surgery. Twelve nonenhanced MR images and six indirect and six direct MR arthrograms were retrospectively reviewed with consensus to determine the presence or absence of recurrent labral or rotator cuff tear. Overall, the accuracy of postoperative MRI was 79% in depicting recurrent labral tears. They determined that MRI, and indirect MR arthrography in particular, were an accurate means of evaluating the shoulder following instability surgery.

Causes of recurrent instability include inadequate or incorrect procedures, and the uncovering of missed

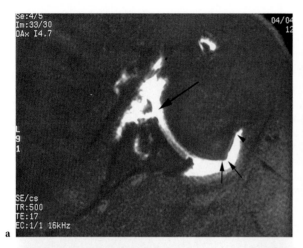

a

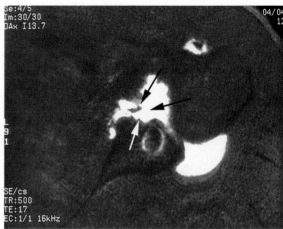

b

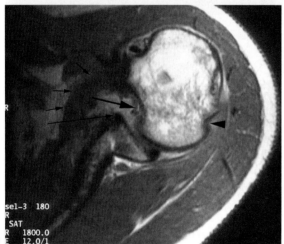

c

Fig. 11.16a–c. Post Bankart repair. Recurrent lesions. Degenerative joint disease. **a, b** MR arthrogram. Axial T1 weighted images with fat suppression. The anterior inferior labrum is detached (*arrows*) in this patient after open Bankart repair. There is a small Hill-Sachs lesion (*arrowhead*). There is some bony erosion of the bony glenoid [*white arrow* in (**b**)]. Note the small osteophyte projecting from the humeral head (*small arrows*) and the early articular cartilage loss, indicating early glenohumeral joint degenerative change. **c** Axial T2 weighted turbo spin echo images. The anterior labrum is blunted (*long thin arrow*). The humeral head is displaced posteriorly, with a wedge-like defect in the anteromedial humeral head (*thicker arrow*), with subjacent marrow edema. These latter two findings were felt to reflect an overtight anterior repair (*shorter thin arrows*), thought to have resulted in secondary posterior laxity/instability. There is joint space narrowing, reflective of glenohumeral joint degenerative change. Also note the small Hill-Sachs lesion of the posterolateral humeral head (*arrowhead*)

anterior or posterior instability with isolated treatment of one. An overtight repair can lead either to degenerative change (ROSENBERG et al. 1995) or may precipitate instability in the other direction (Fig. 11.16). This may be more common in such procedures as the Putti-Platt (OSMOND-CLARKE 1948), or Magnuson-Stack procedure (MAGNUSON and STACK 1943), which may also result in loss of external rotation. In these latter procedures an internal rotation contracture may be present, but may only be apparent if axial images are performed in internal and external rotation. Inferior capsular shifts or other types of capsular plications can also be overtightened. Signs of an overtightened inferior capsular shift may include prominent loss of the axillary pouch. Subtle posterior subluxation of the humeral head relative to the glenoid is another finding of overtightening in an inferior capsular shift, or other shoulder plication. Degenerative arthritis may also occur, if there is persistent instability from inadequate repair (Fig. 11.16). Marginal glenoid cysts may also be present. Misplaced or detached staples or tacks from

labral and capsular repairs (Fig. 11.17) or misplaced screws or coracoid nonunion in a Bristow procedure, may also cause joint derangement. If left unrecognized these may also lead to degenerative changes. These can be identified with MRI but may be better seen with MR arthrography and, if necessary, CT scanning. The presence of coracoid nonunion in the Bristow procedure does not by itself indicate instability, as there is a 5%–10% nonunion rate even in patients who are clinically stable (HELFET 1958; YOUNG and ROCKWOOD 1991; MAY 1970).

In patients after repair of the labrum and capsule the postoperative labrum may be thickened and irregular, due to scar tissue or suture material, but should not be detached. Signal alterations may be present postoperatively and high signal on images with T2 contrast may be present in the earlier postoperative periods due to hyperemic granulation tissue (RAND et al. 1999a). As such outlining the labrum and capsule with intraarticular contrast is the best means of discerning recurrent tears and detachments, by

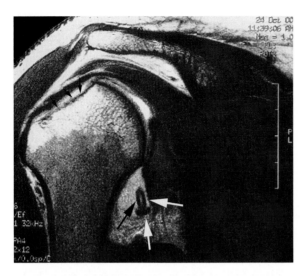

Fig. 11.17. Displaced tack. Coronal oblique image, fast spin echo T1 weighted MR arthrogram, without fat suppression. Note the displaced tack from a prior Bankart repair in the axillary recess (*arrows*). Note the Hill Sachs lesion on the superior humeral head (*smaller arrows*)

outlining any surface irregularities, and revealing any contrast extension into or beneath the labrum (RAND et al. 1996, 1999b). Failed Bankart repairs may show persistence or recurrence of the detached labrum and capsule (Fig. 11.16). This may occur due to breakdown of the fixation, from suture breakage, anchor device pullout, or failure of the reapproximated labral and capsular tissues. The repaired labrum may also become blunted, attenuated or fragmented.

With respect to the joint capsule, postoperatively it may appear thickened and nodular. Measurements of capsular thickening have been described for adhesive capsulitis (EMIG et al. 1994), and can be measured best in the axillary recess on MR arthrography, as a band of low signal adjacent to the hyperintense signal of contrast medially and the hyperintense signal of the fat stripe laterally, on T1 weighted images. A measurement of 4 mm indicates adhesive capsulitis, and one of 2–4 mm is felt to be consistent with the thickening expected after Bankart repair. The glenohumeral ligaments may also appear thickened and nodular post repair. In patients with recurrent instability the repaired capsule may become stretched out and redundant. These changes are best identified by MR arthrography. One criterion suggested for the diagnosis of residual or recurrent capsular stripping may be the presence of a capsular attachment that is more medial than would be expected for a type 3 insertion (RAND et al. 1999a; NEUMANN et al. 1991). TIRMAN et al. recommended measuring the anterior and poste-

rior capsular widths in nonoperated patients using MR arthrography. RAND et al. (1999a) indicate that an anterior capsular width/posterior capsular width ratio of <1 on MR arthrography may predict a good outcome post surgery, particularly if a capsulorraphy, open or arthroscopic approach has been carried out. Imaging patients in abduction and external rotation may be useful to demonstrate any subtle persistent laxity. The glenohumeral ligaments, if abnormal, may appear thin, elongated, irregular and discontinuous.

One potential pitfall even with MR arthrography is the Bankart repair that is partly adherent related to fibrous tissue and granulation tissue, even when the joint is distended with contrast. This may be evident at arthroscopy when this area is probed. Intravenous gadolinium enhancement with T1 weighting and fat suppression may potentially be helpful in such cases by outlining these areas of granulation tissue, which should enhance (RAND et al. 1999a).

Secondary occult impingement and rotator cuff injury can also be an outcome, or cause, of persistent problems with persistent or recurrent instability seen on MRI or MR arthrography. Other postoperative findings on MRI exam include avascular necrosis and paralabral or ganglion cysts (MAGEE et al. 1997) (see Fig. 11.6b).

11.3.2.9
Paralabral Cysts

Paralabral cysts arise in relationship to labral tears and may extend into the spinoglenoid notch (DAUMAS et al. 1995; TIRMAN et al. 1994). The intraarticular portion may be visualized and excised arthroscopically. If it is too large, the visible portion can be unroofed and decompressed (PETERSON et al. 1996, 1998) or it may need to be removed in an open fashion. Failure of this procedure can be due to incomplete removal of the cyst, intraoperative injury to the suprascapular nerve or artery, and continued compression due to hematoma. In patients with incomplete cyst removal or with recurrence, MRI may reveal cyst remnants or a recurrent cyst on images with T2 type contrast, or with MRI arthrography.

11.4
Other Complications of Surgery

Other complications of surgery (Fig. 11.18) include hematoma formation, wound infection, osteomyelitis, septic arthritis, as well as synovitis.

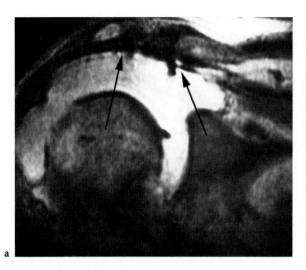

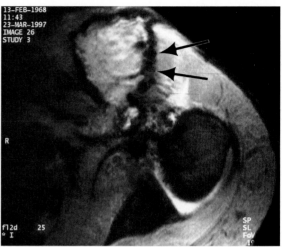

Fig. 11.18a, b. Post operative complications. **a** Coronal oblique T2 weighted image. A large to massive effusion is present in this patient who developed septic arthritis after a rotator cuff repair (*arrows*). **b** Axial two-dimensional T2* gradient echo image. A large anterior hematoma is seen in the deltoid muscle (*arrows*). The patient had an open Bankart repair 2 days prior to this scan

The appearance of a hematoma on MRI will depend on its age. Blood products at the appropriate stage may be bright on T1 and T2 weighted images. Fluid–fluid levels may also be present. Postoperative wound abscess formation may present as a localized cavity with signal characteristics similar to fluid. There may be a rim of inflamed tissue surrounding the abscess cavity, which may be bright on images with T2 type contrast and STIR imaging and enhance with intravenous administration of gadolinium. Osteomyelitis may be best detected with the use of fat suppressed imaging, such as T2 weighted FSE images with fat saturation, or with fast STIR images. Synovitis may also follow surgery. It may be infectious or reactive (HAYGOOD et al. 1993). A joint effusion may then be present. Synovial thickening may be present and synovial proliferation may give rise to a bumpy contour of the inner surface of the joint capsule. Intravenous gadolinium may reveal enhancement. If the synovitis is infectious, joint destruction, including cartilage loss, cysts and erosions may be identified. It may be difficult to differentiate signal alterations seen in infection and inflammation from those that are due to the postoperative status of the patient, particularly in patients with more recent surgery. Interval follow-up is useful in these circumstances (Rand et al. 1999a).

Damage to nerve and vessels such as in the axilla may also occur, but is uncommon. In the rare situation of pseudoaneurysm formation, these may be evaluated with MR angiography. Damage to nerves may cause muscle atrophy and, in the acute phase, muscle edema.

11.5
Conclusion

MRI can be of significant benefit in understanding the alterations of anatomy mediated by surgery in patients with shoulder lesions, particularly those related to rotator cuff disease and shoulder instability. It can successfully diagnose persistent anatomic bony impingement, and progression or recurrence of rotator cuff pathology including partial and full thickness tears. It can uncover pathology that may mimic such pathology, such as paralabral cysts, or uncover lesions of instability that may be mediating such rotator cuff pathology. In patients with recurrent instability, it may reveal the anatomic lesions that are causing such dysfunction, including recurrent Bankart lesions, bony defects, or loosened or misplaced tacks, screws or anchors. It may reveal other complications such as degenerative joint disease, or instability in another direction. MR arthrography is of significant aid in the postoperative patient, by distending the joint and significantly improving overall contrast resolution.

References

Altcheck DW, Warren RF, Skyhar MJ, Ortiz G (1991) T plasty modification of the Bankart procedure for multidirectional instability of the anterior and inferior types. J Bone Joint Surg (Am) 73:105–112

Altchek DW, Russell WF, Wickiewicz TL, Ortiz G (1992)

Arthroscopic labral debridement. A three-year follow-up study. Am J Sports Med 20:702–706

Andrews JR, Broussard TS, Carson WG (1985) Arthroscopy of the shoulder in the management of partial tears of the rotator cuff. A preliminary report. Arthroscopy 1:177–122

Arroyo JS, Flatow EL (1999) Management of Rotator Cuff Disease. Intact and repairable cuff. In: Iannotti JP, Williams GR Jr (eds) Disorders of the shoulder: diagnosis and management, chap 2. Lippincott, Williams and Wilkins, Philadlephia, pp 31–56

Arroyo JS, Hershorn SJ, Bigliani LU (1997) Special considerations in the athletic throwing shoulder. Orthop Clin North Am 28:69–78

Baker CL, Liu SH (1995) Comparison of open and arthroscopically assisted rotator cuff repairs. Am J Sports Med 23:99

Bankart ASB (1923) Recurrent or habitual dislocation of the shoulder joint. Br Med J 2:1132–1133

Bankart ASB (1938) The pathology and treatment of recurrent dislocation of the shoulder. Br J Surg 26:23–39

Beach WR, Caspari RB (1993) Arthroscopic management of rotator cuff disease. Orthopedics 16:1007–1015

Bigliani LU, Morrison DS, April EW (1986) The morphology of the acromion and its relationship to rotator cuff tears. Orthop Trans 10:228

Bigliani LU, Cordasco FA, McIlveen SJ, Musso ES (1992) Operative treatment of failed repairs of the rotator cuff. J Bone Joint Surg (Am) 74:1505–1515

Bigliani LU, Kurzwell PR, Schwartzbach CC et al (1994) Inferior capsular shift procedure for anterior inferior shoulder instability in athletes. Am J Sports Med 22:578–584

Blevins FT, Warren RF, Cavo C, Altchek DW, Dines D, Palletta G, Wickiewicz TL (1996) Arthroscopic assisted rotator cuff repair: results using a mini-open deltoid splitting approach. Arthroscopy 12:50–59

Bokor DJ, Hawkins RJ, Huckell GH, Angelo RL, Schikendantz MS (1993) Results of nonoperative management of full thickness tears of the rotator cuff. Clin Orthop 294:103–110

Budoff JE, Nirschl RP, Guidi EJ (1988) Debridement of partial thickness tears of the rotator cuff without acromioplasty. J Bone Joint Surg (Am) 80:733–748

Burkhart SS (1994) Reconciling the paradox of rotator cuff repair versus debridement: a unified biomechanical rationale for the treatment of rotator cuff tears. Current concepts. Arthroscopy 10:4–19

Burkhart SS (1996) Shoulder arthroscopy. New concepts. Clin Sports Med 15:635–653

Burkhead WZ, Burkhart SS, Gerber C, Harryman DT, Morrison DS, Uthhoff HK, Williams GR Jr (1995) Symposium on the rotator cuff: debridement vs repair, part II. Contemp Orthop 31:313–326

Cain PR, Mutschler TA, Fu FH (1987) Anterior stability of the glenohumeral joint: a dynamic model. Am J Sports Med 15:144–148

Calvert PT, Packer NP, Stoker DJ, Bayley JIL, Kessel L (1986) Arthrography of the shoulder after operative repair of the torn rotator cuff. J Bone Joint Surg (Br) 68:147–150

Caspari RB (1991) Arthroscopic reconstruction for anterior shoulder instability. In: Paulos LE, Tibone JD (eds) Operative techniques in shoulder surgery. Aspen, Gaithersburg MD, pp 57–63

Caspari RB, Savoir B (1990) Arthroscopic reconstruction of the shoulder: the Bankart repair. In: Pariesen JS (ed) Operative arthroscopy. Raven, New York, pp 65–74

Cofield RH (1985) Rotator cuff disease of the shoulder. J Bone Joint Surg (Am) 67:974–979

Daumas JL, Padovani B, Rafelli C et al (1995) Compression du nerf sus-scapulaire dans le defile spinoglenoidien par un kyste synovial. J Radiol 76:25–28

DeOrio JK, Cofield RH (1984) Results of a second attempt at surgical repair of a failed initial rotator-cuff repair. J Bone Joint Surg (Am) 66:563–567

Du Toit GT, Roux D (1956) Recurrent dislocation of the shoulder. J Bone Joint Surg (Am) 38:1–12

Ellman H, Kay SP, Wirth M (1993) Arthroscopic treatment of full-thickness rotator cuff tears: 2- to 7-year follow-up study. Arthroscopy 9:195–200

Emig EW, Schweitzer ME, Karasick D, Lubowitz J (1994) Adhesive capsulitis of the shoulder: MR diagnosis. AJR 164: 1457–1459

Esch J (1993) Rotator cuff disease and Impingement. In: Esch JC, Baker CL (eds) Arthroscopic surgery, chap 11. The shoulder and elbow. Lippincott, Philadelphia, pp 151–175

Farley TE, Neumann CH, Steinbach LS, Jahnke AJ, Peterson SS (1992) Full-thickness tears of the rotator cuff of the shoulder: diagnosis with MR imaging. AJR 158:347–351

Feller JF, Howey TD, Plaga BR (1998) MR imaging of the postoperative shoulder. In: Steinbach LS, Tirman PFJ, Peterfy CG, Feller JF (eds) Shoulder magnetic resonance imaging, chap 10. Lippincott-Raven, Philadelphia, pp 187–221

Field LD, Warren RF, Obrien SJ et al (1995) Isolated closure of rotator interval defects for shoulder instability. Am J Sports Med 23:557–563

Flatow EL, Duralde XA, Nicholson GP, Pollock RG, Bigliani LU (1995) Arthroscopic resection of the distal clavicle from a superior approach. J Shoulder Elbow Surg 4:41–50

Fronek J, Warren RF, Bowen M (1989) Posterior subluxation of the glenohumeral joint. J Bone Joint Surg (Am) 71:205–216

Fu FH, Harner CD, Klein AH (1991) Shoulder impingement syndrome. A critical review. Clin Orthop 269:162–173

Gaenslen ES, Satterlee CC, Hinson GW (1996) Magnetic resonance imaging for evaluation of failed repairs of the rotator cuff. Relationship to operative findings. J Bone Joint Surg (Am) 78:1391–1396

Gartsman GM (1990) Arthroscopic acromioplasty for lesions of the rotator cuff. J Bone Joint Surg (Am) 72:169–180

Gartsman GM, Hammerman SM (1997) Full thickness tears: arthroscopic repair. Orthop Clin North Am 28:83–98

Guanche CA, Quick DC, Sodergren K et al (1996) Arthroscopy vs open reconstruction of the shoulder in patients with isolated Bankart lesions. Am J Sports Med 24:144–148

Gusmer PB, Potter HG, Donovan WD, O'Brien SJ (1997) MR imaging of the shoulder after rotator cuff repair. AJR 168: 559–563

Harryman DT Jr, Mack LA, Wang KY, Jackins SE, Richardson ML, Matsen FA III (1991) Repairs of the rotator cuff. Correlation of functional results with integrity of the cuff. J Bone Joint Surg 73A:982–989

Hashiuchi T, Ozaki J, Sakurai G, Imada K (2000) The changes occurring after the Putti-Platt procedure using magnetic resonance imaging. Arch Orthop Trauma Surg 120:286–289

Hawkins RJ, Misamore GW, Hobeika PE (1985) Surgery for full thickness rotator cuff tears. J Bone Joint Surg (Am) 67: 1349–1355

Hawkins RB (1989) Arthroscopic stapling repair for shoulder instability: a retrospective study of 50 cases. Arthroscopy 5:122–128

Hayashi K, Thabit G III, Bogdanske JJ, Mascio LN, Markel MD (1996) The effect of nonlaser ablative energy on the ultrastructure of joint capsular collagen. Arthroscopy 12:474–481

Haygood TM, Oxner KG, Kneeland JB, Dalinka MK (1993) Magnetic resonance imaging of the postoperative shoulder. MRI Clin North Am 1:143–155

Helfet A (1958) Coracoid transplantation for recurring dislocation of the shoulder. J Bone Joint Surg40B:198–202

Hurley JA, Anderson TE (1990) Shoulder arthroscopy: it's role in evaluating the shoulder disorders in the athlete. Am J Sports Med 18:480–483

Hurley JA, Anderson TE, Dear W, Andrish JT, Bergfeld JA, Weiker GG (1992) Posterior shoulder instability. Surgical versus conservative results with evaluation of glenoid version. Am J Sports Med 20:396–400

Iannotti JP, Zlatkin MB, Esterhai JL, Kressel HY, Dalinka MK, Spindler KP (1991) Magnetic resonance imaging of the shoulder. J Bone Joint Surg (Am) 73:17–29

Kvitne RS, Jobe FW (1993) Diagnosis and treatment of anterior instability in the throwing athlete. Clin Orthop 291: 107–123

Lane JG, Sachs RA, Riehl B (1993) Arthroscopic staple capsulorrhaphy. A long term follow up. Arthroscopy 9:190–194

Longobardi RSF, Rafii M, Minkoff JM (1997) MR imaging of the postoperative shoulder. MRI Clin North Am 5:841–859

Magee TH, Gaenslen ES, Seitz R, Hinson GA, Wetzel LH (1997) MR imaging of the shoulder after surgery. AJR 168: 925–928

Magnuson PB, Stack JK (1943) Recurrent dislocation of the shoulder. JAMA 123:889–892

Matsen FA III, Thomas SC, Rockwood CA, Wirth MA (1998) Glenohumeral instability. In: Rockwood CA, Matsen FA III (eds) The shoulder, 2nd edn. Saunders, Philadelphia, pp 611–754

Matsen FA, Artnz CT, Lippitt SB (1998) Rotator cuff. In: Rockwood CE, Matsen FA (eds) The shoulder, chap 15. Saunders, Philadelphia, pp 755–795

Matthews LS, Pavlovich LJ Jr (1999) Anterior and anteroinferior instability: diagnosis and management, chap 10. In: Iannotti JP, Williams GR Jr (eds) Disorders of the shoulder: diagnosis and management. Lippincott, Williams and Wilkins, Philadlephia, pp 251–294

May VR Jr (1970) A modified Bristow operation for recurrent anterior dislocation of the shoulder. J Bone Joint Surg (Am) 52:1010–1016

McLaughlin HL (1963) Repair of major cuff ruptures. Surg Clin North Am 43:1535–1540

Melilo AS, Savoie FH III, Field LD (1997:Massive rotator cuff tears: debridement versus repair. Orthop Clin North Am 28:117–124

Mitchell MJ, Causey G, Berthoty DP et al (1988) Peribursal fat plane of the shoulder: anatomic study and clinical experience. Radiology 168:699–704

Morgan C (1991) Arthroscopic transglenoid Bankart suture repair. Oper Techn Orthop 1:171–179

Morgan CD, Bodenstab AB (1987) Arthroscopic Bankart suture repair. Technique and early results. Arthroscopy 3: 111–122

Mumford EB (1941) Acromioclavicular dislocation. A new operative treatment. J Bone Joint Surg 23:799–802

Needell SD, Zlatkin MB (1997) Comparison of fat-saturation fast spin echo versus conventional spin-echo MRI in the detection of rotator cuff pathology. JMRI 7:674–677

Neer CS Jr (1972) Anterior acromioplasty for the chronic impingement syndrome of the shoulder: a preliminary report. J Bone Joint Surg (Am) 54A:41–50

Neer CS Jr (1983) Impingement lesions. Clin Orthop 173: 70–77

Neer CS Jr, Foster CR (1980) Inferior capsular shift for involuntary inferior and multidirectional instability of the shoulder. A preliminary report. J Bone Joint Surg (Am) 62:897–908

Neumann CH, Peterson SA, Jahnke AH et al (1991) MRI in the evaluation of patients with suspected instability of the shoulder joint including CT arthrography. Fortschr Roentgenstr 154:593–600

Neviaser JS, Neviaser RJ, Neviaser TJ (1978) The repair of chronic massive ruptures of the rotator cuff. J Bone Joint Surg (Am) 60:681–684

Nobuhara K, Ikeda H (1987) Rotator interval lesion. Clin Orthop 223:44–50

Norwood L, Fowler FH (1989) Rotator cuff tears. A shoulder arthroscopy complication. Am J Sports Med 17:837–841

O'Driscoll S, Evans D (1993) Long term results of staple capsulorrhaphy for anterior instability of the shoulder. J Bone Joint Surg 75A:249–258

Ogilvie-Harris D, Wiley A, Sattarian J (1990) Failed acromioplasty for impingement syndrome. J Bone Joint Surg (Br) 72:1070–1072

Osmond-Clarke H (1948) Habitual dislocation of the shoulder. The Putti-Platt operation. J Bone Joint Surg (Br) 30:19–25

Owen RS, Iannotti JP, Kneeland JB, Dalinka MKD, Deren JA, Oleaga L (1993) Shoulder after surgery. MR imaging with surgical validation. Radiology 186:443–447

Oxner KG (1997) Magnetic resonance imaging of the musculoskeletal system. Clin Orthop 334:354–373

Ozaki J, Fujimoto S, Masuhara K et al (1986) Reconstruction of chronic massive rotator cuff tears with synthetic materials. Clin Orthop 202:173–183

Pagnani MJ, Warren RF, Altcheck DW et al (1996) Arthroscopic shoulder stabilization using transglenoid sutures: a four year minimum follow up. Am J Sports Med 24:459–567

Paulos LE, Franklin JL (1990) Arthroscopic shoulder decompression development and application: a five year experience. Am J Sports Med 18:235–244

Perthes G (1906) Über Operationen der habituellen Schulterluxation. Dtsche Z Chir 85:199

Peterson CA, Altcheck DW, Warren RF (1998) Shoulder arthroscopy. In: Rockwood CA, Matsen ED (eds) The shoulder, chap 8. Saunders, Philadelphia

Peterson CA Jr, Altchek DW (1996) Arthroscopic treatment of rotator cuff disorders. Clin Sports Med 15:715–736

Rafii M, Firooznia H, Golimbu C, Weinreb J (1993) Magnetic resonance imaging of glenohumeral instability. MRI Clin North Am 1:87–104

Ramsey ML, Klimkiewica JJ (1999) Posterior instability: diagnosis and management. In: Iannotti JP, Williams GR Jr (eds) Disorders of the shoulder: diagnosis and management, chap 10. Lippincott, Williams and Wilkins. Philadlephia pp 295–319

Rand T, Trattnig S, Breitenseher M, Feilinger W (1996) Postoperative MR arthrography of the shoulder joint. Radiologe 36:966–970

Rand T, Trattnig S, Breitenseher M, Wurnig C, Marchner B, Imhof H (1999a) The postoperative shoulder. Top Magn Reson Imaging 10:203–213

Rand T, Feilinger W, Breitenseher M et al (1999b) Magnetic resonance arthrography (MRA) in the postoperative shoulder. Magn Reson Imaging 17:843–850

Rockwood CA, Lyons FR (1993) Shoulder impingement syndrome. Diagnosis, radiographic evaluation, and treatment with a modified Neer acromioplasty. J Bone Joint Surg (Am) 75:409–424

Rosenberg BN, Richmond JC, Levine WN (1995) Long term follow up of Bankart reconstruction. Incidence of late glenohumeral arthrosis. Am J Sports Med 23:538–544

Rowe CR, Patel D, Southmayd WW (1978) The Bankart procedure. A long-term end-result study. J Bone Joint Surg (Am) 60:1–16

Rowe CR, Zarins B, Ciullo JV (1984) Recurrent anterior dislocation of the shoulder after surgical repair. Apparent cause of failure and treatment. J Bone Joint Surg (Am) 66:159–168

Snyder SJ, Stafford BB (1993) Arthroscopic management of instability of the shoulder. Orthopedics 16:993–1002

Snyder SJ, Pachelli AF, Del Pizzo W, Friedman MJ, Ferkel RD, Patten G (1991) Partial thickness rotator cuff tears: results of arthroscopic treatment. Arthroscopy 7:1–7

Speer KP, Warren RF, Pagnani M, Warner JJ (1996) An arthroscopic technique for anterior stabilization of the shoulder with a bioabsorbable tack. J Bone Joint Surg (Am) 78:1801–1807

Speilman AL, Forster BB, Kokan P, Hawkins RH, Janzen DL (1999) Shoulder after rotator cuff repair: MR imaging findings in asymptomatic individuals initial experience. Radiology 213:705–708

Sugimoto H, Suzuki K, Mihara K, Kubota H, Tsutsui H (2002) MR arthrography of shoulders after suture-anchor Bankart repair. Radiology 224:105–111

Tirman PF, Feller JF, Janzen DL et al (1994) Association of glenoid labral cysts and tears and glenohumeral instability. Radiololgical findings and clinical significance. Radiology 190:653–658

Tirman PFJ, Stauffer AE, Crues JV et al (1993) Saline magnetic resonance arthrography in the evaluation of glenohumeral instability. Arthroscopy 9:550–559

Wagner SC, Schweitzer ME, Morrison WB, Fenlin JM Jr, Bartolozzi AR (2002) Shoulder instability: accuracy of MR imaging performed after surgery in depicting recurrent injury – initial findings. Radiology 222:196–203

Weber SC (1997) All arthroscopic versus mini open repair in the management of complete tears of the rotator cuff. Arthroscopy 13:368–372

Wolf E, Walk R, Richmond J (1992) Arthroscopic Bankart repair using suture anchors. Operv Techn Orthop 1:184–191

Young DC, Rockwood CA Jr (1991) Complications of failed Bristow procedure and their management. J Bone Joint Surg (Am) 73:969–981

Zanetti MD, Jost B, Hodler J (1999) MR findings in asymptomatic patients after supraspinatus reconstruction. Radiology 213:157

Zlatkin MB (2000) Arthro-IRM de l'epaule. In: Laredo JD (ed) Arthrographie, arthroscanner, arthro-IRM, chap 6. Masson, Paris, pp 93–117

Zlatkin MB (2002) MRI of the postoperative shoulder. Skeletal Radiol 31:63–80

Zlatkin MB, Iannotti JP, Roberts MC et al. (1989) Rotator cuff disease. Diagnostic performance of MR imaging: comparison with arthrography and correlation with surgery. Radiology 172:223–229

12 The Postoperative Shoulder 2: Arthroplasty, Arthrodesis and Osteotomy

T. H. Berquist

CONTENTS

12.1
Indications

Shoulder arthroplasty (glenohumeral joint) has become the technique of choice for patients with articular damage and pain that does not respond to more conservative measures (ARNTZ et al. 1993; BELL and GESCHWEND 1986). The procedure is performed to relieve pain and improve function. The most frequent causes of symptoms are rheumatoid arthritis, osteoarthritis, avascular necrosis and trauma (COFIELD 1983; FRIEDMAN et al. 1989).

Regardless of the underlying disorder, the prognosis and selection of operative approach varies with the extent of joint, bone and soft tissue involvement (COFIELD 1984; FRIEDMAN et al. 1989; HASAN et al. 2002).

T. H. BERQUIST, MD, FACR
Diagnostic Radiology, Mayo Clinic, 4500 San Pablo Road, Jacksonville, FL 32224, USA

12.2
Preoperative Evaluation

Both clinical and imaging data must be carefully reviewed prior to selection of components and approaches for shoulder arthroplasty.

The University of California at Los Angeles scoring system is commonly used to grade pain, function and strength pre- and postoperatively (AMSTATZ et al. 1988). The system uses a 10-point scale for each of the areas. Scores in each category are graded as excellent (9–10 points), good (6–8 points), fair (4–5 points) and poor (1–3 points). Patients with severe pain (1–3 points) are likely to experience the greatest improvement (FRIEDMAN et al. 1989).

Preoperative imaging may require a multimodality approach. True AP (anteroposterior), axillary and scapular "Y" views are required to evaluate the joint spaces and osseous abnormalities (Fig. 12.1). Bone changes may be more accurately assessed with computed tomography (CT), especially changes in the glenoid. Significant bone loss and need for bone grafting must be appreciated preoperatively. Magnetic resonance imaging (MRI) is useful for evaluating soft tissue support. Arthrograms and/or preoperative aspirations or diagnostic injections are not commonly employed (BERQUIST 1992; FIGGIE et al. 1988). Templates are used with radiographs to serve as a guide for component selection and sizing (Fig. 12.2).

12.3
Component Selection

Design choices for shoulder arthroplasty include constrained, semi-constrained, and anatomic or non-constrained systems (ALIBRADI et al. 1988; AMSTATZ et al. 1988; BECKER 1991; COFIELD 1983; LETTIN et al. 1982; POST and JABLON 1979; McFARLAND et al. 2002). Constrained components are used for patients with a deficient rotator cuff and inadequate

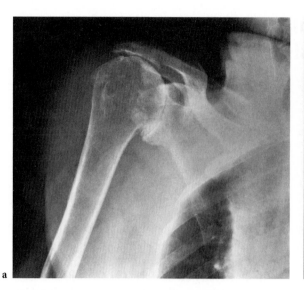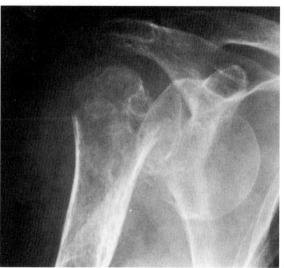

a b

Fig. 12.1a, b. Preoperative radiographs. **a** Anteroposterior view of the shoulder shows advanced degenerative arthritis with loss of humeral acromial space due to a chronic rotator cuff tear. **b** Displaced fracture of the humeral head with high incidence of avascular necrosis. Indication for hemiarthroplasty

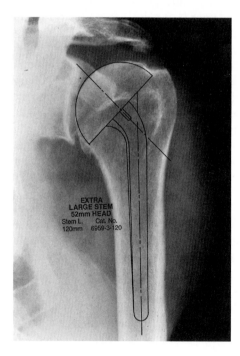

EXTRA
LARGE STEM
52mm HEAD
Stem L,   Cat. No.
120mm   6959-3-120

Fig. 12.2. Anteroposterior radiograph with overlaid humeral component template

soft tissue support (Post 1987; Grammont and Baulot 1993; Rittmeister and Kerschbaumer 2001). These systems have limited indications and an unacceptably high rate of loosening so they are rarely used today (Post 1979). Therefore, we will emphasize nonconstrained designs.

12.3.1
Humeral Components

Humeral component design has progressed from metal or silicone cups in the 1980s to new components used today. The Neer prosthesis has multiple head sizes and 14 types of stems. Bipolar components were designed by Swanson in 1975 for patients with rotator cuff disease. The larger head and unflexed cup distribute deltoid muscle forces over a larger area of the acromion (Swanson et al. 1989).

Modular humeral components are popular today. These systems provide flexibility in matching head and stem configurations needed for a given patient. With some variation, all humeral components have proximal holes for suturing soft tissue or bone fragments (Fig. 12.3).

12.3.2
Glenoid Components

Glenoid components may be configured completely of polyethylene or have polyethylene articular surfaces with metal backing. Fixation is accomplished using pegs, fins, a keel or cancellous screws. Neer et al. (1982) suggested metal backed components for younger, more active patients. Hooded glenoid components are designed for patients with deficient rotator cuffs (Fig. 12.4) (Amstatz et al. 1988).

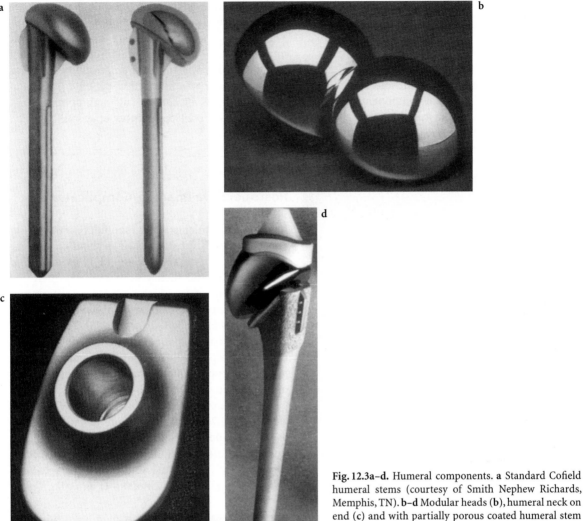

Fig. 12.3a–d. Humeral components. a Standard Cofield humeral stems (courtesy of Smith Nephew Richards, Memphis, TN). b–d Modular heads (b), humeral neck on end (c) and with partially porous coated humeral stem assembled (d) Biomodular Total Shoulder (Courtesy of Biomet, Warsaw, IN)

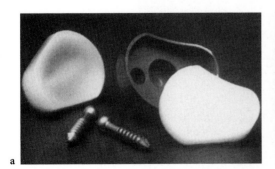
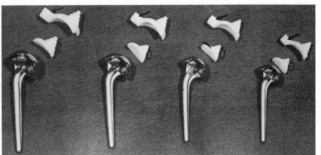

Fig. 12.4a, b. Glenoid components. a Metal backed glenoid component with fixation screws and two thicknesses of polyethylene insert (courtesy of Biomet, Warsaw, IN). b D.A.N.A (designed after natural anatomy; Howmedica, Rutherford, N.J.) total shoulder with non-modular humeral components and hooded (arrows) and standard (open arrows) polyethylene glenoid components

12.4
Hemiarthroplasty versus Total Shoulder Arthroplasty

Numerous humeral components have been developed for hemiarthroplasty (no glenoid component). Bipolar or modular humeral components are commonly used (Fig. 12.5). Hemiarthroplasty is more often selected for patients with avascular necrosis (AVN) (Fig. 12.6), complex humeral head and neck

fractures (see Fig. 12.1) and certain patients with osteoarthritis (INGLIS 1989).

Function and pain relief is most consistently improved with total shoulder arthroplasty. Range of motion is improved more dramatically in patients with osteoarthritis compared to patients with rheumatoid arthritis or rotator cuff arthropathy (BELL and GESCHWEND 1986; BRENNER et al. 1989).

12.5
Postoperative Imaging/Complications

Imaging of patients after shoulder arthroplasty plays a significant role in their evaluation. Routine radiographs are obtained 2, 6 and 12 months after the procedure and then yearly assuming there are no indications of complications. Most authors suggest AP, axillary and scapular "Y" views for screening (AMSTATZ et al. 1988; BERQUIST 1996). This series is adequate for most patients with hemiarthroplasty. However, proper evaluation of the glenoid component and certain humeral components is suboptimal unless the shoulder is fluoroscopically positioned to provide optimal evaluation of implant bone interfaces (Fig. 12.7). Serial radiographs are still the most useful method for evaluating subtle changes over time (BERQUIST 1996). In patients with suspected complications, additional studies may be indicated (WESTHOFF et al. 2002), SPELING et al. 2002).

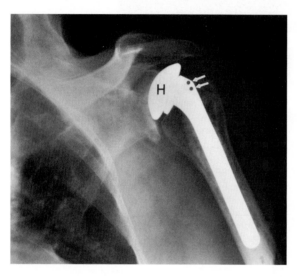

Fig. 12.5. Anteroposterior view of the shoulder after hemiarthroplasty with a modular humeral component. Head size (*H*) can be modified. Note the two holes for soft tissue attachment (*arrows*)

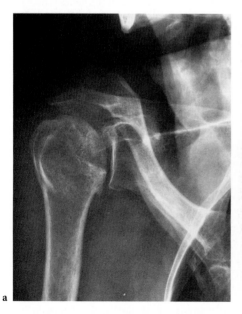
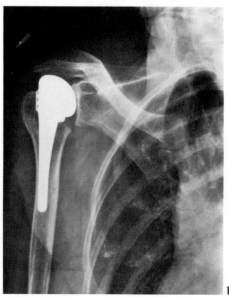

a   b

Fig. 12.6. a Anteroposterior view of the shoulder shows avascular necrosis of the humeral head. The glenoid shows no major defects. **b** Hemiarthroplasty was performed using a modular component

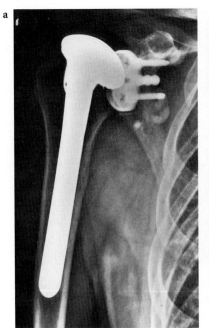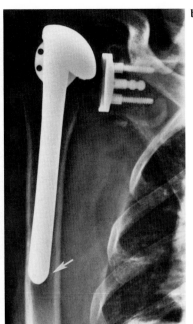

Fig. 12.7a, b. Cofield total shoulder arthroplasty. **a** The anteroposterior (AP) view does not adequately demonstrate the glenoid component interfaces. **b** Fluoroscopically positioned AP shows the glenoid position optimally. Note slight lucency at the humeral tip (*arrow*) raising the question of toggling due to humeral component loosening

Complications related to shoulder arthroplasty vary with the type of prosthesis (constrained, semi-constrained, unconstrained, hemiarthroplasty) and underlying condition (bone, soft tissue integrity) (BARRETT et al. 1987; COFIELD 1984; FRICH et al. 1991; NEER et al. 1982). Table 12.1 summarizes complications of total shoulder arthroplasty. Complication rates in various reports range from 9%–38% (WEISS et al. 1990).

Table 12.1. Complications of total shoulder arthroplasty

Complication	Incidence (%)
Glenoid component loosening	3–15
Humeral component loosening	5
Humeral subsidence	7
Subluxation/dislocation	6
Superior migration of humerus	22
Neural injury	1–2
Infection	1–3
Humeral fracture	1.6

12.5.1
Loosening

Glenoid component loosening is the most frequent complication of shoulder arthroplasty (3%–15% for unconstrained components; average 4.7%) (BELL and GESCHWEND 1986; COFIELD 1984; FRANKLIN et al. 1988) (Fig. 12.8). Humeral component loosening occurs in about 5% (range 1%–7%) of patients (see Fig. 12.7). Lucent lines at the bone cement interface are common with component loosening (Fig. 12.8). Lucent lines alone may not be significant. Serial radiographs that demonstrate lucent lines that progress or exceed 2 mm in width are a more accurate indication of loosening. Progressive superior humeral migration has also been associated with increased incidence of glenoid component loosening (BERQUIST 1996; CRAIG 1988; WEISS 1990).

12.5.2
Humeral Component Migration

Subsidence (sinking of the humeral component into the shaft) occurs in about 7% of cases (ALIBRADI et al. 1988). Superior migration (Fig. 12.9), subluxation and dislocation of the humeral head (Fig. 12.10) have all been reported. Subluxation or dislocation occurs in up to 6% of patients (range 1%–18%). Superior humeral migration occurs in 22%–53% of patients. Humeral migration does not necessarily cause symptoms. It may be related to rotator cuff deficiency or failed cuff repair (Fig. 12.9) (BARRETT et al. 1987; BOYD et al. 1991). Rotator cuff tears are confirmed in about one fourth of patients (BOYD et al. 1991).

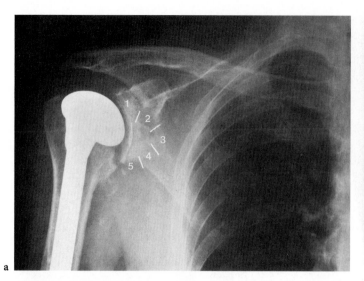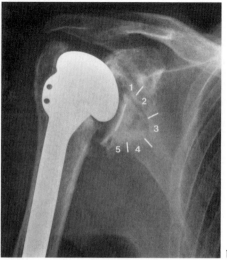

a   b

Fig. 12.8a, b. Glenoid component loosening. **a** Total shoulder arthroplasty demonstrating the five zones evaluated for loosening. Lucent lines are common in *1* and *5*, but more significant in *2–4*. **b** Same patient 6 years later; there is increased width of lucent line on zones *1–3* due to loosening

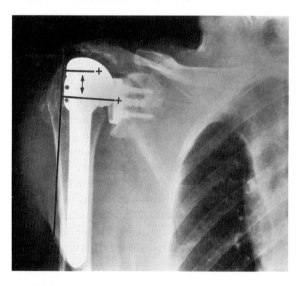

Fig. 12.9. Shoulder arthroplasty with progressive superior humeral migration and reduced humero-acromial space. Consistent measurement assures evaluation of progression on serial radiographs. The center of the humeral head (+) and glenoid (+) are connected by horizontal lines to a line perpendicular to the humeral component to measure change

12.5.3
Infection

Infection is an uncommon complication of shoulder arthroplasty. Deep infection occurs in less than 1% of unconstrained and 2%–3% of constrained prosthesis. Infection after hemiarthroplasty is rare (ALIBRADI et al. 1988; COFIELD 1991).

Routine radiographic features of infection include areas of bone destruction, obvious loosening, endosteal scalloping and periosteal new bone formation (Fig. 12.11) (BERQUIST 1992). Radionuclide scans are also useful. Technetium–99m scans may be positive in normal patients for up to 1 year after surgery. Combined technetium-99m with labeled white blood cells (indium-111 or technetium) is more accurate. Combined arthrography with intra-articular technetium-99m sulfur colloid may be even more useful. Joint aspiration can be performed as part of the latter procedure (MAXON et al. 1989; MAGNUSON et al. 1988).

12.5.4
Nerve Injury

Nerve injury is more common in patients with previous trauma or surgery where scar tissue compromises surgical dissection (CRAIG 1988). The incidence is nevertheless still low (1%–2%) (COFIELD 1991). Imaging may be accomplished with MRI depending upon the type of implant and extent of metal artifact.

12.5.5
Fractures

Fractures of the humeral shaft are uncommon (1.6%) (BONUTTO and HAWKINS 1992). Fractures occur during or after surgery. Conservative therapy

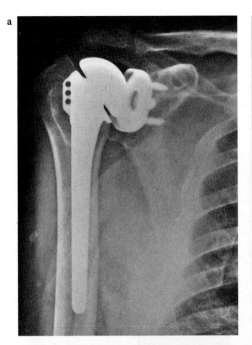

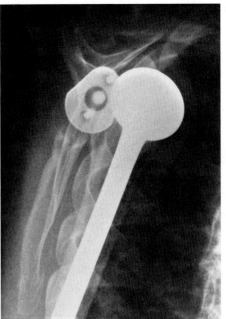

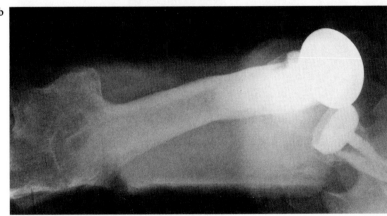

Fig. 12.10a–c. Dislocation. Modular total shoulder arthroplasty with anterior dislocation seen on anteroposterior (a), axillary (b) and scapular "Y" views (c)

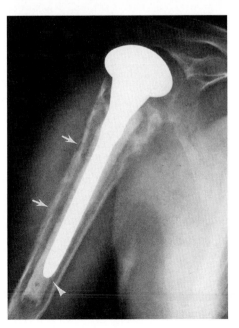

Fig. 12.11. Infected, loose hemiarthroplasty. Anteroposterior view demonstrates irregular lucency at the bone cement interface around the entire component. There is periosteal new bone (arrows) and a cement fracture (arrowhead) due to loosening

or banding with Dall-Miles cables or plastic bands is usually adequate (Figs. 12.12, 12.13). Complications of humeral fractures include radial nerve injury (6%–25%) and non-union (1%–13%) (COFIELD 1991; BOYD et al. 1992). Routine radiographs are adequate for fracture diagnosis. Non-union or nerve injury may be confirmed by MRI. The smooth humeral component causes minimal image distortion. More artifact may be evident when Dall-Miles cables are in place.

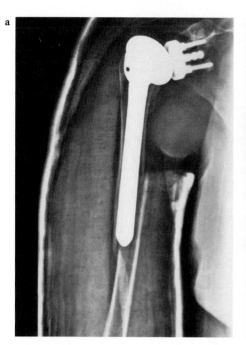

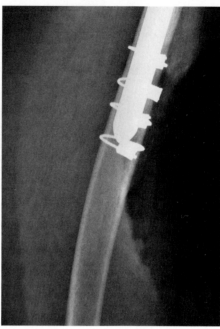

Fig. 12.12. a Antero-posterior view of a Cofield arthroplasty with fracture at the tip of the humeral stem. b After reduction with Dall-Miles cables

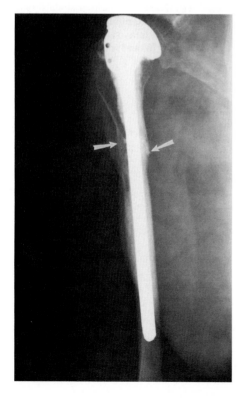

Fig. 12.13. Anteroposterior view of a healed proximal humeral fracture (*arrows*) revised with a long stem humeral component

References

Alibradi P, Weissman BN, Thornhill T, Nippoor N, Sosman JL (1988) Evaluation of a nonconstrained total shoulder prosthesis. AJR 151:1169–1172

Amstatz HC, Thomas BJ, Kabo JM, Jinnah RH, Dorey FJ (1988) The Dana total shoulder arthroplasty. J Bone Joint Surg (Am) 70:1174–1182

Arntz CT, Jackins S, Matsen FA III (1993) Prosthetic replacement of the shoulder for treatment of defects in the rotator cuff and the surface of the glenohumeral joint. J Bone Joint Surg (Am) 75:485–491

Barrett WP, Franklin JL, Jackins SE, Wyss CR, Matsen FA III (1987) Total shoulder arthroplasty. J Bone Joint Surg (Am) 69:865–872

Becker DA (1991) Prosthetic design, surgical technique and rehabilitation. In: Morrey BF, ed. Joint replacement arthroplasty. New York: Churchill Livingstone

Bell SN, Geschwend N (1986) Clinical experience with total arthroplasty and hemiarthroplasty of the shoulder using a Neer prosthesis. Int Orthop 10:217–222

Berquist TH (1992) Imaging of orthopedic trauma. Philadelphia: WB Saunders

Berquist TH (1996) Imagine Atlas of Orthopedic Appliances and Prosthesis. New York, Raven Press

Bonutto PM, Hawkins RJ (1992) Fracture of the humeral shaft associated with total replacement of the shoulder. J Bone Joint Surg (Am) 74:617–618

Boyd AD Jr, Alibradi P, Thornhill TS (1991) Postoperative proximal migration in total shoulder arthroplasty. J Arthroplasty 6:31–37

Boyd AD, Thornhill TS, Barnes CL (1992) Fractures adjacent to humeral prosthesis. J Bone Joint Surg (Am) 74:1498–1504

Brenner BC, Ferlic DC, Clayton ML, Dennis DA (1989) Survivorship of unconstrained total shoulder arthroplasty. J Bone Joint Surg (Am) 71:1289–1296

Cofield RH (1991) Results and complications. In: Morrey BF, ed. Joint replacement arthroplasty. New York: Churchill Livingstone: 437

Cofield RH (1983) Unconstrained total shoulder prosthesis. Clin Orthop 173:97–108

Cofield RH (1984) Total shoulder arthroplasty with the Neer prosthesis. J Bone Joint Surg (Am) 66:899–906.

Craig EV (1988) Total shoulder replacement. Orthopedics 11:125–136

Figgie HE, Inglis AE, Goldberg VM, Ranawat CS, Figgie MP, Wile JM (1988) Analysis of factors affecting the long term results of total shoulder arthroplasty in inflammatory arthritis. J Arthroplasty 3:123–130

Franklin JL, Barrett WP, Jackins SE, Matsen FA III (1988) Glenoid loosening in total shoulder arthroplasty. J Arthroplasty 3:39–46

Frich LH, Sojbjerg JO, Sneppen O (1991) Shoulder arthroplasty in complex and chronic proximal humeral fractures. Orthopedics 14:949–954

Friedman FJ, Thornhill TS, Thomas WH, Sledge CB (1989) Non-constrained total shoulder replacement in patients who have rheumatoid arthritis and class IV function. J Bone Joint Surg (Am) 71:494–498

Grammont PM, Baulot E (1993) Delta shoulder prosthesis for rotator cuff rupture. Orthopaedics 16:65–88

Hasan SS, Leith JM, Campbell B, Kapil R, Smith KL, Matse FA (2002) Characteristics of unsatisfactory shoulder arthroplasties. J Shoulder Elbow Surg 11:431–441

Inglis AE (1989) Advances in implant arthroplasty. Clin Exp Rheumatol 7:141–144

Lettin AW, Copeland SA, Scales JT (1982) The Stanmore total shoulder arthroplasty. J Bone Joint Surg (Br) 64:47–51

Magnuson JE, Brown ML, Hauser MF, Berquist TH, Fitzgerald RH, Klee GG (1988) In-111-labeled leukocyte scintigraphy in suspected orthopedic prosthesis infection: comparison with other imaging modalities. Radiology 168:235–239

Maxon HR, Schneider HJ, Hopson CN, Miller EH, Von Stein DE, Kereuakes JG, Cummings DD, McDevitt RM (1989) A comparative study of indium-111 DTPA radionuclide and iotholamate meglumine roentgenographic arthrography in the evaluation of painful hip arthroplasty. Clin Orthop 245:156–159

McFarland EG, Chronopoulos E, Kim T-K (2002) New trends in shoulder arthroplasty. Curr Opin Orthop 13:275–280

Neer CS II, Watson KC, Stanton FJ (1982) Recent experience in total shoulder replacement. J Bone Joint Surg (Am) 64:319–337

Post M (1987) Constrained arthroplasty of the shoulder. Orthop Clin North (Am) 18:455

Post M, Jablon M (1979) Constrained total shoulder arthroplasty. A critical review. Clin Orthop 144:130–150

Rittmeister M, Kerschbaumer F: Grammont reverse total shoulder arthroplasty in patients with rheumatoid arthritis and nonreconstructible rotator cuff lesions (2001) J Shoulder Elbow Surg 10:17–22

Sperling JW, Potter HG, Craig EV, Flatow E, Warren RF (2002) Magnetic resonance imaging of painful shoulder arthroplasty. J Shoulder Elbow Surg 11:315–321

Swanson AB, Swanson GD, Sattel AB, Cendo RD, Hynes D, Jarning W (1989) Bipolar implant shoulder arthroplasty. Clin Orthop 249:227–247

Weiss A-PC, Adams MA, Moore JR, Weiland AJ (1990) Unconstrained shoulder arthroplasty. Clin Orthop 257:86–90

Westhoff B, Wild A, Werner A, Schneider T, Kahl V, Krauspe R (2002) The value of ultrasound after shoulder arthroplasty. Skeletal Radiol 31:695–701

13 Arthritis

N. Lektrakul, C. B. Chung, D. Resnick

CONTENTS

13.1 Introduction

Arthritis has been classically described as a joint disorder resulting from inflammation. This term has been applied to many individual disease processes, including infection, metabolic disorders, and trauma. Arthritis is a significant public health issue with approximately 350 million people affected worldwide, 37 million people in United States alone. This translates to both significant morbidity for the involved patient population, as well as a significant expenditure of health care dollars for diagnosis and treatment.

The radiographic evaluation of the shoulder joint in the context of arthritis presents both technical and diagnostic challenges with respect to imaging findings and the development of differential diagnostic considerations. These challenges will be discussed in the following text.

N. Lektrakul, MD; C. B. Chung, MD; D. Resnick, MD
Radiology Department, Veterans Affairs San Diego Healthcare System, University of California, San Diego, 3350 La Jolla Village Drive, San Diego CA 92161, USA

13.2 Technical Considerations

Radiography has been used as a gold standard in the evaluation of arthritis because of its advantages of wide availability, low cost, reproducibility, and extensive experience with its use. There are, however, certain disadvantages with this technique including relatively poor contrast for soft tissues, no means for direct visualization of the articular cartilage, synovium, joint fluid and capsulolabral structures, and relative insensitivity to the early detection of bone erosions.

The distance between apposing articular cortices on radiographs has been used as an indirect measure for cartilage thickness in many joints (Buckland-Wright et al. 1995), but is valid only where the articular cartilage surfaces are directly in contact with each other. In the knee and (less accurately) the hip, this can be accomplished by obtaining the image while the patient is standing. Applying an appropriate load to the glenohumeral joint is more difficult and not practical. Moreover, beam centering must be tangential to the joint line, which in the shoulder requires 40° posterior-oblique positioning (Brower 1988). In addition, the clinician must correct for magnification effects

Arthrography can offer a partial solution by delineating the articular cartilage surfaces in the glenohumeral joint, revealing regions of cartilage loss. Due to the curved nature of the articular surface of the humeral head and the orientation of the glenoid cavity, this means of evaluation offers limited visualization of the entirety of the articular surface of this joint. Furthermore, it offers no real means to analyze the soft tissues and is an invasive procedure.

Bone scintigraphy may be helpful in the evaluation of articular disease. It may confirm the presence of disease, demonstrate the distribution of disease, and even help to evaluate the activity of the disease. It is widely accepted as a very sensitive but nonspecific technique with poor resolution limiting its application.

Computed tomography (CT) provides excellent contrast resolution and has the advantage of allowing cross sectional display of anatomic regions. CT of the shoulder is limited to a direct axial plane of section. Although reconstructed images are routinely available on most scanners, the approximation of the articular surface is not adequate for detection of subtle osseous changes. The soft tissue contrast is certainly superior to that of conventional radiography, but not optimal when compared to other imaging techniques. For these reasons, CT is not generally required in the evaluation of arthritis. The main indication for this imaging method is the detection of small intraarticular bodies seen in cases of advanced osteoarthritis. When combined with intraarticular contrast material, this technique offers excellent evaluation of the surface of the glenohumeral articular cartilage and capsulolabral structures. CT arthrography is invasive, however, and does not provide visualization of intrasubstance changes that may precede morphologic changes in these structures.

Ultrasonography can offer direct multiplanar imaging capability and sufficient soft tissue contrast to visualize the articular cartilage, synovium, joint fluid, and other important articular structures. In numerous recent studies, it has proven more sensitive and specific than magnetic resonance (MR) imaging for the evaluation of changes in the synovium, although it has proven less effective in the assessment of early erosive changes in bone (KOSKI 1991; ALASAARELA et al. 1997; BACKHAUS et al. 1999). Studies are currently under way to evaluate the role of contrast agents in conjunction with ultrasonography for synovial analysis. Ultrasonography of the glenohumeral joint can be somewhat challenging due to the acoustic shadowing that results from the coracoacromial arch and portions of the scapula. The dynamic nature of this study, requiring the patient to place the shoulder in different positions to completely visualize all parts of the joint, can be advantageous, allowing the examiner to identify symptomatic areas. Ultrasonography could also prove problematic for obtaining a complete examination in patients with a limited range of shoulder motion. In addition, the performance and interpretation of the examination are highly dependent on the experience and expertise of the operator.

MR imaging is especially well suited to evaluation of the shoulder owing to multiplanar imaging capability and excellent soft tissue contrast. As previously mentioned, it offers an excellent way to evaluate the synovium, although it is less sensitive and specific than ultrasonography. It has proven to be the optimal means to detect the presence of early erosive change in inflammatory processes and has been incorpo-

rated into some scoring systems for rheumatoid arthritis. When used in conjunction with the intravenous administration of contrast material, it has also been used to distinguish active inflammatory pannus from inactive fibrous pannus, a distinction that could have significant implications for diagnosis as well as monitoring progression of disease. In addition, this imaging technique has emerged as an excellent way to evaluate articular cartilage, subchondral bone, and marrow edema, all implicated in the pathogenesis of osteoarthritis.

13.3
Specific Abnormalities

13.3.1
Joint Effusion and Synovial Inflammation

A joint effusion represents a non-specific response to a variety of articular insults. Routine radiography is relatively insensitive in the detection of an early effusion. MR imaging can readily assess joint fluid by its location and by its low to intermediate signal intensity on T1-weighted and proton density-weighted images and its high signal intensity on T2-weighted images. WINALSKI et al. (1993) have shown that a joint effusion gradually enhances after intravenous gadolinium administration with the peripheral fluid enhancing first. This phenomenon is important to recognize because the peripheral rim of enhancing joint fluid may be misinterpreted as enhanced, thickened synovium; thus, noninflammatory joint effusion may be mistakenly diagnosed as synovitis.

The synovial membrane is a highly vascular tissue that lines portions of synovial joints, bursae, and tendon sheaths. Synovial inflammation and proliferation are believed to be responsible for joint destruction and have been monitored clinically in patients with rheumatoid arthritis to determine the need for or response to therapy. The findings can be difficult to quantify, but can be done with specific software packages that calculate the synovial volume when MR imaging is performed in conjunction with the intravenous administration of contrast material. Plain radiographs, CT, and non-contrast-enhanced MR images can not easily differentiate between synovial thickening and joint fluid (BJÖRKENGREN et al. 1990).

Most synovial tissue exhibits a slightly shorter T1 than joint fluid, but under normal circumstances, the contrast on T1-weighted images is relatively poor.

Intravenous gadolinium administration can improve synovial contrast by enhancing this highly vascular tissue on T1-weighted images and allows the differentiation of active synovial inflammation from joint effusion. Synovial enhancement is present within minutes, plateaus after 30 min, and persists for at least 1 h. Thus, MR images must be obtained immediately after intravenous gadolinium injection and compared with non-contrast-enhanced MR images to allow differentiation between synovial enhancement and delayed enhancement of synovial fluid (WINALSKI et al. 1993).

Gadolinium-enhanced MR imaging has also been used to grade the severity of synovial inflammation (BJÖRKENGREN et al. 1990). A rapid synovial enhancement rate and high maximal enhancement following bolus intravenous injection of gadolinium correlate with severe synovial inflammation and hyperplasia, whereas sluggish enhancement corresponds to chronic fibrotic synovium. This may be useful for monitoring therapeutic response and optimizing therapeutic regimens in individual patients (PETERFY et al. 1998).

13.3.2
Bone Erosion

Bone erosions are the earliest and most prognostically important radiographic changes in rheumatoid arthritis, appearing within the first 2 years after the onset of symptoms in about 90% of patients (BROOK and CORBETT 1977). Radiography can be used to determine the extent of bone damage but is of limited usefulness because the disease must be relatively advanced before bone changes become apparent (LANNUZZI et al. 1983). MR imaging has been shown to be more sensitive than radiography for detecting bone erosions in rheumatoid arthritis. Bone erosions appear on T1-weighted MR imaging as subcortical areas of low signal in the marrow adjacent to the bony margin or beneath the chondral surface.

Because the synovial inflammatory tissue within the bone erosions enhances so intensely, a gadolinium-enhanced fat-suppressed spoiled gradient recalled acquisition in the steady state (SPGR) sequence was considered to be more sensitive than any other sequence in the detection of such erosion. However, pannus enhancement is sometimes so intense that bone anatomy was actually obscured by it. In these instances, T1-weighted images give the clearest demonstration of the shape and size of individual bone erosions (ROMINGER et al. 1993).

13.3.3
Articular Cartilage Loss

The humeral head is round and covered by articular cartilage with the exception of the bare area on its posterior aspect (NOTTAGE 1995). This area is more prone to cartilage and bone erosion in early rheumatoid arthritis (RIEDERER et al. 1999). If cartilage damage occurs, the patient's condition has progressed beyond the phase of reversible inflammation into that of irreversible joint destruction (HARRIS 1990). The detection of subtle chondral changes has become increasingly important as more sophisticated treatment options for cartilage damage become available. Ultrasonography and MR imaging have been proven useful for evaluation of articular cartilage.

With ultrasonography, the articular cartilage typically appears as a thin hypoechoic, homogeneous layer between two curvilinear, echoic, smooth lines that are associated with the anterior cartilage–soft tissue and posterior cartilage–subchondral bone interfaces (Fig. 13.1). Blurring of the normal sharp anterior articular margin, loss of cartilage clarity, narrowing of joint cartilage, and increased intensity of the posterior bone–cartilage interface are sonographic features of osteoarthritis (GRASSI et al. 1999).

A variety of MR sequences have been proposed for the evaluation of articular cartilage. Unfortunately, most of them are inadequate related to the complexity of articular cartilage, which is not a uniform structure with regard to its cellularity or collagen fiber composition (RESNICK 1994). Three-dimensional (3D) SPGR sequences obtained with fat suppression are currently considered the best clinically applicable sequence to evaluate articular cartilage. DISLER et al. (1996) showed 85% sensitivity and 97% specificity for detecting articular damage using this sequence. This sequence can provide high spatial resolution and a high contrast-to-noise ratio between cartilage and fluid and between cartilage and bone. Although conventional spin-echo images are not sensitive for the detection of abnormalities of articular cartilage, proton density-weighted and T2-weighted fast spin-echo images with fat suppression have been shown to be highly sensitive, with similar results as those achieved for 3D SPGR imaging (BRODERICK et al. 1994; BREDELLA et al. 1999; POTTER et al. 1998) (Figs. 13.2, 13.3).

A vast amount of research time and money has been dedicated to the evaluation of articular cartilage, in particular to cartilage imaging. The current direction of imaging appears to be emphasizing

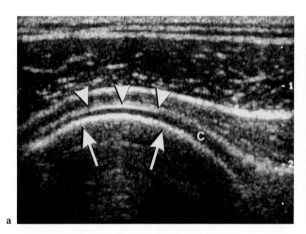
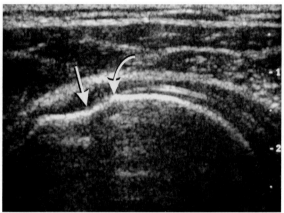

Fig. 13.1a, b. Ultrasound of the left shoulder. **a** The normal cartilage appears as a homogeneously anechoic band easily differentiated from adjacent tissue. *C*, cartilage; *arrowheads*, cartilage–soft tissue interface; *arrows*, posterior bone–cartilage interface. **b** The humeral head is covered by the articular cartilage (*curved arrow*) except in the bare area (*straight arrow*) on the posterolateral aspect which is more prone to bony erosion in early rheumatoid arthritis

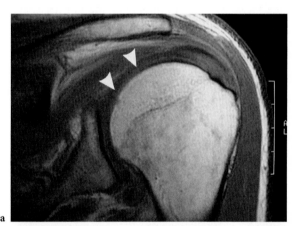

Fig. 13.2a–c. Articular cartilage of left shoulder. **a** Coronal oblique T1-weighted spin echo (566/12.2) magnetic resonance (MR) image shows the poor contrast between the cartilage (*arrowheads*) and adjacent structures. **b, c** Axial fat-suppressed intermediate-weighted (2550/10.6) fast spin-echo (**b**) and three-dimensional fat-suppressed spoiled gradient recalled acquisition in the steady state (SPGR) (60/5/40) (**c**) MR images demonstrate the articular cartilage (*arrowheads*) as a high signal intensity structure contrasted against the low signal intensity of the suppressed marrow fat

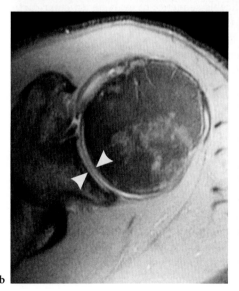
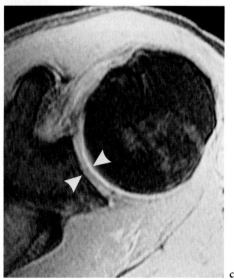

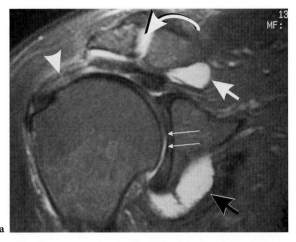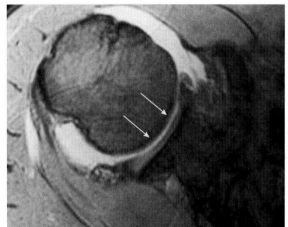

Fig. 13.3a, b. Articular cartilage loss. Coronal oblique fat-suppressed T2-weighted fast spin echo (3500/64) (**a**) and axial fat-suppressed gradient echo (600/20/20) (**b**) MR images demonstrate loss of articular cartilage at the inferior surface of the humerus (*double arrows*). A tear of the supraspinatus tendon (*arrowhead*), fluid in the subacromial bursa (*white straight arrow*) and a joint effusion (*black straight arrow*) are seen. Note the osteoarthritis changes at the acromioclavicular joint (*curved arrow*)

novel imaging sequences, attaining an optimal signal-to-noise ratio by use of higher field strength magnets and local gradient coils, and exploring functional imaging with the help of the administration of contrast material in conjunction with MR imaging.

In MR images, cartilage defects due to osteoarthritis are distinguished from sites of chondral injury. In osteoarthritis, there are usually multiple such defects or diffuse cartilage thinning. The defects are variable in size and depth. The margins of the cartilaginous defects are typically broadly obtuse in angulation, whereas chondral defects resulting from injury are acutely marginated. In addition to this, MR images of cases of osteoarthritis show features of extrinsic repair such as osteophyte formation and subchondral bone sclerosis (DISLER et al. 2000).

13.3.4
Marrow Edema

Marrow edema can sometimes be seen subjacent to the areas of articular cartilage loss in arthritic joints. Such marrow edema is depicted with high sensitivity using short tau inversion recovery (STIR) or fast spin-echo STIR sequences. Fat suppressed T2-weighted fast spin-echo sequences are also highly sensitive; they offer the advantage of higher resolution and improved contrast for articular cartilage with elimination of fat-induced motion and chemical-shift artifacts. However, spectral fat suppression can be difficult to use in the shoulder

because of magnetic field heterogeneities associated with shoulder anatomy.

13.3.5
Intraarticular Bodies

Intraarticular bodies can relate to a variety of articular insults. In the glenohumeral joint, they can be found in the subscapular recess as a typical finding of osteoarthritis. These bodies may consist of cartilage alone, cartilage and bone together, or rarely bone alone (RESNICK 1994). They are usually round or ovoid and smoothly marginated and may appear laminated. Routine radiography, ultrasonography, and CT alone or combined with arthrography are useful techniques in the assessment of intraarticular bodies. MR imaging lacks sensitivity in this particular diagnosis (RESNICK 1994).

13.3.6
Rotator Cuff Tear

Complete rupture of the rotator cuff is a common late complication in a number of conditions affecting the glenohumeral joint, such as osteoarthritis, mechanical trauma, or inflammatory disorders. Such ruptures may go clinically unrecognized because of preexisting pain and immobility. With chronic cuff disruption, conventional radiography reveals the secondary sign of abnormal alignment of the shoulder with a high riding humeral head. Arthrography, ultrasonography, CT arthrography, and MR imaging are more sensitive methods for the detection of tears of the rotator cuff.

13.4
Specific Diseases

13.4.1
Osteoarthritis

Osteoarthritis is common, especially in the elderly (HAMERMAN 1995), and women are affected more frequently than men. The abnormalities predominate in the cartilaginous and osseous tissue, whereas alterations in the synovial membrane are generally mild. Degenerative changes in the acromioclavicular joint are far more common than in the glenohumeral joint. Articular degeneration may result from either abnormal concentration of force on a normal joint or normal concentration of force on an abnormal joint (RESNICK and NIWAYAMA 1995a). As the glenohumeral joint is clearly not a weight-bearing articulation, the diagnosis of osteoarthritis necessitates the consideration of a predisposing primary process such as trauma, chronic repetitive microtrauma, metabolic disorders, osteonecrosis, rotator cuff tear, crystal deposition diseases such as calcium pyrophosphate dihydrate (CPPD) arthropathy, or neuropathic disorders.

Radiographically, the typical findings of osteoarthritis include joint space narrowing, osteophytosis, bony eburnation, subchondral cyst formation, and intraarticular osteochondral bodies (Fig. 13.4). Joint space narrowing appears to be a relatively late manifestation of glenohumeral joint osteoarthritis (KERR et al. 1985) The most frequent degenerative abnormality is the formation of osteophytes along the articular margin of the humeral head and the line of attachment of the labrum to the glenoid, which are best seen when radiographs are obtained with external rotation of the humerus (Fig. 13.5). Focal or global eburnation of the articular surface of the humeral head is manifested radiographically as subchondral sclerosis. It is most evident in the middle and superior parts of the humeral head, those surfaces in contact with glenoid fossa when the arm is abducted between 60–100°. Osteophytes that project inferiorly at the acromioclavicular joint commonly exert mass effect on the rotator cuff and contribute to the external shoulder impingement syndrome.

13.4.2
Rheumatoid Arthritis

Rheumatoid arthritis is a common, chronic disease characterized by bilateral, symmetrical joint involvement. It predominates in women between 25 and 55 years of age. The major abnormalities of rheumatoid arthritis appear in the synovial joints of the appendicular skeleton, particularly the small joints of the hand and foot, the wrist, the knee, and the elbow. Rheumatoid arthritis of shoulder is not uncommon (KIEFT et al. 1990). It can affect the synovium within the glenohumeral and acromioclavicular joints, the distal third of the clavicle, rotator cuff tendons, bursae, and surrounding muscles (RESNICK and NIWAYAMA 1995b). Synovial inflammation may appear as fibrous nodules that resemble grains of polished rice, commonly referred to as *rice bodies* (CHEUNG et al. 1980; POPERT et al. 1982) (Fig. 13.6).

Radiographically, the typical findings of rheumatoid arthritis include marginal bone erosions without bone apposition, osteoporosis, and soft tissue swelling (BELTRAN et al. 1987) (Figs 13.7, 13.8). Changes in the glenohumeral joint are joint space narrowing, bony sclerosis, and cyst formation. The diminution of articular space can be accompanied by marginal erosions, which are most prominent along the superolateral portion of the humerus, adjacent to the greater tuberosity. Such erosions may resemble a Hill Sach lesion. A deep bony erosion may develop on the medial aspect of the surgical neck of the humerus, related to abnormal pressure exerted by the adjacent glenoid margin; rarely, a pathologic fracture of the

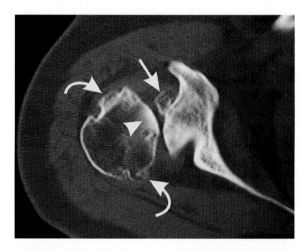

Fig. 13.4. Axial computed tomogram of the right shoulder demonstrate the intraarticular bodies (*straight arrow*). Note the osteophyte formation at the inferior aspect of the humeral head (*curved arrow*) and subchondral sclerosis (*arrowhead*)

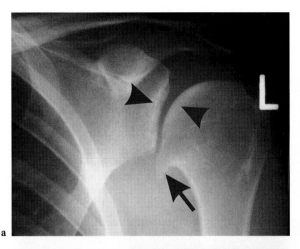

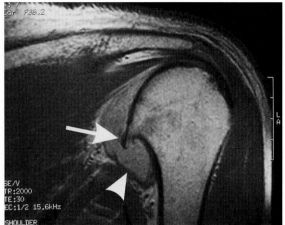

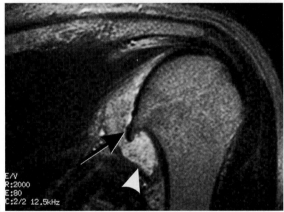

Fig. 13.5a–c. Osteoarthritis. **a** Radiograph of the left shoulder demonstrates narrowing of the glenohumeral joint with subchondral sclerosis (*arrowheads*). Note the osteophyte (*arrow*) at the inferior aspect of the humeral head. **b, c** Coronal oblique intermediate-weighted (2000/30) (**b**) and T2-weighted (2000/80) spin echo (**c**) MR images demonstrate the osteophyte (*arrow*) at the inferior aspect of the humeral head. A joint effusion (*arrowhead*) is also seen

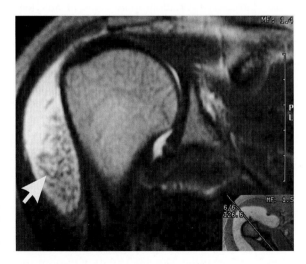

Fig. 13.6. Rheumatoid arthritis. Coronal oblique T2-weighted spin echo (2000/80) MR image of the shoulder demonstrates multiple fibrous nodules, or rice bodies (*arrow*), in the subacromial–subdeltoid bursa

humeral neck may result. At the acromioclavicular joint, the early findings are soft tissue swelling and erosions, which tend to be more prominent on the clavicular side of the joint. Destruction of the large portion of the distal clavicle may be seen as a late manifestation.

13.4.3
Seronegative Spondyloarthropathies

Rheumatoid arthritis and seronegative spondyloarthropathies have many similar radiographic and pathologic features. Both may cause considerable inflammation of synovial articulations, bursae, and tendon sheaths. However, there are some differences between these two entities, especially in the distribution and morphology of the abnormalities. Alterations in spondyloarthropathies characteristi-

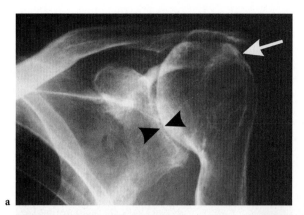

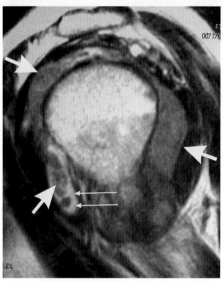

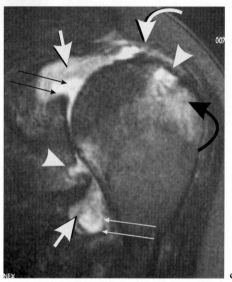

Fig. 13.7a–c. Rheumatoid arthritis. **a** Conventional radiograph of the left shoulder demonstrates narrowing of the glenohumeral joint (*arrowheads*). A high riding of the humeral head is seen, suggestive of rotator cuff tear. Note the bony erosion at the posterolateral aspect of the humeral head (*arrow*). **b, c** Sagittal oblique intermediate-weighted spin echo (3000/16) (**b**) and coronal oblique fat-suppressed T2-weighted fast spin echo (3000/99.2) (**c**) MR images demonstrate lower signal intensity of synovial proliferation (*white straight arrow*) than joint effusion, representing pannus. Tear of the supraspinatus at musculotendinous junction (*white curved arrow*) is seen. Bone erosion (*arrowhead*) in the posterolateral aspect of the humerus and inferior aspect of glenoid is noted. Adjacent marrow edema (*black curved arrow*) is also seen

cally occur in synovial and cartilaginous joints as well as at sites of tendon and ligament attachment to bone, called entheses. The two major seronegative spondyloarthropathies afflicting the shoulder are ankylosing spondylitis and psoriatic arthropathy, which have several similar pathologic and imaging features including the presence of erosive abnormalities, osseous proliferation, and intraarticular osseous ankylosis. Osteoporosis may be absent. The degree of inflammation in synovial articulations, bursae, and tendon sheaths is generally less severe than in rheumatoid arthritis.

Ankylosing spondylitis typically has an insidious onset in patients between the ages of 15 and 35 years; men are affected 4 to 10 times more often than women (RESNICK and NIWAYAMA 1995b). The disease has predilection for involvement of the axial skeleton. The shoulder is affected in one third of patients with chronic ankylosing spondylitis (EMERY et al. 1991). The shoulder abnormalities usually are bilateral, and include derangement in the glenohumeral,

acromioclavicular, and coracoclavicular joints. The most characteristic radiographic signs of ankylosing spondylitis in the shoulder include prominent erosive defects that occur at the superolateral aspect of the humeral head, termed the hatchet deformity (Fig. 13.9), as well as enthesophytes that occur at the acromial attachment of the coracoacromial ligament, termed a bearded acromion. Scalloping of inferior surface of clavicle at or near the site of attachment of the coracoclavicular ligament may be secondary to inflammatory enthesopathy, bursitis, or mechanical changes. Destructive articular changes in the acromioclavicular joint are identical to those in rheumatoid arthritis (RESNICK and NIWAYAMA 1995b).

Psoriatic arthritis has a similar age of onset as rheumatoid arthritis, and no sex predilection. Psoriatic arthritis is commonly asymmetric or even unilateral in distribution. The small joints of the foot and hand are the primary target sites. When the glenohumeral, acromioclavicular, and sternoclavicular joints are affected, the characteristic radiographic findings

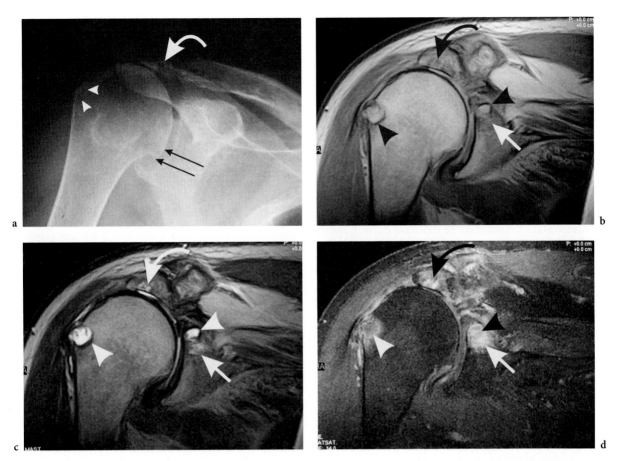

Fig. 13.8a–d. Rheumatoid arthritis. **a** Radiograph of the right shoulder demonstrates a high riding of humerus related to rotator cuff tear. Erosion of the inferior aspect of the clavicle (*curved arrow*), small osteophyte at the inferior aspect of the humeral head (*double arrows*), and subchondral cysts in the humeral head (*arrowheads*) are seen. **b–d** Coronal oblique intermediate-weighted MR image (2000/16) (**b**), T2-weighted MR image (2000/80) (**c**), and fat-suppressed T1-weighted (645/14) spin echo MR image (**d**) with intravenous gadolinium administration demonstrate increased enhancement of pannus within the bone erosion in the inferior aspect of the clavicle (*curved arrow*) and superior aspect of glenoid (*straight arrow*). The rim enhancement in the lateral aspect of the humerus and superior aspect of the glenoid suggests the presence of a subchondral bone cyst (*arrowhead*). Note the high riding humerus related to rotator cuff tear

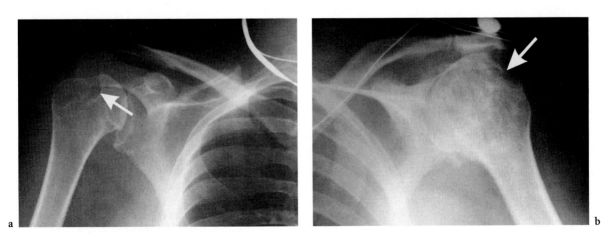

Fig. 13.9a, b. Hatchet deformity. Radiographs of two different patients with ankylosing spondylitis demonstrate prominent bone erosion in the superolateral aspect of the humerus (*arrow*)

are a combination of bone proliferation, periarticular osseous erosion, and joint space narrowing (BOUTIN and WEISSMAN 1997).

13.5
Summary

Recent advances in the treatment of arthritis including osteochondral grafting, autologous chondrocyte implantation, and the use of chondroprotective drugs, have necessitated accurate early diagnosis of articular disease and an assessment of its extent. Some imaging methods, such as ultrasonography and MR imaging, are critical to early diagnosis and may allow monitoring of the progression of disease as well as its response to therapy. Despite this emphasis on more sophisticated means of imaging, the role for conventional radiographic evaluation of the shoulder joint as an initial screening examination should not be underestimated.

References

Alasaarela E, Takalo R, Tervonen O, Hakala M, Suramo I (1997) Sonography and MRI in the evaluation of painful arthritic shoulder. Br J Rheumatol 36:996–1000

Backhaus M, Kamradt T, Sandrock D et al (1999) Arthritis of the finger joints: a comprehensive approach comparing conventional radiography, scintigraphy, ultrasound, and contrast-enhanced magnetic resonance imaging. Arthritis Rheum 42:1232–1245

Beltran J, Caudill JL, Herman LA et al (1987) Rheumatoid arthritis: MR imaging manifestations. Radiology 165: 153–157

Björkengren AG, Geborek R, Rydholm U, Holt_s S, Petterson H (1990) MR imaging of the knee in acute rheumatoid arthritis: synovial uptake of gadolinium-DOTA. AJR 155: 329–332

Boutin RD, Weissman BN (1997) MR imaging of arthritides affecting the shoulder. MR Clin North Am 5:861–879

Bredella MA, Tirman PFJ, Peterfy CG et al (1999) Accuracy of T2-weighted fast spin-echo MR imaging with fat saturation in detecting cartilage defects in the knee: comparison with arthroscopy in 130 patients. AJR 172:1073–1080

Broderick LS, Turner DA, Renfrew DL et al (1994) Severity of articular cartilage abnormalities in patients with osteoarthritis: evaluation with fast spin-echo MR vs arthroscopy. AJR 162:99–103

Brook A, Corbett M (1997) radiographic changes in early rheumatoid disease. Ann Rheum Dis 36:71–73

Brower AC (1988) Imaging techniques and modalities. In: Arthritis in black and white. Saunders, Philadelphia, pp 1–30

Buckland-Wright JC, Macafrlane DG, Lynch JA, Jasani MK, Bradshaw CR (1995) Joint space width measures cartilage

thickness in osteoarthritis of the knee: high resolution plain film and double contrast macroradiographic investigation. Ann Rheum Dis 54:263–268

Cheung HS, Ryan LM, Kozin F, McCarty DJ (1980) Synovial origins of rice bodies in joint fluid. Arthritis Rheum 23: 72–76

Disler DG, McCauley TR, Kelman CG et al (1996) Fat-suppressed three-dimensional spoiled gradient echo MR imaging of hyaline cartilage defects in the knee: comparison with standard MR imaging and arthroscopy. AJR 167: 127–132

Disler DG, Recht MP, McCauley TR (2000) MR imaging of articular cartilage. Skeletal Radiol 29:367–377

Emery RJH, Ho EKW, Leong JCY (1991) The shoulder girdle in ankylosing spondylitis. J Bone Joint Surg (Am) 73: 1526–1531

Grassi W, Lamanna G, Farina A, Cervini C (1999) Sonographic imaging of normal and osteoarthritic cartilage. Semin Arthritis Rheum 28 :398–403

Hamerman D (1995) Clinical implications of osteoarthritis and aging. Ann Rheum Dis 54:82–85

Harris ED (1990) Rheumatoid arthritis: pathophysiology and implications for therapy. N Engl J Med 322:1277–1289

Kerr R, Resnick D, Pineda C, Haghighi P (1985) Osteoarthritis of the glenohumeral joint: a radiologic-pathologic study. AJR 144:967–972

Kieft GJ, Dijkmans BAC, Bloem Jl, Kroon HM (1990) Magnetic resonance imaging of the shoulder in patients with rheumatoid arthritis. Ann Rheum Dis 49:7–11

Koski JM (1991) Validity of axillary ultrasound scanning in detecting effusion of the glenohumeral joint. Scand J Rheumatol 20:49–51

Lannuzzi L, Dawson N, Zein N, Kurshner I (1983) Does drug therapy slow radiographic deterioration in rheumatoid arthritis? N Engl J Med 309:1023–1028

Nottage WM (1995) Arthroscopic anatomy of the glenohumeral joint and subacromial bursa. Orthop Clin North Am 24:27–32

Peterfy CG, Mow VC, Bigliani LU (1998) Evaluating arthritic changes in the shoulder with MRI. In: Steinbach LS, Tirman PFL, Peterfy CG, Feller JF (eds) Shoulder magnetic resonance imaging. Lippincott-Raven, Philadelphia, pp 221–235

Popert AJ, Scott DL, Wainwright AC, Walton KW, Williamson N, Chapman JH (1982) Frequency of occurrence, mode of development, and significance of rice bodies in rheumatoid joints. Ann Rheum Dis 41:109–117

Potter HG, Linklater JM, Allen AA, Hannafin JA, Haas SB (1998) Magnetic resonance imaging of articular cartilage in the knee: an evaluation with use of fast-spin-echo imaging. J Bone Joint Surg Am 80:1276–1284

Resnick D (1994) Magnetic resonance imaging of articular abnormalities. Acta Radiol Portuguesa 6:23–25

Resnick D, Niwayama G (1995a) Degenerative disease of extraspinal locations. In: Resnick D (ed) Diagnosis of bone and joint disorders, 3rd edn. Saunders, Philadelphia, pp 1263–1371

Resnick D, Niwayama G (1995b) Rheumatoid arthritis and the seronegative spondyloarthropathies: radiographic and pathologic concepts. In: Resnick D (ed) Diagnosis of bone and joint disorders, 3rd edn. Saunders, Philadelphia, pp 807–865

Riederer B, Chhem RK, Cardinal E, Petroon P (1999) Shoulder: nonrotator cuff disorders. In: Chhem RK, Cardinal E (eds) Guideline and gamuts in musculoskeletal ultrasound. Wiley-Liss, New York, pp 1–37

Rominger MB, Bernreuter WK, Kenny PJ et al (1993) MR imaging of the hands in early rheumatoid arthritis: preliminary results. Radiographics 13:37–46

Winalski CS, Aliabadi P, Wright JR et al (1993) Enhancement of joint fluid with intravenously administered gadopenetetate dimeglumine: technique, rationale, and implications. Radiology 187:179–185

14 Infection

S.-T. Quek, W. C. G. Peh, V. N. Cassar-Pullicino

CONTENTS

14.1
Introduction

Infections around the shoulder are an uncommonly encountered but important clinical problem because of the serious morbidity that may result (GELBERMAN et al. 1980). They are more common in the paediatric age group, occur more frequently in certain disease states, e.g. diabetes mellitus, immuno-compromised host, sickle cell disease, drug abuse etc., and are easily overlooked in the elderly population. Several predisposing factors have been implicated with the major ones being altered host immunity

S.-T. Quek, MBBS, FRCR
Consultant, Department of Diagnostic Radiology, National Cancer Centre, Singapore 169610
W. C. G. Peh, MBBS, MD, FRCPG, FRCPE, FRCR
Senior Consultant, Department of Diagnostic Radiology, Singapore General Hospital, Singapore 169608
V. N. Cassar-Pullicino, MD, FRCR
Consultant and Clinical Director , Department of Diagnostic Radiology, The Institute of Orthopaedics, Robert Jones and Agnes Hunt Orthopaedic Hospital, Oswestry, Shropshire UK SY10 7AG

and the virulence of organisms gaining access to the joint. Prognosis depends on a number of factors, with a favourable outcome being most often dependent on early diagnosis coupled with aggressive and appropriate treatment.

14.2
Mechanism of Spread/Route of Infection

The infection may be confined to the joint or it may involve the bone or surrounding soft tissues resulting in osteomyelitis, bursitis, cellulitis or pyomyositis. Regardless of whether it affects the joint, bone or soft tissues, there are four basic routes (Fig. 14.1) through which infection may occur (RESNICK and NIWAYAMA 1995), namely:

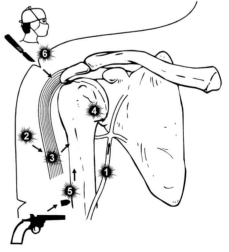

Fig. 14.1. Mechanisms of route of spread of infection. Haematogenous spread (*1*) is the commonest route causing septic arthritis and osteomyelitis. Cellulitis (*2*), pyomyositis (*3*) and osteomyelitis (*4*) may remain confined or co-exist through adjacent spread. Metaphyseal osteomyelitis (*4*) can rupture into the joint causing septic arthritis. Penetrating injury (*5*), diagnostic and surgical techniques (*6*) can also introduce infection in the shoulder

1. Haematogenous spread of infection

   Spread via the bloodstream is the most common mode of contamination. This often arises from foci of infection elsewhere, e.g. the genitourinary or respiratory systems. However, it should be noted that in some cases, no primary source of infection can be identified.

2. Spread from an adjacent source of infection

   Musculoskeletal infections may also result from spread from an adjacent contaminated source. A primarily extra-skeletal infective source such as cellulitis or soft tissue infection can subsequently involve the neighbouring osseous and articular structures. Similarly as the intra-articular growth plate lies within the shoulder capsule, septic arthritis may occur from direct extension of a metaphyseal focus of infection when a metaphyseal abscess ruptures into the joint cavity.

3. Direct implantation

   This usually occurs following trauma to the area whereby organisms are introduced via a penetrating injury or puncture wound. In the shoulder, infection may also result from joint aspiration or injection following a diagnostic or therapeutic procedure (LESLIE et al. 1989).

4. Post-operative infection

   Although often the result of direct implantation of organisms during surgery, this is such an important route of spread that it is often considered in a category of its own. The increasing frequency and complexity of orthopaedic procedures, such as arthroscopy and joint replacement surgery, has resulted in a corresponding increase in the number of post-operative infections encountered. In addition to the usual risk factors for developing infection such as systemic disease and the use of steroids, other factors predisposing to infection following surgery include prolonged operative time, prior surgery, as well as the complexity of the surgical procedure (Goss 1993).

Scant information is available with regard to infection rate following surgery to the shoulder but a rate of approximately 2% following total shoulder arthroplasty (TSA) for constrained systems, and a rate of less than 1% for unconstrained systems or for humeral prosthetic placement alone has been suggested (COFIELD 1991; SILLIMAN and HAWKINS 1994). Infection may occur in the early post-operative period, or as long as months or years following the initial surgery. The former is usually the result of direct implantation during the surgery itself whereas the latter is often due to haematogenous spread from a systemic focus elsewhere (AHLBERG et al. 1978).

14.3
Organisms

Bacterial infections account for the majority of cases with *Staphylococcus aureus* (MADER et al. 1999) being the most common organism implicated. Patients with sickle cell anaemia have a propensity for infection with *Salmonella* organisms, while *Haemophilus influenzae* is occasionally seen in the paediatric age group. Gonococcal arthritis, which not infrequently affects certain other joints, is less commonly encountered in the shoulder.

Tuberculous infection is of particular importance. The disease itself is still endemic in many countries and, consequently, musculoskeletal involvement is not uncommon. Even in the developed countries where the incidence of the disease is low, the changing pattern of disease brought about by the spread of AIDS has resulted in an increasing number of cases seen. In comparison, fungal, parasitic and viral infections around the shoulder are rare and are probably more likely to occur in immuno-compromised patients with disseminated disease (CUELLAR et al. 1992).

14.4
Clinical Presentation

The onset can be acute, sub-acute or chronic. Patients with septic arthritis or osteomyelitis classically present acutely with localised pain and swelling, joint stiffness, low-grade fever, chills, anorexia and malaise. There may however be considerable variation in the presentation depending on the causative agent, the immune status of the patient and the presence of pre-existing joint or bone abnormality.

The onset of symptoms in tuberculous infections is usually indolent and tends to follow a more protracted clinical course than pyogenic ones. In immuno-compromised patients or those with chronic debilitating disease, the symptoms may be partially masked by the inability to mount a proper immune response or the use of steroids. The presence of pre-existing joint abnormality, e.g. crystal or rheumatoid arthropathy, may also lead to confusion between relapse of the underlying arthropathy and superimposed septic arthritis. Likewise, in patients with sickle cell disease, it may be difficult to distinguish bone infarcts from infection and, in some cases, the two conditions may co-exist. Finally, the clinical features of septic arthritis or osteomyelitis may sometimes mimic other conditions such as bursitis or tendinitis.

Cellulitis, fasciitis and pyomyositis are usually clinically apparent. The findings include local features such as pain/tenderness, erythema, skin swelling, "wooden" feel of the soft tissues or muscles, or fluctuance, if there is abscess formation. A discharging sinus may occur with progression of infection. Systemic signs include fever, chills, rigors and malaise.

The age of the patient also plays a role in clinical presentation. In children the normal developmental anatomical changes influence the manifestations of osteomyelitis. In neonates the vascular connections of diaphyseal, metaphyseal and epiphyseal vessels across the cartilaginous growth plate result in an increased tendency to epiphyseal and articular infection. The vascular connection across the physis is obliterated at around 1 year, which is why childhood osteomyelitis usually commences and is located in the metaphysis. The vascular continuity with the epiphysis is restored following physeal closure re-introducing the risk of articular and epiphyseal spread (KOTHARI et al. 2001).

14.5
Types of Infection and Imaging Features

14.5.1
Septic Arthritis Pyogenic/Tuberculous

Septic arthritis is usually pyogenic and represents a surgical emergency as a delay in diagnosis has a profound effect on the prognosis of both articular morphology and function. Even in this era of modern antibiotics, the incidence of septic arthritis appears to be increasing (LESLIE et al. 1989). It can occur at any age, but is most common in children under 3 years of age. The increased incidence is in part due to the aging population and in part to the prolonged survival of patients with chronic debilitating or immuno-deficiency diseases. However, compared to the other major joints, septic arthritis affecting the shoulder is still relatively uncommon. The involvement is usually mono-articular (90%) with positive blood cultures in around 30%, while aspirate cultures are positive in about 60% (SHETTY and GEDALIA

1998). Tuberculosis on the other hand can present insidiously with a long history of joint symptoms (CHILDS 1996).

Conventional radiography is often the initial imaging modality employed. Unfortunately, it is not reliable in making an early diagnosis as the changes are often confined to the soft tissues. This reflects the initial pathological response of the inflamed synovium that consists of synovial hypertrophy and joint effusion (PHEMISTER 1924). Early radiographic findings include widening of the joint space, peri-articular soft tissue swelling and osteopenia, all of which are often subtle and difficult to appreciate. With progression there is joint space loss, ill-defined peri-articular erosions and periosteal reaction (Fig. 14.2).

The time course for these changes is dependent on the infective organism. Rapid cartilage and bone destruction is often the rule in bacterial infections due to the release of cytokines and proteolytic enzymes (Fig. 14.3), whereas in tuberculous and fungal infections, the changes are more insidious (Goss 1993). In tuberculous infections, the findings may be limited mainly to peri-articular osteopenia and marginal osseous erosions, with relative preservation of the joint space. Periosteal reaction is not as frequently seen as in pyogenic infections. When peri-ostitis occurs, it tends to be linear and parallel the bone contour in contrast to the interrupted or perpendicular varieties more frequently encountered in aggressive bone tumours. With progression, frank bone destruction, sequestration, sinuses or fistulae, soft-tissue abscesses (Figs. 14.4, 14.5, 14.6) and fibrous ankylosis may develop. Tuberculous arthritis may go unnoticed and unsuspected for months and years, particularly in the elderly. The development is insidious, systemic involvement is usually not noted, and the presentation is late with significant osteoarticular destruction. It may present as a draining abscess in the arm with chronic sinus formation (Figs. 14.6, 14.7) (MILLER and MOORE 1983).

Due to the lag period between the initial infection and radiographic changes, further assessment by another imaging modality is often required. 99m-Tc bone scintigraphy is highly sensitive in the detection of infection (TUMEH 1996). Increased activity is seen in the affected joint in the flow, blood pool and delayed phases before radiographic changes become apparent. However, the findings are not specific as increased isotope uptake may be present in a number of other conditions, notably the inflammatory arthropathies which may mimic septic arthritis clinically. The use of other agents (DATZ and MORTON 1993) such as Gallium-67 citrate, labelled

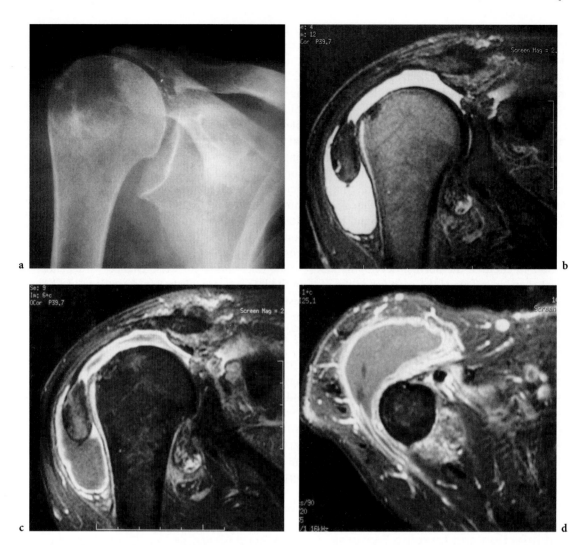

Fig. 14.2a–d. Septic arthritis (*Staphylococcus aureus*) in a 77-year-old man of the gleno-humeral joint extending into the sub-acromial and sub-deltoid bursa. There is superior migration of the humeral head (**a**) with absence of the supraspinatus tendon, fluid and debris in the bursa and gleno-humeral joint (**b**). There is intense rim enhancement of the synovium within the bursa on the coronal (**c**) and axial (**d**) fat suppressed T1 post Gadolinium DTPA sequences

leucocytes or immuno-globulins have not significantly improved diagnostic capability as these all show increased isotope uptake in both inflammatory and septic arthropathies.

MRI is more sensitive and capable of demonstrating changes early in the course of the disease but, like scintigraphy, it tends to lack specificity. Effusions are readily seen as areas of low signal on T1-weighted and high signal on T2-weighted sequences but it is difficult, if not impossible, to distinguish septic effusions from reactive ones, even with intravenous MR contrast administration (Deely and Schweitzer 1997). Contrast-enhanced MRI is useful in showing marked rim enhancement of a thickened abscess wall or inflamed synovium

(see Figs. 14.2, 14.4). In both septic and reactive synovitis there is an effusion with enhancement of the proliferating synovium. The demonstration of signal abnormalities in the adjacent bone marrow on fat-suppressed Gd-DTPA enhanced T1 and T2 images is a good predictor of septic arthritis as it is not seen in reactive synovitis (see Fig. 14.17) (Lee et al. 1999).

With sonography, this distinction may sometimes be possible. It is thought that effusions with large amounts of intrinsic particulate material (as reflected by increased echoes within the collection) are more likely to be septic, but again this is not a specific sign. In addition associated osteomyelitis is not reliably detected. Thus, while MRI, sonography and

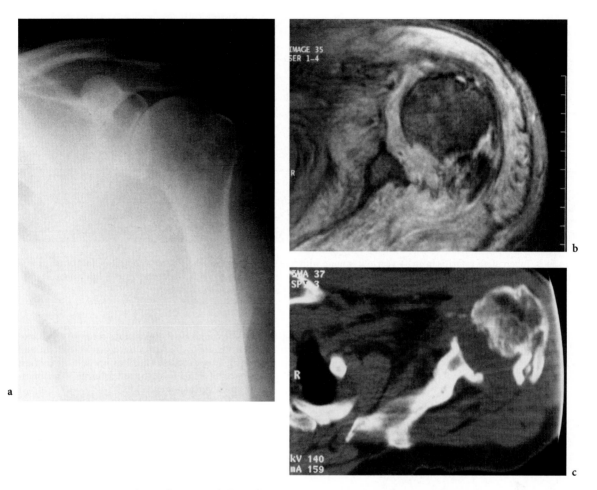

Fig. 14.3. a–c Pyogenic arthritis showing early loss of joint space (**a**), with subsequent joint destruction and debris outlined by intra-articular fluid on the axial T2 (**b**) MR image and CT (**c**)

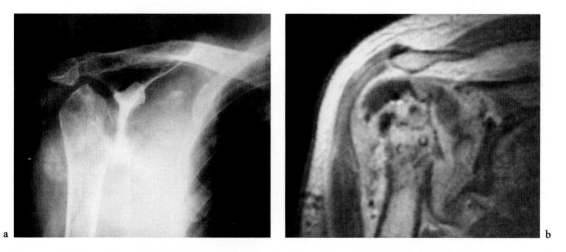

Fig. 14.4a, b. Tuberculous arthritis in an 84-year-old woman, presenting with swelling and a discharging sinus. Note the bone and joint destruction and debris (**a**) with extension into the sub-deltoid bursa highlighted by the rim enhancement following IV Gadolinium DTPA on the coronal T1 MR image (**b**)

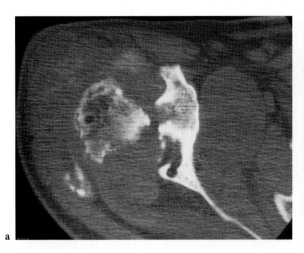
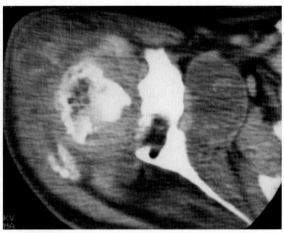

Fig. 14.5a, b. Tuberculous arthritis in an 84-year-old woman with free spread into the subscapularis and subdeltoid bursa as well as abscess formation in the muscles. Axial CT (bone windows) (**a**) shows osteo-articular destruction with bony debris while, post-contrast CT (soft tissue windows) (**b**) shows rim enhancement around the abscess formations

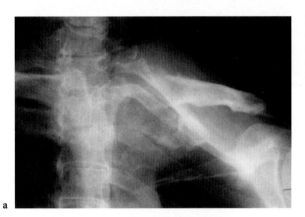

Fig. 14.6. a Tuberculous discharging sinus secondary to osteo-articular destruction of the (left) sternoclavicular joint and clavicle in a patient with diabetes mellitus. **b, c** Note the contrast enhancement of the sinus track (**b**) and fistulous communication with the joint at sinography (**c**)

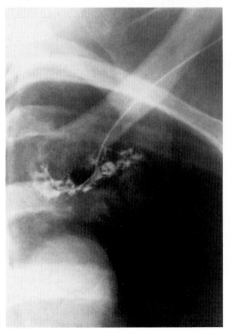
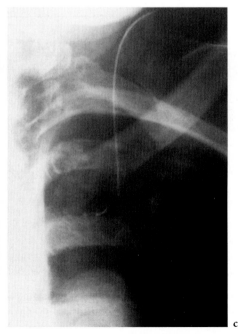

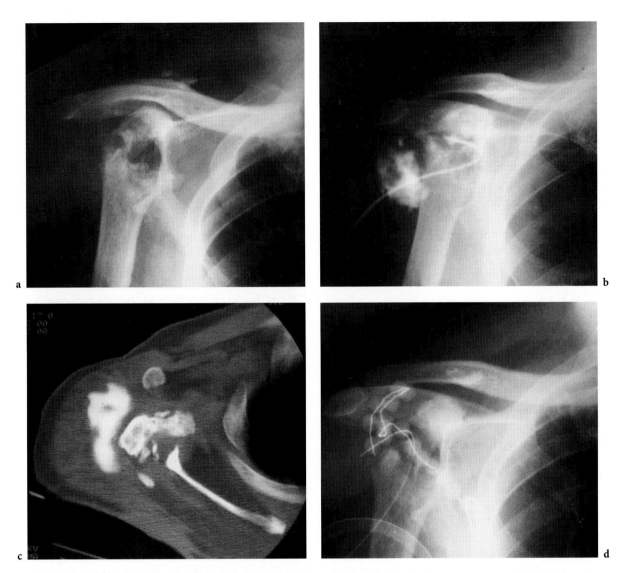

Fig. 14.7a–d. Re-activation of tuberculosis 30 years after initial diagnosis, in a 71-year-old man presenting with a shoulder mass and a persistent discharge. Pre- (**a**) and post- (**b**) sinogram radiographs of the shoulder showing osteo-articular disintegration and a contrast filled sub-deltoid cavity, which are well depicted on the post sinogram axial CT (**c**). **d** Post-operative radiograph showing antibiotic beads in situ following surgical debridement and sinus track excision

scintigraphy are more sensitive than conventional radiography in detecting early septic arthritis, they are not more specific. Their role in early assessment is often to confirm that there is indeed a joint pathology when the radiographs are still unremarkable, and to direct a joint aspiration to make a definitive diagnosis. In this regard, sonography provides a cheap and reliable means of guiding joint aspiration and synovial biopsy (CRAIG 1999). Infection in the acromio-clavicular joint has an increased frequency in immuno-compromised patients and drug addicts. A normal sonographic appearance of the gleno-humeral joint in a patient clinically suspected to have

septic arthritis, requires evaluation of the acromio-clavicular joint and aspiration using sonography (WIDMAN et al. 2001).

In patients with TSA, the detection of septic arthritis is further complicated by the use of metallic prostheses and radiopaque cement. The effectiveness of MRI and scintigraphy in the early detection of disease is often marred by the artifacts that are present, and by the fact that the joint may normally show increased isotope uptake for a period of time following the surgery. On conventional radiographs, infection may be confused with loosening of the prosthesis as both conditions may result in a radiolucent zone at the bone–cement, or less commonly, at the cement–prosthesis interfaces. This problem may be exacerbated by the fact that a zone of lucency may sometimes develop in the normal post-operative state, possibly due to heat-induced bone necrosis from the exothermic bone-cement polymerisation reaction, inadequate cement packing or micromotion (MITCHELL et al. 1988)

In the absence of overt cortical or medullary bone destruction, a definitive distinction between infection and loosening is achieved by analysis of the joint aspirate. Arthrography may also demonstrate prosthetic loosening with extension of the contrast agent into the space between the bone and cement or between the cement and prosthesis.

14.5.2
Osteomyelitis

Osteomyelitis usually involves the proximal humerus and is less commonly seen in the scapula and clavicle. As with septic arthritis, the early radiographic finding is predominantly that of non-specific soft tissue swelling related to inflammation, and regional hyperemia with resultant fat plane obliteration (Fig. 14.8). This is followed by permeative osteolysis, cortical erosion and periosteal reaction, all of which may be evident only several days (7–10) to a couple of weeks after the onset of disease (SCHAUWECKER et al. 1990). Loss of 30%–50% of bone mineralisation is a prerequisite to radiographic detection. These features may resemble and sometimes be confused with aggressive bone tumours or even reflex sympathetic dystrophy, transient regional osteoporosis or stress/healing fractures (RESNICK and NIWAYAMA 1995). In the sub-acute and chronic stages where there is bony sequestration, involucrum formation, mature periosteal reaction and bony deformity, the appearances are more diagnostic. CT and MRI can demonstrate these signs of chronicity. A sinus tract appears typically as a linear/curvilinear zone of high T2 signal which may enhance with Gd-DTPA.

Technetium 99 m bone scintigraphy facilitates the early diagnosis of osteomyelitis by showing increased isotope uptake. It may also be useful in distinguishing osteomyelitis from cellulitis. Although the overall sensitivity is high (>90%) (GOLD et al. 1991), false-negative diagnosis may occur, especially in the developing skeleton where the increased metaphyseal uptake in infection may be partially masked by the normal increased activity seen in the adjacent growth plate.

In the shoulder girdle, CT is a useful adjunct to conventional radiography as it is able to depict the complex cross-sectional anatomy better. In selected patients where the changes of osteomyelitis may be difficult to visualise on conventional radiography (e.g. in the scapula where it may be partially obscured by overlapping bones), CT may be of value in depicting early cortical erosion, bone fragmentation, sequestration and cloacae, and in guiding percutaneous bone biopsy. Contrast-enhanced CT may also aid in demonstrating the presence of abscess (see Figs. 14.5, 14.7).

MRI is the most sensitive technique for the early detection of osteomyelitis. The marrow abnormality is seen as an area of low signal on T1-weighted, and high signal on T2-weighted and short tau inversion-recovery sequences (STIR) (MORRISON et al. 1993). This is due to replacement of the bone marrow by inflammatory cells and exudate. Although not as helpful as CT in demonstrating the cortical disruption sequestrum, formation and periosteal reaction, it is better for depicting the soft tissue changes and abscess formation (see Figs. 14.2–14.4). This, coupled with its multi-planar capability, provides for good demonstration of sinus tracts which is useful in pre-operative surgical planning (MORRISON et al. 1995), especially when limited resection is contemplated.

Sonography is not routinely used in imaging of osteomyelitis although some studies have shown that the sonographic findings of a breach in the cortex, periosteal thickening and soft tissue swelling (Figs. 14.8, 14.9) may be visualised before the radiographic changes become evident (MAH et al. 1994). It has however been suggested that it may be useful in children for detecting sub-periosteal abscesses (KAISER and ROSENBORG 1994). In young patients, the periosteum is relatively loosely attached to the bone compared to adults, and the increase in pressure in the bone marrow that develops with osteomyelitis can force the inflammation to extend outwards to form a sub-periosteal abscess. Detection of this collection is important as it needs to be drained surgically. This differs from uncomplicated osteomyelitis, which can be treated with antibiotics.

14.5.3
Osteomyelitis in Sickle Cell Disease

Some mention should be given to an uncommon but interesting type of osteomyelitis caused by *Salmonella* infection. This is usually encountered in patients with sickle cell disease. Bone infarcts may

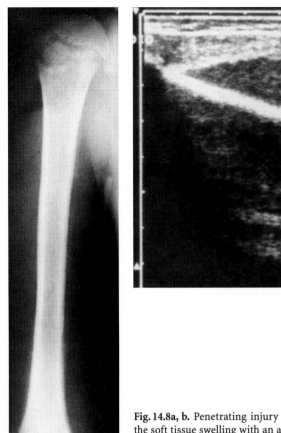

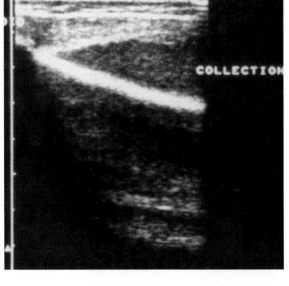

Fig. 14.8a, b. Penetrating injury producing soft tissue and bone infection in a farmer's son. Note the soft tissue swelling with an air–fluid level (*arrow*) and diffuse periosteal reaction in (a) with an extensive sub-deltoid abscess seen on the ultrasound examination (b)

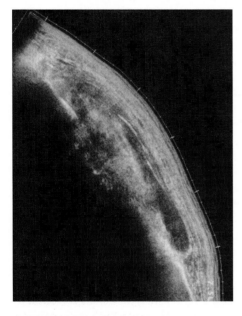

Fig. 14.9. Osteomyelitis of the humerus. Longitudinal sonogram, showing a cortical breach, an overlying heterogeneous soft tissue mass and large abscess cavity

develop as a complication of the disorder and serve as a nidus for infection. Although any organism may be implicated, these patients often develop *Salmonella* infections (Fig. 14.10). This is probably due to micro-infarctions of the bowel which permit the intestinal flora including the *Salmonella* organisms to gain access to the circulation resulting in haematogenous spread of infection. While the radiological features are similar to those of other pyogenic infections, the site of involvement is frequently in the diaphysis (corresponding to the site of bone infarction) rather than in the metaphysis or epiphysis, is more likely to be multi-focal, and is associated with significant sequelae. Less frequently, infarction with subsequent infection may also occur at the ends of long bones. The annual incidence of osteomyelitis in sickle cell patients is around 0.36% (PIEHL et al. 1993). The humerus is the commonest affected bone and multiple causative organisms can colonise the infarcted bone. The infection is clinically and radiologically indistinguishable from bone infarction, especially as infarction is about 50 times more likely to occur

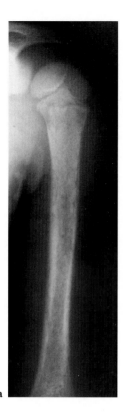

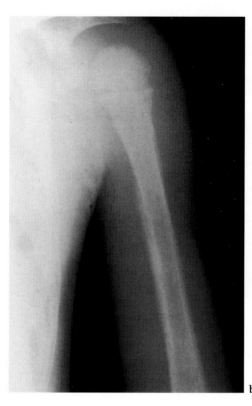

Fig. 14.10a, b. Salmonella osteomyelitis in a child with sickle cell disease. Note the extensive soft tissue swelling, extensive diaphyseal involvement (**a**) with a permeative destructive appearance 2 weeks later (**b**)

(STARK et al. 1991) and the diagnosis relies heavily on aspiration and biopsy.

14.5.4
Chronic Recurrent Multi-focal Osteomyelitis

This distinct entity, usually found in children and young adults, encompasses recurrent and relapsing bouts of aseptic osteitis, with spontaneous remissions (KING et al. 1987). In the upper limb the clavicle is commonly involved, especially its sternal end. Involvement can be symmetrical, and although multi-focal lesions are common, some may be asymptomatic (MANDELL 1996). Skin lesions (palmo-plantar pustulosis, psoriasis) are associated with chronic recurrent multi-focal osteomyelitis (CRMO) and as a result it is often grouped under the unifying term SAPHO (synovitis, acne, pustulosis, hyperostosis, osteitis.) The aetiology is unknown as culture is usually negative. Altered immune response and seronegative arthropathy have been postulated as possible causes. Imaging characteristically shows mixed areas of lysis and sclerosis, periosteal new bone formation, with no abscess, sinus or sequestrum formation (Fig. 14.11). Scintigraphy is essential in depicting multi-focal disease especially in excluding the

clinically asymptomatic lesions. MRI shows areas of marrow oedema in the active sites, while the marrow signal is restored to normal with healing (JURIK and EGUND 1997). The changes in the clavicle may persist for several years, with areas of relapse seen as radiolucent on CT and as hyper-intense marrow on STIR or fat-suppressed T2 sequences.

14.5.5
Hydatid Disease

Hydatid bone disease is rare with skeletal involvement seen in only 1%–2% of all hydatid infections. It results from ingestion of the parasite's eggs and subsequent penetration of the embryos through the intestinal mucosa into the circulatory system. In the skeleton, due to the slow growth of the parasite, the classical signs of localised pain and deformity may not be apparent for some time. Occasionally, the initial presentation may be a pathological fracture. The early changes include poorly defined lucencies in the affected bone. These are often multiple and may coalesce giving rise to lytic lesions traversed by residual bone strands. There may be bony expansion, thinning of the cortex and sclerosis at the margins of the lesion (Fig. 14.12). Periosteal reaction is rare in the

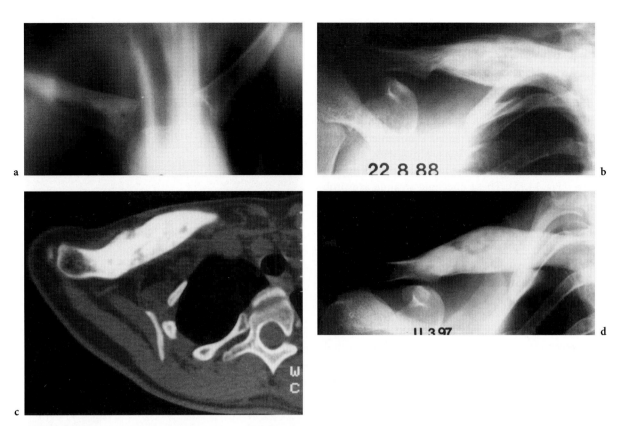

Fig. 14.11a–d. Natural history of clavicular involvement in a child with chronic recurrent multi-focal osteomyelitis (CRMO). Coronal tomogram (**a**) showing a mixed lytic and sclerotic appearance in the medial end of the (right) clavicle, progressing to a sclerotic hyperostotic appearance with spread of osteitis 6 months later (**b**). The CT shows sparing of the lateral end of the clavicle with a few lytic areas within the sclerotic and hyperostotic clavicle (**c**) while the appearances persist albeit in an asymptomatic state 11 years later (**d**)

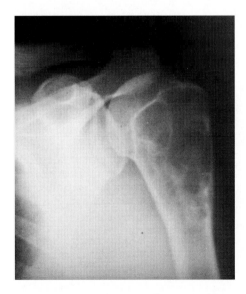

Fig. 14.12. Hydatid disease in the proximal humerus of a 47-year-old abattoir worker shown as an expanded lytic lesion in the metaphysis and diaphysis. (Courtesy of Professor PD Corr, University of Natal, South Africa)

absence of a pathological fracture. The appearances are unlike those of pyogenic osteomyelitis and it is often mistaken for other bone lesions such as giant cell tumour, aneurysmal bone cyst or even fibrous dysplasia. The diagnosis is often based on careful history-taking and biochemical tests such as specific IgG ELISA AbB (antigen B-rich fraction), immuno-electrophoresis or latex agglutination tests.

14.5.6
Cellulitis, Fasciitis and Pyomyositis

These conditions are usually clinically apparent and do not normally require imaging. However, if there is clinical suspicion of associated abscess formation, sonography provides a quick and cheap means of detecting this complication and may also aid in guiding diagnostic or therapeutic aspiration. Striated muscle is inherently resistant to bacterial infection and suppuration usually is associated with damaged muscle (MIYAKE 1904), malnutrition, concurrent illness (malignancy, diabetes mellitus), steroid treatment, HIV infection or immuno-suppression. Pyomyositis usually involves one muscle, is less common in the upper than the lower limb, but is multi-focal in 40% of cases (RODGERS et al. 1993).

On sonography, cellulitis is demonstrated as diffuse thickening and increased echogenicity of the skin and subcutaneous layer often with anechoic strands within it giving rise to a cobblestone appearance (Fig. 14.13). These anechoic strands are probably due to small amounts of inflammatory exudates/interstitial fluid (LOYER et al. 1995). With pyomyositis, two sonographic appearances have been described (BELLI et al. 1992). The initial appearance is that of diffuse non-specific muscle oedema which appears as alteration of the normal muscle echo-texture with poorly-defined areas of hypo-echogenicity. In this early stage, full resolution can be achieved with antibiotic treatment alone (CANOSO and BARZA 1993) However, if inadequately treated, a focal hypoechoic

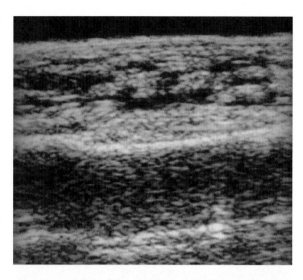

Fig. 14.13. Cellulitis of the subcutaneous fat plane shown sonographically as oedema in the interstitium with streaky anechoic areas. The underlying humeral cortex is intact

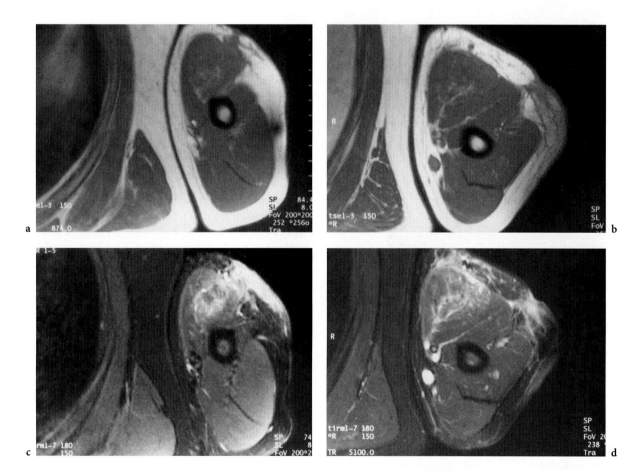

Fig. 14.14a–d. Cellulitis with multiple sinus tracts and pyomyositis of the biceps muscle following iatrogenic steroid injection in a 28-year-old body builder. T1 axial images (**a, b**) and STIR sequences (**c, d**) showing the altered soft tissue signal in the involved areas

area denotes an intra-muscular abscess that requires surgical or percutaneous drainage may develop.

MRI is a more costly means of imaging these conditions; it may however be useful in demonstrating the extent of involvement in necrotising fasciitis and also to look for possible spread to the adjacent bone. In some cases of pyomyositis where the clinical presentation may mimic a soft tissue sarcoma, MRI may also be useful to distinguish between the two entities (HALL et al. 1990). On MRI, pyomyositis is demonstrated as enlargement of the affected muscles. There is slightly increased T1-weighted signal (compared to normal muscles) which becomes higher on the T2-weighted sequences (see Figs. 14.14, 14.15). A central low T1 and hyper-intense T2 fluid collection consistent with an abscess may sometimes be present (GORDON et al. 1995).

14.5.7
Bursitis

Although more commonly related to trauma and chronic overuse syndromes (especially in sports requiring repetitive over-arm movement), bursitis may also occasionally result from infection. In most cases involving the shoulder, this may be associated with, and possibly even be secondary, to joint involvement. Even in the occasional case where the infection appears to be limited to the subacromial/sub-deltoid (SASD) bursa (Figs. 14.13, 14.14), it is often shown at operation that the infection is initially intra-articular but eventually communicates with the bursa through a full-thickness tear of the rotator cuff (see Fig. 14.2).

Imaging with sonography or MRI is therefore useful as it may reveal associated rotator cuff and joint abnormality in addition to the bursal pathology. Bursitis is demonstrated as a well-defined fluid collection in the expected anatomic site of the bursa (Fig. 14.16), although sometimes it may appear relatively solid due to thickening of the bursal wall in chronic cases (ZEISS et al. 1993).

Tuberculosis of the sub-deltoid bursa is well documented without articular involvement (Fig. 14.17) (ALKALAY et al. 1980). Corpora oryzoidea (rice bodies or melon seed-like bodies) are typically found, but these are nonspecific as they merely illus-

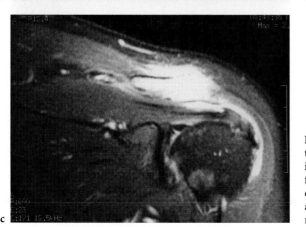

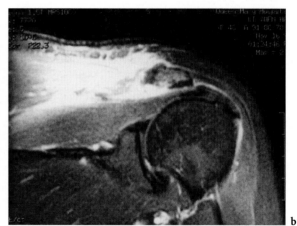

Fig. 14.15a–c. Pyomyositis (*Staphylococcus aureus*) of the (left) trapezius muscle in a 48-year-old woman shown as T2 hyper-intense areas on the initial coronal fast spin-echo T2-weighted fat-suppressed MR image (**a**), as well as intense enhancement on the coronal spin-echo T1-weighted fat-suppressed image after IV Gadolinium DTPA injection (**b**). Improvement is noted after antibiotic treatment (**c**)

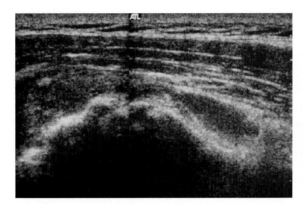

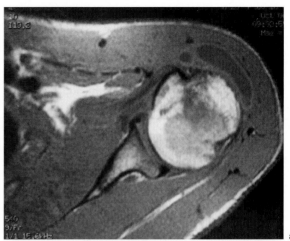

Fig. 14.16. Sonography of sub-deltoid bursitis seen as a fluid filled bursa, with intact outlines of the bone and deltoid muscle

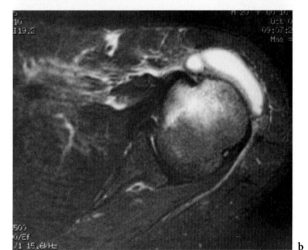

trate the presence of fibrinous inflammation which can also occur in rheumatoid disease (Fig. 14.18) (KARKOV 1994).

14.6
Imaging Approach

In practice, the diagnosis of bone or joint infection may be difficult to establish clinically. MRI is probably the most important clinical modality in the diagnosis and exclusion of infection in and around the shoulder (Fig. 14.19). Septic arthritis may mimic other forms of arthropathy. Initial assessment by conventional radiography is often inadequate and further imaging (preferably using MRI or, if unavailable, using CT or bone scintigraphy or even sonography in the case of septic arthritis) is often required. In patients with suspected septic arthritis, joint aspiration is usually mandatory to establish the definitive diagnosis.

In cases of soft tissue infection, e.g. cellulitis/pyomyositis, the diagnosis can often be confidently made on clinical examination and imaging serves mainly to look for associated complications. These include:

1. The development of intra-/inter-muscular abscesses which are best assessed with either sonography or MRI

2. Looking for possible spread to the adjacent bone or joint

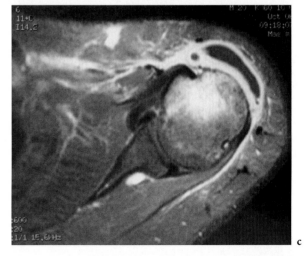

Fig. 14.17. a–c Tuberculous sub-deltoid bursitis in a 20-year-old man showing purulent fluid as low T1 (**a**) and high T2 signal (**b**), with rim enhancement of the thickened bursal wall after IV Gadolinium DTPA enhancement (**c**). Note the adjacent bone marrow oedema on the T2 fat suppressed (**b**) and post-contrast T1 fat suppressed MR image (**c**)

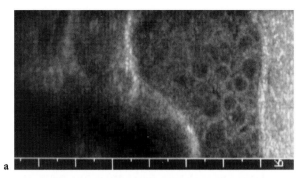

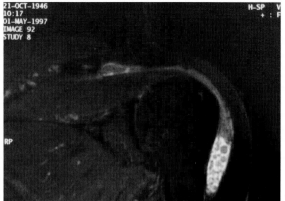

Fig. 14.18. Rice Bodies within an inflamed and enlarged sub-acromial/sub-deltoid bursa appearing as multiple discrete filling defects at sonography (**a**) and coronal STIR sequences (**b**). Tuberculosis needs to be excluded in this setting but rice bodies can also be seen in rheumatoid disease

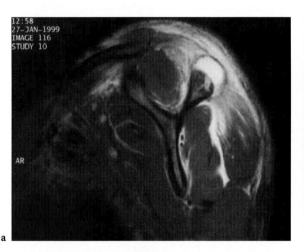

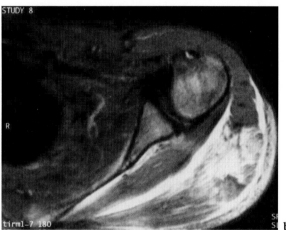

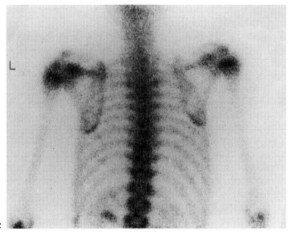

Fig. 14.19. Acute osteomyelitis with a large sub-periosteal abscess arising from the spine of the scapula in a 13-year-old boy. The multi-planar capability and soft tissue contrast resolution of MR are well shown (**a**) on the axial STIR and (**b**) para-sagittal STIR sequence. Note the associated inter-muscular fluid collection, muscle involvement, and signal changes within the subcutaneous tissues. In contrast, only the bony changes are seen on the scintigram (**c**)

14.7 Conclusion

Although relatively rare, infections of the shoulder are important because of their associated morbidity. The diagnosis is often not apparent clinically. A high index of suspicion and an understanding of the imaging approach are required to establish an early diagnosis so that the appropriate treatment may be instituted.

References

Ahlberg A, Carlsson AS, Lindberg L (1978) Hematogenous infection in total joint replacement. Clin Orthop 137:69–75

Alkalay I, Kaufman T, Suprun H (1980) Tuberculosis of the subdeltoid bursa. A case report. Isr J Med Sci 16:853–855

Belli L, Reggiori A, Cocozza E, Riboldi L, Tacconi L (1992) Ultrasonographic study of tubercular effusions. Apropos of 12 cases. Radiol Med (Torino) 83:659–661

Canoso JJ, Barza M (1993) Soft tissue infections. Rheum Dis Clin North Am 19:293–309

Childs SG (1996) Osteoarticular Mycobacterium tuberculosis. Orthop Nurs 15:28–33

Cofield RH (1991) The shoulder: results of complications. In: Morey BF, Cooney WP III (eds) Joint replacement arthroplasty. Churchill Livingstone, New York, pp 437–453

Craig JG (1999 Infection: ultrasound-guided procedures. Radiol Clin North Am 37:669–678

Cuellar ML, Silveira LH, Espinoza LR (1992) Fungal arthritis. Ann Rheum Dis 51:690–697

Datz FL, Morton KA (1993) New radiopharmaceuticals for detecting infection. Invest Radiol 28:356–365

Deely DM, Schweitzer ME (1997) MR imaging of bone marrow disorders. Radiol Clin North Am 35:193–212

Gelberman RH, Menon J, Austerlitz MS, Weisman MH (1980) Pyogenic arthritis of the shoulder in adults. J Bone Joint Surg (Am) 62:550–553

Gold RH, Hawkins RA, Katz RD (1991 Bacterial osteomyelitis: findings on plain radiography, CT, MR, and scintigraphy. AJR 157:365–370

Gordon BA, Martinez S, Collins AJ (1995) Pyomyositis: characteristics at CT and MR imaging. Radiology 197:279–286

Goss TP (1993) Shoulder infections. In: Bigliani LU (ed) Complications of shoulder surgery. Williams and Wilkins, Baltimore, pp 202–213

Hall RL, Callaghan JJ, Moloney E, Martinez S, Harrelson JM (1990 Pyomyositis in a temperate climate. Presentation, diagnosis, and treatment. J Bone Joint Surg (Am) 72:1240–1244

Jurik AG, Egund N (1997) MRI in chronic recurrent multifocal osteomyelitis. Skeletal Radiol 26:230–238

Kaiser S, Rosenborg M (1994) Early detection of subperiosteal abscesses by ultrasonography. A means for further successful treatment in pediatric osteomyelitis. Pediatr Radiol 24: 336–339

Karkov JN (1994) Corpora oryzoidea – rice bodies or melon seed-like bodies. Ugeskr Laeger 156:3638–3639

King SM, Laxer RM, Manson D, Gold R (1987) Chronic recurrent multifocal osteomyelitis: a noninfectious inflammatory process. Pediatr Infect Dis J 6:907–911

Kothari NA, Pelchovitz DJ, Meyer JS (2001) Imaging of musculoskeletal infections. Radiol Clin North Am 39:653–671

Lee SK, Suh KJ, Kim YW, Ryeom HK, Kim YS, Lee JM, Chang Y, Kim YJ, Kang DS (1999) Septic arthritis versus transient synovitis at MR imaging: preliminary assessment with signal intensity alterations in bone marrow. Radiology 211:459–465

Leslie BM, Harris JM III, Driscoll D (1989) Septic arthritis of the shoulder in adults. J Bone Joint Surg (Am) 71:1516–1522

Loyer EM, Kaur H, David CL, DuBrow R, Eftekhari FM (1995) Importance of dynamic assessment of the soft tissues in the sonographic diagnosis of echogenic superficial abscesses. J Ultrasound Med 14:669–671

Mader JT, Shirtliff M, Calhoun JH (1999) The host and the skeletal infection: classification and pathogenesis of acute bacterial bone and joint sepsis. Baillieres Best Pract Res Clin Rheumatol 13:1–20

Mah ET, LeQuesne GW, Gent RJ, Paterson DC (1994) Ultrasonic features of acute osteomyelitis in children. J Bone Joint Surg (Br) 76:969–974

Mandell GA (1996) Imaging in the diagnosis of musculoskeletal infections in children. Curr Probl Pediatr 26:218–237

Miller KD, Moore ME (1983) Tuberculous arthritis of the shoulder: delayed diagnosis aided by arthrography. Clin Rheumatol 2:61–64

Mitchell M, Howard B, Haller J, Sartoris DJ, Resnick D (1988) Septic arthritis. Radiol Clin North Am 26:1295–1313

Miyake H (1904) Beitrage AUR, Kenntnis der Sogenenten. Myositis infectiosa. Mitt Grenzgeb Med Chir 13:155

Morrison WB, Schweitzer ME, Bock GW, Mitchell DG, Hume EL, Pathria MN, Resnick D (1993) Diagnosis of osteomyelitis: utility of fat-suppressed contrast-enhanced MR imaging. Radiology 189:251–257

Morrison WB, Schweitzer ME, Wapner KL, Hecht PJ, Gannon FH, Behm WR (1995) Osteomyelitis in feet of diabetics: clinical accuracy, surgical utility, and cost-effectiveness of MR imaging. Radiology 196:557–564

Phemister DB (1924) Changes in the articular surfaces in tuberculosis and pyogenic infections of joints. AJR 12:1–14

Piehl FC, Davis RJ, Prugh SI (1993) Osteomyelitis in sickle cell disease. J Pediatr Orthop 13:225–227

Resnick D, Niwayama G (1995) Osteomyelitis, septic arthritis and soft tissue infection: mechanisms and situations. In: Resnick D (ed) Diagnosis of bone and joint disorders, 3rd edn. Saunders, Philadelphia, pp 2325–2418

Rodgers WB, Yodlowski ML, Mintzer CM (1993) Pyomyositis in patients who have the human immunodeficiency virus. Case report and review of the literature. J Bone Joint Surg (Am) 75:588–592

Schauwecker DS, Braunstein EM, Wheat LJ (1990 Diagnostic imaging of osteomyelitis. Infect Dis Clin North Am 4: 441–463

Shetty AK, Gedalia A (1998) Septic arthritis in children. Rheum Dis Clin North Am 24:287–304

Silliman JF, Hawkins RJ (1994) Complications following shoulder arthroplasty. In: Friedman RJ (ed) Arthroplasty of the shoulder. Thieme, New York, pp 242–253

Stark JE, Glasier CM, Blasier RD, Aronson J, Seibert JJ (1991) Osteomyelitis in children with sickle cell disease: early diagnosis with contrast-enhanced CT. Radiology 179: 731–733

Tumeh SS (1996) Scintigraphy in the evaluation of arthropathy. Radiol Clin North Am 34:215–231

Widman DS, Craig JG, van Holsbeeck MT (2001) Sonographic detection, evaluation and aspiration of infected acromioclavicular joints. Skeletal Radiol 30:388–392

Zeiss J, Coombs RJ, Booth RL Jr, Saddemi SR (1993) Chronic bursitis presenting as a mass in the pes anserine bursa: MR diagnosis. J Comput Assist Tomogr 17:137–140

15 Osteonecrosis and Marrow Disorders

B. C. Vande Berg and V. Baudrez

CONTENTS

Imaging of the bone marrow of the shoulder girdle has been less extensively developed than imaging of the proximal femur. Most likely, this is due to the lower incidence of fractures secondary to osteonecrosis or marrow lesions in the shoulder than in the femur because of the lack of weight-bearing stresses in the upper limb. This chapter focuses on the normal magnetic resonance (MR) anatomy of the proximal humerus and on the patterns of ischemic and neoplastic marrow lesions that involve the shoulder.

15.1
Marrow Anatomy of the Proximal Humerus

Accurate interpretation of marrow appearance on MR images requires knowledge of normal variations

B. C. Vande Berg, MD, PhD
Department of Radiology, Cliniques Universitaires St Luc, University Catholique de Louvain, Avenue Hippocrate 10, Brussels, 1200, Belgium
V. Baudrez, MD
Department of Radiology, Clinique Universitaire de Mont-Godinne, University Catholique de Louvain, Yvoir, 5530, Belgium

in red and yellow marrow distribution and appearance (Vogler and Murphy 1988). MR appearance of the proximal humerus varies with age and sex in a relatively predictable manner (Taccone et al. 1995; Jaramillo et al. 1991). At birth, the diaphysis contains highly cellular marrow that is responsible for very low signal intensity on T1- and T2-weighted images. The epiphysis lacks ossified matrix and contains no hematopoietic tissue. With aging, a progressive increase in signal intensity of the medullary cavity appears on T1-weighted images that parallels an increase in the proportion of fatty marrow (Fig. 15.1). This progressive transformation of red to yellow marrow, namely red marrow conversion starts in the diaphysis and proceeds both centrifugally and centripetally, although at a higher pace distally.

By the age of 25, the adult pattern of red marrow distribution is established. Red marrow predominates in metaphyseal and diaphyseal areas and yellow marrow predominates in the epiphysis and trochiter. Within the same decade of age, there is a wide interindividual variation in the amount of humeral red marrow with no significant gender variation in the metaphyseal area (Mirowitz 1993). There is a common pattern of focal subchondral red marrow in the medial aspect of the humeral head (Fig. 15.2). This finding is more prominent in women than in males, most frequently presenting between the third and six decade of life (Mirowitz 1993; Richardson and Patten 1994). Distribution of red and yellow marrow is similar between left and right sides (Richardson and Patten 1994). Hence, examination of the controlateral side when an uncommon pattern is observed might help to decide whether or not a focal lesion is present. Finally, there is no relationship between marrow distribution pattern in the proximal humerus and the presence of rotator cuff disease (Richardson and Patten 1994), and marrow changes in relation to rotator cuff disorders appear to be a relatively rare finding (McCauley et al. 2000).

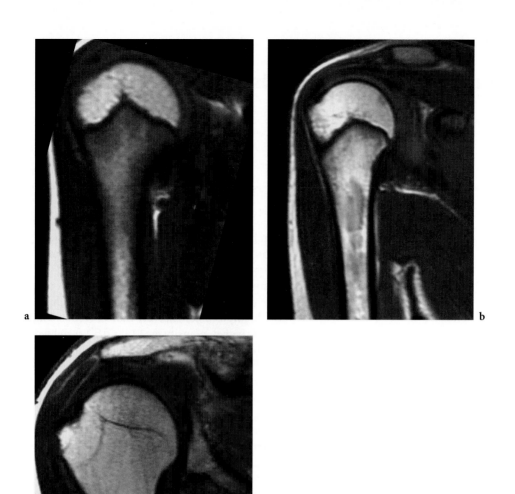

Fig. 15.1. a–c Coronal T1-weighted magnetic resonance images of (**a**) a 4-year-old patient, (**b**) a 10-year-old patient, and (**c**) a 55-year-old patient show changes in marrow appearance with age. The humeral head contains fatty marrow and the amount of red marrow decreases with age in the metaphyses and diaphyses

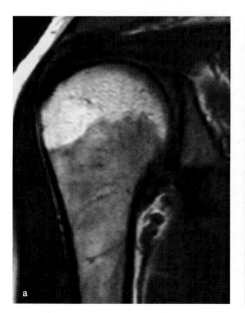
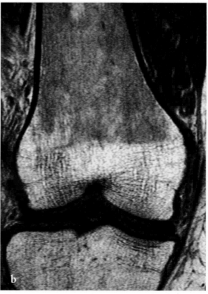

Fig. 15.2. (a) Coronal T1-weighted magnetic resonance (MR) image of the right shoulder of a 36-year-old woman shows a large amount of red marrow in the meta-diaphyseal area of the humerus. The subchondral area of the humeral head has intermediate signal intensity that probably reflects the presence of red marrow (**b**). Coronal T1-weighted MR image of her knee shows benign hematopoietic marrow hyperplasia with a large amount of red marrow in the distal femoral metaphysis

15.2
Epiphyseal Osteonecrosis

15.2.1
Introduction

The term *epiphyseal osteonecrosis* is used to describe an irreversible clinical and radiological condition characterized by altered joint function and collapse of the epiphysis on radiographs. We use the term *bone infarct* to describe a most frequently asymptomatic condition characterized by the presence of a well-delineated area of bone and marrow necrosis on MR images or radiographs wherever it develops, including in an epiphysis (VANDE BERG et al. 2001).

The clinical history and radiographic findings of humeral head osteonecrosis parallel those in the femoral head. However, stress magnitude and distribution on the articular surfaces differ between proximal ends of the humerus and femur because of differences in shape and of the lack of weight-bearing stresses in the humeral head. Hence, the natural history of ischemic lesions of the proximal humerus, that remains to be assessed, is most likely different from that of ischemic lesions of the proximal femur.

Ischemic disorders of the proximal humerus may result from traumatic disruption of the humerus vasculature at a relative distance from the subchondral area or from local alteration of bone and marrow perfusion. The relative prevalence of non-traumatic and post-traumatic osteonecrosis of the humeral head is a matter of patient recruitment. In a series of 200 cases of shoulder osteonecrosis, steroid therapy was involved in 112 shoulders, trauma in 37, Gaucher's disease in three, radiation therapy in one and no evident cause in 44 (HATTRUP and COFIELD 1999).

15.2.2
Nontraumatic Osteonecrosis

The pattern of changes that develop in the humeral head parallels that observed in other epiphyses. At an early stage, the radiographic and MR appearance of ischemic bone and marrow remains normal. At a largely ignored delay after the development of histologic changes, yellow marrow infarct may develop, as a subchondral area of normal fatty signal intensity delineated by a rim of low signal intensity on T1-weighted images. On T2-weighted images, this peripheral interface shows the double-line sign with an outer low and inner high signal intensity line that probably results from a chemical-shift misregistration artifact (DUDA et al. 1993) (Fig. 15.3). The radiographs show the focal lesion after a longer time delay than with MR imaging because the reactive interface needs to be calcified to become visible on radiographs.

At a later stage of the disease, fracture of the humeral head develops and the lesion generally becomes symptomatic. Fracture of the epiphysis appears on radiographs as a mild depression or marked collapse of the epiphysis or as a subchondral cleft that reflects the extent of the fracture in the

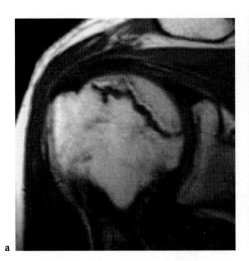
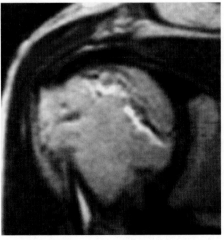

a   b

Fig. 15.3. a Coronal T1-weighted magnetic resonance (MR) image of the right shoulder of a 41-year-old man with a marrow infarct that appears as a subchondral area of normal signal intensity surrounded by a low signal intensity line. **b** On the corresponding T2-weighted MR image, increased signal intensity is present in the interface and the signal of the marrow infarct remains equivalent to that of normal fatty marrow

subchondral bone (Fig. 15.4). Areas of sclerosis and resorption develop in the subchondral lesion. At MR imaging, the subchondral bone fracture appears as a deformity of the epiphyseal contour or as a high signal intensity line on T2-weighted images extending under the subchondral bone plate. At this time, the signal intensity of the necrotic tissue is either equivalent to that of fat or more heterogeneous with subchondral low signal intensity areas on T1-, T2-, and enhanced T1-weighted images reflecting the presence of mummified fat or eosinophilic necrosis, respectively (LANG et al. 1988; VANDE BERG et al. 1992). Signal alterations in marrow area adjacent to the lesion can be prominent findings on MR images with low signal intensity on T1-weighted and high signal intensity on T2-weighted images. In the proximal femur, these marrow changes adjacent to the lesion are more frequent in symptomatic than asymptomatic lesions (KOO et al. 1999) and are more likely to be related to the development of the epiphyseal fracture than to the presence of the infarct itself (SAKAI et al. 2000). These signal changes in marrow adjacent to the lesion are occasionally prominent and may cause confusion with other processes because the infarct and the reactive interface are swamped in reactive changes.

In the final stage of the disease, articular cartilage that was initially spared becomes abnormal because of articular incongruity. Bone changes on radiographs and marrow changes on MR images are heterogeneous and depend on the balance between ischemic changes, repair process and degenerative disease.

15.2.3
Post-traumatic Osteonecrosis

The blood supply of the humeral head derives from vessels that penetrate the marrow cavity at the level of the bicipital groove, the base of the neck and at the tendinous insertion of the rotator cuff tendon (LAING 1956). Following displaced fracture of the humeral neck or severe fracture-dislocation, necrosis of a large segment of the epiphysis can develop in those areas with vulnerable blood supply secondary to lesions to the vasculature.

The radiographic diagnosis of post-traumatic shoulder osteonecrosis can be difficult and is usually delayed until osteoporosis of the adjacent viable bone creates a relatively increased density of the avascular epiphysis (Fig. 15.6). This finding may become apparent within 2–3 months following injury. The initial radiographic stage of increased radiological density due to the lack of participation of the bone in the hyperemia and osteoporosis subsequent to the fracture (relative sclerosis) is followed by a stage of absolute increased bone density secondary to the healing process, to passive deposition of calcium salts in the necrotic area or to compression of necrotic

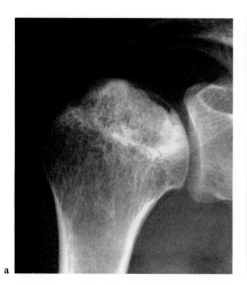
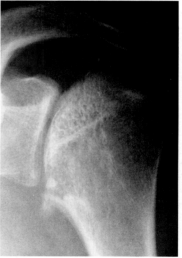

a   b

Fig. 15.4. a Radiograph of the right shoulder of a 43-year-old patient with chronic steroid therapy shows a subchondral cleft fracture as a radiolucent line parallel to the subchondral bone plate. **b** Radiograph of the left shoulder of the same patient shows marked epiphyseal collapse indicating epiphyseal osteonecrosis

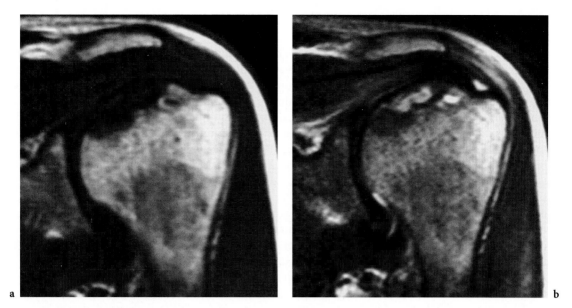

Fig. 15.5. a Coronal T1-weighted magnetic resonance (MR) image of the left shoulder of a 37-year-old patient with a subchondral low signal intensity area associated with mild depression of the humeral head. **b** On the corresponding T2-weighted image, most of the lesion has high signal intensity that is related to the presence of the repair process. Irregularities of the humeral head remain discrete and are best shown on radiographs

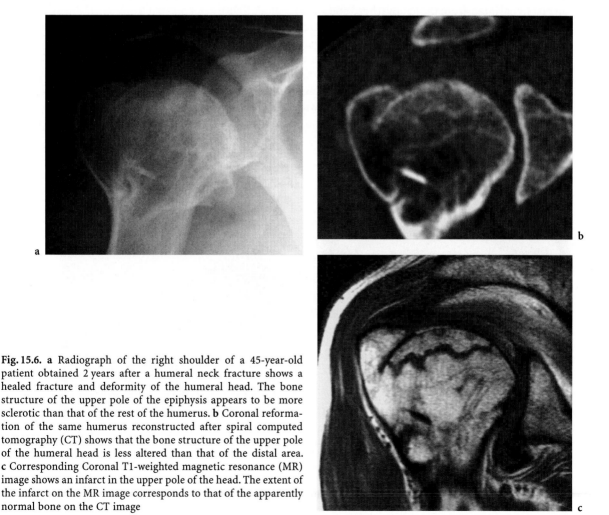

Fig. 15.6. a Radiograph of the right shoulder of a 45-year-old patient obtained 2 years after a humeral neck fracture shows a healed fracture and deformity of the humeral head. The bone structure of the upper pole of the epiphysis appears to be more sclerotic than that of the rest of the humerus. **b** Coronal reformation of the same humerus reconstructed after spiral computed tomography (CT) shows that the bone structure of the upper pole of the humeral head is less altered than that of the distal area. **c** Corresponding Coronal T1-weighted magnetic resonance (MR) image shows an infarct in the upper pole of the head. The extent of the infarct on the MR image corresponds to that of the apparently normal bone on the CT image

trabeculae (MALGHEM and MALDAGUE 1981). The phase of relative densification might be more easily detected on conventional radiographs than on computed tomography (CT) images, because of a summation effect. Conversely, the participation of the humeral head in the localized osteoporosis related to the fracture and the healing process is best detected on CT images than on conventional radiographs and is a good prognostic sign indicating adequate blood supply to the bone. Collapse of the humeral head secondary to a post-traumatic infarct may develop at a delay after the lesion that varies according to numerous parameters. In the femoral head, a 12-month follow-up is generally accepted as a time interval sufficient to establish the presence or absence of osteonecrosis (MALGHEM and MALDAGUE 1981).

MR patterns of post-traumatic osteonecrosis of the humeral head have barely been reported and general principles must be derived from post-traumatic osteonecrosis of the femoral head. MR images obtained within a few days after the fracture show normal signal intensity of the femoral head and signal alterations that remain localized in the fracture area, due to impaction of the fracture, hemorrhage, edema and cellular necrosis (SPEER et al. 1990; LANG et al. 1993). Consequently, routine MR imaging does not detect epiphyseal marrow changes at an early stage. In preliminary limited investigation of patients with femoral neck fracture at risk for epiphyseal osteone-

crosis, LANG et al. showed that gadolinium enhanced MR imaging was useful to detect altered perfusion in femoral head with normal signal intensity (LANG et al. 1993). At a time delay after the causative trauma, marrow infarct may develop in the subchondral area of the humeral head with elementary changes that are probably very similar to those observed in nontraumatic osteonecrosis (Fig. 15.6).

15.3
Marrow Lesion Patterns of Bone Marrow Changes

Patterns of marrow alteration in proximal humerus are similar to those observed elsewhere in the long bone extremities. Marrow changes can be focal or diffuse and the intensity of the decrease in signal intensity observed on T1-weighted images generally parallels the decrease in fatty amount (VANDE BERG et al. 1998).

Reactive marrow infiltration is an ill-delimited area of moderate decrease in signal intensity on T1-weighted images and of increased signal intensity on T2-weighted images. These changes probably reflect the presence of marrow edema, hemorrhage, or fibrosis. Presence of reactive marrow infiltration or edema is a sign that an abnormal process is under way but

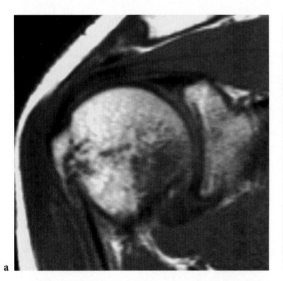
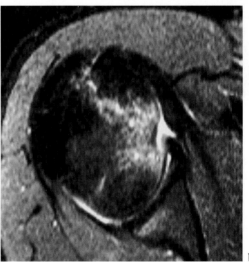

Fig. 15.7. a Coronal T1-weighted image of the right shoulder of a 29-year-old male after apparent minor ski trauma. The bone marrow of the medial aspect of the proximal end of the humerus shows an ill defined area of decreased signal intensity. **b** On the axial fat-saturated intermediate-weighted magnetic resonance image, the lesion has high signal intensity which indicates that the lesion probably corresponds to an area of "bone marrow edema". The deformity of the anterior humeral head contour and the presence of a similar lesion involving the posterior aspect of the glenoid bone indicates that this patient has had a spontaneously reduced posterior dislocation of the shoulder

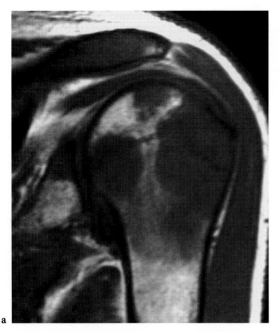
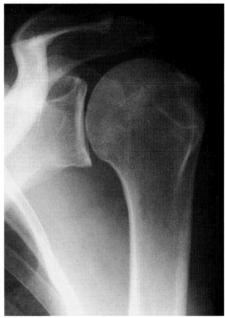

a   b

Fig. 15.8. a Coronal T1-weighted magnetic resonance image of the left shoulder of a 44-year-old man shows multiple areas of decreased signal intensity that correspond to areas of marrow replacement. Biopsy of a pelvic lesion demonstrated bone lymphoma. (**b**) The corresponding anteroposterior radiograph shows disease destruction of the greater tuberosity

it is not a diagnosis. Bone marrow edema can be secondary to a fracture (after shoulder dislocation), to a tumor (osteoid osteoma, chondroblastoma), or to an infection (arthritis, osteomyelitis) (Fig. 15.7). Occasionally, subtle bone marrow infiltration remains occult on T1-weighted images and shows up on fat-saturated T2-weighted images or on fat-saturated T1-weighted images after gadolinium injection. This pattern of marrow alteration can be encountered in adhesive capsulitis, in association with thickening of the synovial membrane and capsule.

Focal or diffuse marrow replacement occurs when the fatty component of the bone marrow is completely replaced by another process. This lesion pattern occurs in bone metastasis, multiple myeloma (Fig. 15.8), lymphoma and other less common disorders including sarcoïdosis, tuberculosis and primary bone tumors.

References

Duda SH, Laniado M, Schick F et al (1993) The double-line sign of osteonecrosis: evaluation on chemical shift MR images. Eur J Radiol 16:233–238

Hattrup SJ, Cofield RH (1999) Osteonecrosis of the humeral head: relationship of disease stage, extent, and cause to natural history. J Shoulder Elbow Surg 8:559–564

Jaramillo D, Laor T, Hoffer FA et al (1991) Epiphyseal marrow in infancy: MR imaging. Radiology 180:809–812

Koo KH, Ahn IO, Song HR et al (1999) Bone marrow edema and associated pain in early stage osteonecrosis of the femoral head: prospective study with serial MR images. Radiology 213:715–722

Laing PG (1956) The arterial supply of the adult humerus. J Bone Joint Surg (Am) 38:1105–1112

Lang P, Jergesen HE, Moseley ME et al (1988) Avascular necrosis of the femoral head: high-field-strength MR imaging with histologic correlation. Radiology 169:517–524

Lang P, Mauz M, Schörner W et al (1993) Acute fracture of the femoral neck: assessment of femoral head perfusion with gadopentetate dimeglumine-enhanced MR imaging. AJR 160:335–341

Malghem J, Maldague B (1981) Radiologic aspects of epiphyseal necrosis and pathogenetic implications. Acta Orthop Belg 47:200–224

McCauley TR, Disler DG, Tam MK (2000) Bone marrow edema in the greater tuberosity of the humerus at MR imaging: association with rotator cuff tears and traumatic injury. Magn Reson Imaging 18:979–984

Mirowitz SA (1993) Hematopoietic bone marrow within the proximal humeral epiphysis in normal adults: investigation with MR imaging. Radiology 188:689–693

Richardson ML, Patten RM (1994) Age-related changes in marrow distribution in the shoulder: MR imaging findings. Radiology 192:209–215

Sakai T, Sugano N, Nishii T et al (2000) MR findings of necrotic lesions and the extralesional area of osteonecrosis of the femoral head. Skeletal Radiol 29:133–141

Speer KP, Spritzer CE, Harrelson JM et al (1990) Magnetic

resonance imaging of the femoral head after acute intracapsular fracture of the femoral neck. J Bone Joint Surg (Am) 72:98–103

Taccone A, Oddone M, Dell'Acqua A et al (1995) MRI "roadmap" of normal age-related bone marrow. Pediatr Radiol 25:596–606

Vande Berg BC, Malghem J, Labaisse MA et al (1992) Avascular necrosis of the hip: comparison of contrast-enhanced and nonenhanced MR imaging with histologic correlation.

Work in progress. Radiology 182:445–450

Vande Berg BC, Malghem J, Lecouvet FE et al (1998) Classification and detection of bone marrow lesions with magnetic resonance imaging. Skeletal Radiol 27:529–545

Vande Berg BC, Malghem J, Lecouvet FE et al (2001) Magnetic resonance imaging and differential diagnosis of epiphyseal osteonecrosis. Semin Musc Radiol 5:57–67

Vogler JBI, Murphy WA (1988) Bone marrow imaging. Radiology 168:679–693

16 Tumours and Tumour-Like Lesions

A. M. Davies and D. Vanel

CONTENTS

A. M. DAVIES, MD
Consultant Radiologist, MRI Centre, Royal Orthopaedic Hospital, Birmingham B31 2AP, United Kingdom
D. VANEL, MD
Department of Radiology, Institut Gustav Roussy, 39 rue Camille Desmoulins, Villejuif 94805, France

16.1 Introduction

Tumours arising from the bones or the shoulder girdle or adjacent tissues rank second in incidence only to tumours around the knee joint. The commonest site for bone tumours in the shoulder is the proximal humerus (70%), particularly in adolescents in whom this is a site of rapid bone growth. Despite this, the proportion of tumours that occur in the proximal humerus is frequently less than 10% of all cases of individual tumour types (Table 16.1). Approximately 20% of shoulder girdle tumours arise in the scapula and 10% in the clavicle. The purpose of this chapter is to discuss the basic principles of the detection, diagnosis and surgical staging of tumours in or around the shoulder. Only those tumour types with a predilection for the shoulder will be discussed in any detail. Unless otherwise stated, incidence data quoted has been calculated combining results from several authoritative texts on the subject (MULDER et al. 1993; UNNI 1996; CAMPANACCI 1999).

Table 16.1. Proportion of individual bone tumours arising in the proximal humerus in descending order of incidence [figures obtained by combining results from MULDER et al. (1993), UNNI (1996) and CAMPANACCI (1999)]

Benign bone tumours	(%)	Malignant bone tumours	(%)
Simple bone cyst	43	Parosteal osteosarcoma	11
Chondroblastoma	20	Chondrosarcoma	9
Osteochondroma	16	Conventional osteosarcoma	8
Chondroma	7.3	Paget's sarcoma	7.9
ABC	5.4	MFH/fibrosarcoma	7.5
Giant cell tumour	4.7	Radiation sarcoma	7.4
FCD/NOF	3.6	Lymphoma of bone	6.3
Osteoid osteoma	3.1	Ewing's sarcoma	5.7

16.2 Detection

The past 25 years have seen major advances in both imaging and the management of bone and soft tissue tumours, but a successful outcome, namely a cure with preservation of function, can only be anticipated with early detection and prompt diagnosis. The method of detection has changed little for the vast majority of patients heavily reliant on clinical examination and radiography. The radiograph remains the preliminary and single most important imaging investigation. Frequently, the diagnosis may be obvious to the trained eye and further imaging, if required, is then directed towards staging the lesion. Alternatively, if an abnormality is present on the film and the precise nature is not immediately apparent, certain features will indicate a differential diagnosis and other forms of imaging can then be employed to assist in establishing a more definitive radiological diagnosis. If the initial radiograph is normal, however, with persisting and increasing symptoms a repeat radiograph in due course may be indicated

Early signs of a bone tumour, or infection for that matter, include subtle areas of ill-defined lysis or sclerosis, cortical destruction, periosteal new bone formation and soft tissue swelling (ROSENBERG et al. 1995). Not surprisingly, bone lesions are frequently missed or overlooked on the initial radiograph. In an audit performed at one of the author's institutions (AMD) neither the clinician nor the radiologist at the referring centre detected the bone tumour on the initial radiographs in approximately 20% of cases , although evidence was present on retrospective review of the films (GRIMER and SNEATH 1990). This is a bigger problem with tumours of flat bones, such as the scapula, or where there is overlapping of structures as with the clavicle. Fortunately, tumours are much less common at both these sites than the humerus (see Sect. 16.7). The pathological process may be well established even in the presence of a normal radiograph. At least 40%–50% of trabecular bone must be destroyed before a discrete area of lucency can be discerned on the radiographs (ARDRAN 1951; EDELSTYN et al. 1967). Erosion or destruction of the cortex is more readily apparent. In the presence of a normal radiograph, referred pain needs to be considered. Shoulder pain may be referred from tumours infiltrating the cervical spine, brachial plexus and chest wall. If referred pain is suspected then radiographs of these other areas are indicated.

Both bone scintigraphy and magnetic resonance (MR) imaging are significantly more sensitive in detecting early marrow change. A minority of radiographically occult lesion cases may, therefore, be detected by either of these techniques (Fig. 16.1). It is important to stress that MR imaging all too frequently reveals abnormalities of doubtful significance. An increasing number of shoulder MR scans are performed each year for a variety of conditions. Incidental medullary abnormalities will be revealed in the proximal humeral meta-diaphysis in a small percentage of cases which frequently prove to be innocuous chondromas. Increased T2 signal in the distal clavicle is a relatively common finding and in most cases is of no clinical significance (FIORELLA et al. 2000).

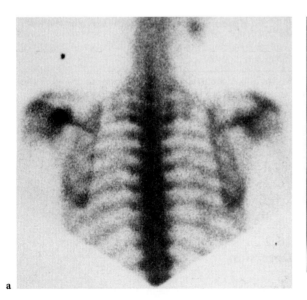

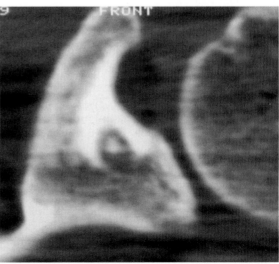

Fig. 16.1a, b. Osteoid osteoma base of coracoid process. **a** The tumour is detected on the posterior bone scan of the trunk. **b** The diagnosis is confirmed by the axial CT

16.3
Diagnosis

16.3.1
Diagnosis of Bone Tumours

Once an osseous abnormality has been detected around the shoulder, the next objective of imaging is to attempt to characterise the lesion and, in doing so, indicate an appropriate differential diagnosis to the referring clinician. At this stage important maxims that should be appreciated include not overtreating a benign lesion, not undertreating a malignant lesion and not misdirecting the approach to biopsy which might prejudice subsequent surgical management (MOSER and MADEWELL 1987). Before assessing the imaging the prudent radiologist should establish some basic facts regarding the patient. By recognising the relevance of certain clinical details an extensive differential diagnosis may be significantly reduced even before the imaging is considered. Important factors to be considered include:

1. Age: The age of the patient is arguably the single most useful piece of information as it frequently influences the differential diagnosis. Many musculoskeletal neoplasms exhibit a peak incidence at different ages (Figs. 16.2 and 16.3). For osteosarcoma this is in the second and third decades. Metastases and myeloma should always be con-

sidered in a patient over 40 years of age. Similarly, metastatic neuroblastoma should be in the differential at 2 years of age or under. Conversely, a tumour arising in adolescence or early adult life is unlikely to be a metastasis.

2. Family History: There is little evidence of a familial predisposition to the formation of musculoskeletal neoplasms in most instances. The exception includes certain congenital bone conditions which may undergo malignant transformation e.g., diaphyseal aclasis.

3. Multiplicity: It is critical early in the management of a patient to establish whether a lesion is solitary or multiple as it will influence the differential diagnosis. Frequently this question will not be definitively answered until the staging imaging is performed.

It is at this stage that attention should now turn to the imaging. The radiograph remains the most accurate of all the imaging techniques currently available in determining the differential diagnosis of a bone lesion (KRICUN 1983). Although many lesions will be instantly recognisable it is prudent to analyse the radiographic features present. The analysis can be performed by answering the following questions: Which bone and what part of the bone is involved? What is the tumour doing to the bone (pattern of destruction)? What form of periosteal reaction, if

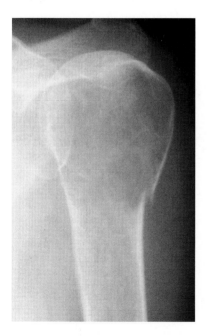

Fig. 16.2. Giant cell tumour in a 28-year-old male. The AP radiograph shows a pathological fracture through a lytic subarticular tumour

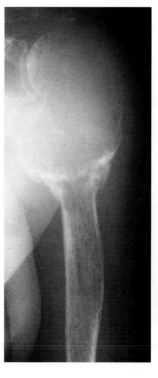

Fig. 16.3. Expansile metastasis from a thyroid primary in a 66-year-old female. A giant cell tumour might give a similar appearance but the patient's age would be against this diagnosis. Note the "herring-bone" appearance of the disuse osteoporosis in the distal humerus

any, is present? What type of matrix mineralisation, if any, is present?

16.3.1.1
Site in Skeleton

As the second commonest site, after the knee, many different benign and malignant bone tumours may arise in the proximal humerus (Table 16.1). Common benign conditions include simple bone cyst (Fig. 16.4), chondroblastoma (Fig. 16.5) and osteochondroma. Some conditions are sufficiently rare in the proximal humerus to be effectively excluded from the routine differential diagnosis. These include: Langerhans cell histiocytosis, chondromyxoid fibroma, haemangioma of bone, adamantinoma and high grade surface and periosteal osteosarcomas. In the first two decades the commonest tumours to be seen in the scapula are Langerhans cell histiocytosis, aneurysmal bone cyst (ABC) and Ewing's sarcoma. The prevalence of a condition as well as its incidence at a particular site need to also be considered. For example, only 0.8% of cases of osteosarcoma arise in the scapula as compared with 3% for Ewing's sarcoma. However, the incidence of osteosarcoma in the general population is slightly more than twice that of

Ewing's sarcoma so that one can expect to see only twice as many cases of Ewing's sarcoma in the scapula and not four times as many.

16.3.1.2
Location in Bone

The precise site of origin of a bone tumour is an important parameter of diagnosis (MADEWELL et al. 1981). Frequently, it reflects the site of greatest cellular activity. During the adolescent growth spurt the most active areas are the metaphyses around the knee and in the proximal humerus. Tumour originating from marrow cells may occur anywhere along the bone. Conventional osteosarcoma will tend, therefore, to originate in the metaphysis or meta-diaphysis, whereas Ewing's sarcoma originates in the metaphysis or, more distinctively, in the diaphysis. In the child the differential diagnosis of a lesion arising within an epiphysis can be realistically limited to chondroblastoma (Fig. 16.5), epiphyseal abscess (pyogenic or tuberculous) and rarely eosinophilic granuloma. Following skeletal fusion subarticular lesions, analogous in the adult to the epiphyseal lesions, include giant cell tumour (GCT) (Fig. 16.2), clear cell chondrosarcoma and intraosseous ganglion. The latter two are rare in the proximal humerus. With the exception of epiphyseal abscess most osteomyelitis will arise within the metaphysis of a long bone, less common in the proximal humerus than the proximal tibia or distal femur.

It is also helpful to identify the origin of the tumour with respect to the transverse plane of the bone. Is

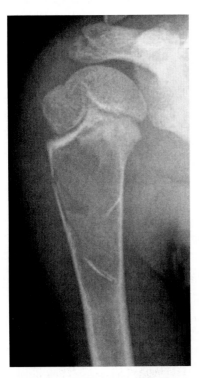

Fig. 16.4. Simple bone cyst. Undisplaced fracture of the lateral wall of the cyst with two "fallen fragments"

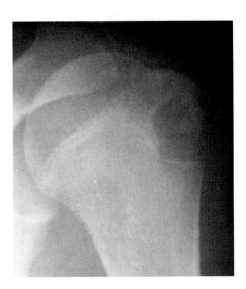

Fig. 16.5. Chondroblastoma. Well defined lytic lesion in the lateral aspect of the proximal humeral epiphysis

the tumour central, eccentric or cortically based? For example, a simple bone cyst (Fig. 16.4), fibrous dysplasia and Ewing's sarcoma will tend to be centrally located. Osteochondroma and fibrous cortical defect/nonossifying fibroma are typically eccentric (Fig. 16.6). Lesions that usually arise in an eccentric position may appear central if the tumour is particularly large or the involved bone is of a small calibre. Therefore, most tumours arising in the clavicle will

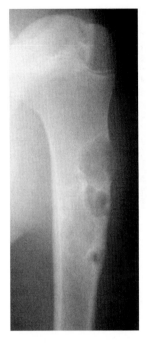

Fig. 16.6. Non-ossifying fibroma. Well defined, lobulated, eccentric lytic lesion

appear "central". There are numerous surface lesions of bone which are related to the outer cortex (KENAN et al. 1993a; SEEGER et al. 1998). The majority of the malignant surface lesions of bone arising around the shoulder will be either a peripheral chondrosarcoma or a parosteal osteosarcoma (Fig. 16.7). By identifying the origin of a bone tumour in both the longitudinal and transverse planes it is possible to narrow down the differential diagnosis significantly.

16.3.1.3
Pattern of Bone Destruction

Analysis of the interface between tumour and host bone is a good indicator of the rate of growth of the lesion. A sharply marginated lesion usually denotes slower growth than a non-marginated lesion. The faster the growth the more aggressive the pattern of destruction and the wider the zone of transition between tumour and normal bone. Aggressivity per se does not conclusively indicate malignancy but the malignant tumours tend to be faster growing than their benign counterparts. Geographic bone destruction is the term applied to bone lesions that appear well marginated with a thin zone of transition. The thicker the sclerotic border the longer the host bone has had to respond to the lesion and therefore, by implication, the slower the rate of growth of the lesion. The vast majority of bone tumours in children showing a geographic pattern of destruction are benign such as simple bone cyst (SBC) (Fig. 16.4), aneurysmal bone cyst (ABC), fibrous dysplasia and enchondroma.

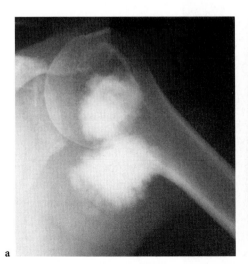
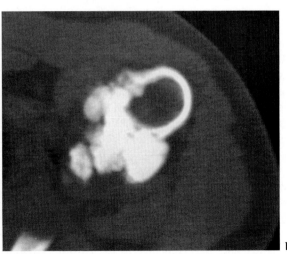

a   b

Fig. 16.7a, b. Parosteal osteosarcoma. Radiograph (a) and axial CT (b). The CT shows breaching of the cortex with early intramedullary spread of tumour

Moth-eaten and permeative bone destruction are terms used to describe bone destruction in which there are multiple tiny cortical lucencies with an ill-defined zone of transition. These patterns indicate the aggressive nature of these lesions in contrast to those with a geographic pattern. The rapid growth of these lesions does not allow the host bone sufficient time to react and produce a response. Typically malignancies, including osteosarcoma, Ewing's sarcoma (Fig. 16.8) and neuroblastoma metastasis exhibit a moth-eaten or permeative pattern of bone destruction. Acute osteomyelitis is the "benign" condition which may also give a moth-eaten appearance. Disuse osteoporosis in the upper limb may give a "herringbone" appearance to the humerus simulating an infiltrative process (Fig. 16.9) (KEATS and ANDERSON 2001).

16.3.1.4
Periosteal Reaction

The periosteum is normally radiolucent but will mineralise when stimulated by an adjacent osseous or paraosseous process. The rate of mineralisation is partly dependent on the age of the patient. The younger the patient the more rapid the appearance of radiographic change and vice versa. Periosteal reaction, otherwise known as periosteal new bone formation, may occur in any condition which elevates the periosteum whether it be blood, pus or tumour. The appearance and nature of a periosteal reaction is frequently valuable in narrowing down the differential diagnosis of a bone tumour.

A 'shell' is used to describe a lytic lesion with bone expansion. The shell is the periosteal new bone laid in response to the growing tumour. The thicker the shell the slower growing the lesion and vice versa. Shells in the proximal humerus are typically found in benign lesions such as SBC (Fig. 16.4), ABC (Fig. 16.10), and fibrous dysplasia. It may also be seen with a telangiectatic osteosarcoma which frequently mimics an ABC. In the older age group shells are found in expansile metastases (renal and thyroid) (Fig. 16.3) and plasmacytoma.

A lamellar periosteal reaction is seen in many traumatic and inflammatory conditions. The lamellated periosteal reaction, otherwise known as onion-skin, is seen in Ewing's sarcoma, osteosarcoma, eosinophilic granuloma, and acute osteomyelitis. A spiculated periosteal reaction occurs when the mineralisation is oriented perpendicular to the cortex and denotes a more rapidly evolving process. It is typical of malignant tumours such as osteosarcoma

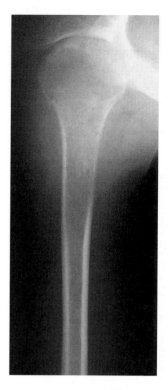

Fig. 16.8. Ewing's sarcoma. Extensive, permeative, lytic tumour

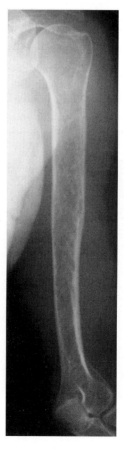

Fig. 16.9. Disuse osteoporosis of the humerus. The "herring-bone" appearance simulates infiltration such as might be seen with myeloma

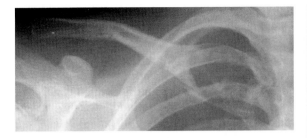

Fig. 16.10. Aneurysmal bone cyst medial clavicle. Lytic expansion with a thin peripheral shell

and Ewing's sarcoma (Fig. 16.11). It may be seen in benign tumours such as haemangioma of bone and non-neoplastic conditions such as thalassaemia and thyroid acropachy, but not in relation to the shoulder.

16.3.1.5
Matrix

A number of tumours produce a matrix, the intercellular substance, that can calcify or ossify. The radiodense foci should be differentiated from other causes of calcifications such as fracture callus, sclerotic response adjacent to a tumour, necrotic debris and dystrophic calcification. Radiodense tumour matrix is either osteoid or chondroid. The exception is fibrous dysplasia where the collagenous matrix may be sufficiently dense to give a ground-glass appearance. Tumour osteoid is typified by solid (sharp-edged) or cloud to ivory-like (ill-defined edge) patterns (Figs. 16.7, 16.11). Tumour cartilage is variously described as stippled, flocculent, ring-and-arc and popcorn in appearance (Fig. 16.12). Identifying the pattern of matrix calcification will significantly reduce the differential diagnosis but matrix per se has no influence as to whether the lesion is benign or malignant. The distribution can be helpful. For example, both enchondroma and medullary infarction may show calcification of a similar nature. The distribution in enchondroma is typically central and peripheral in medullary infarction (Fig. 16.12).

16.3.2
Diagnosis of Soft Tissue Tumours

The lack of contrast resolution is a well-recognised limitation of radiography, but the value of the examination should not be underestimated in the evaluation of soft tissue masses. It may not identify

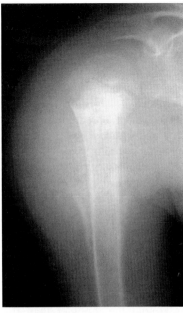

Fig. 16.11. Osteosarcoma. Extensive tumour with a spiculated periosteal reaction proximally, lamellar distally with Codman's angles at the interface. There is some dense malignant osteoid overlying the growth plate

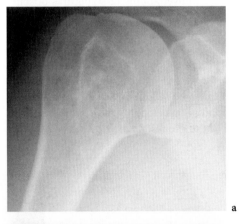

a

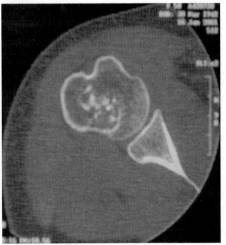

b

Fig. 16.12a, b. Enchondroma. AP radiograph (a) and axial CT (b). The popcorn calcification indicating a chondroid lesion is more conspicuous on the CT

the precise diagnosis, in all but a minority of cases, but can still provide valuable information, e.g. the presence of calcification and bone involvement. The absence of any bony abnormality in the presence of a clinically palpable mass immediately indicates that the pathology is of soft tissue origin, albeit with a large differential diagnosis.

The radiodensity of most soft tissue masses approximates to that of water and is similar to that of muscle and they are, therefore, only revealed by virtue of mass effect. In a minority of cases, part or all of the tumour may exhibit a radiodensity sufficiently different to that of water for it to be visualised directly on radiographs. Lipomas, the commonest of all soft tissue tumours, produce a low radiodensity between that of muscle and air. For this reason lipomas are typically well-demarcated from the surrounding soft tissues and can be diagnosed on radiographs with moderate confidence (Fig. 16.13). It is more difficult to identify lipomas around the shoulder than the extremities due to overlapping of structures obscuring the relatively low attenuation fat.

Increased radiodensity may be seen in the tissues due to haemosiderin, calcification or ossification. Haemosiderin deposition typically occurs in synovial tissues exposed to repeated haemorrhage such as seen in pigmented villonodular synovitis (PVNS) and haemophiliac arthropathy, although both are uncommon in the shoulder. Calcification or ossifica-

tion in the soft tissues is a feature of a large spectrum of pathologies including congenital, metabolic, endocrine, traumatic and parasitic infections. Primary soft tissue tumours are one of the less common causes of calcification that the general radiologist can expect to come across in his or her routine practice.

Ultrasound is an important technique in the initial assessment of a suspected soft tissue mass. First, it can confidently confirm/exclude the presence of a mass. Second, it can to a degree characterise the lesion by distinguishing purely cystic lesions, such as an enlarged subacromial/subdeltoid bursa, from solid tumours. Doppler ultrasound can be employed to assess the vascularity of a lesion and ultrasound is ideally suited for image-guided biopsy.

16.3.3
CT and MR Imaging in Diagnosis

The principal role of CT and MR imaging in the management of the patient with a suspected musculoskeletal tumour is in staging (see Sect. 16.4). In selected cases both techniques can be useful in establishing a differential diagnosis. The CT features that should be assessed are similar to those described above when evaluating the radiographs. This reflects the fact that both are radiographic techniques relying on the attenuation of an X-ray

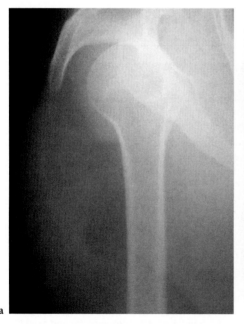
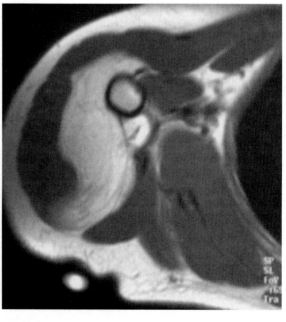

a   b

Fig. 16.13a, b. Lipoma. The radiograph (**a**) shows a low attenuation soft tissue mass lying on the lateral aspect of the proximal humerus which is high signal intensity on the T1-weighted image (TR/TE = 500/15) (**b**)

source. Cortical breaching, soft tissue extension and faint mineralisation are all more readily appreciated on CT scans than radiographs (Fig. 16.12). Assessment of CT attenuation values will allow distinction between fat-containing and fluid-containing masses. CT images of the shoulder are frequently suboptimal, particularly in heavily built individuals, due to beam hardening artefacts.

Although the physical basis of MR imaging is very different, similar morphological information can be easily identified. The exception are the signal voids of fine mineralisation which can be easily missed on MR imaging. Potentially misleading MR features seen that might suggest a bone sarcoma are prominent marrow oedema and soft tissue oedema (HAYES et al. 1992). These are, however, common with osteoid osteoma, osteoblastoma, chondroblastoma, Langerhans cell histiocytosis, stress fractures and infection. Of these conditions, chondroblastoma is the commonest in the proximal humerus (Fig. 16.14). Many soft tissue sarcomas will appear well defined on MR imaging due to the presence of a pseudocapsule, whereas inflammatory processes, such as abscesses will appear poorly defined due to the surrounding inflammatory exudate.

The majority of tumours will have prolonged T1 and T2 relaxation times, thereby showing low to intermediate signal on T1-weighted and high signal on T2-weighted sequences. T1 shortening, with a high signal intensity, will be seen in fat-containing tumours, subacute haemorrhage and gadolinium chelate enhancement. A low signal intensity on T2-weighted images is seen with dense mineralisation, hypocellular/fibrous tumours, signal voids from flowing blood, haemosiderin deposition, surgical implants and bone cement. Fluid–fluid levels are well demonstrated on both CT and MR imaging in a large number of different musculoskeletal conditions. In the immature with the appropriate radiographic appearances fluid–fluid levels in the bones of the shoulder girdle are most commonly seen in ABCs (Fig. 16.15) (DAVIES and CASSAR-PULLICINO 1992).

Dynamic contrast-enhanced MR imaging has been used to differentiate benign from malignant bone lesions using the slope of the derived time–intensity curves (VERSTRAETE et al. 1994). Benign bone lesions tend to show a low slope as compared with the high or steep slope of malignant lesions. Although many of the studies show a statistically significant difference in slope values of benign and malignant lesions, there is considerable overlap such that this technique is of limited value in routine practice. For example, highly vascularised or perfused lesions such as ABC, Langerhans cell histiocytosis, osteoid osteoma and acute osteomyelitis may all show slope values in the malignant tumour range. Similarly, in the soft tissues, early myositis ossificans will show a steep slope mimicking malignancy.

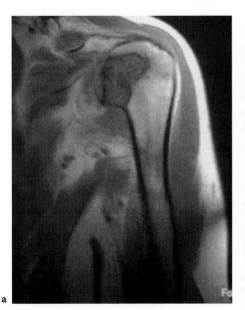 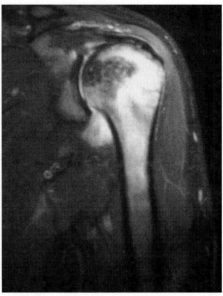

a   b

Fig. 16.14a, b. Chondroblastoma. Coronal T1-weighted (TR/TE = 769/14) (**a**) and coronal STIR (TR/TE = 4460/27) (**b**) images. There is a well defined epiphyseal lesion containing signal voids indicating chondroid mineralisation. There is a reactive shoulder joint effusion and marked marrow oedema

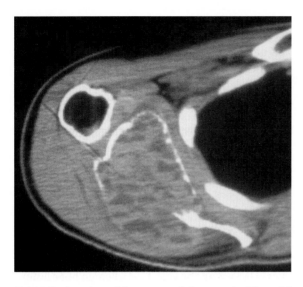

Fig. 16.15. Aneurysmal bone cyst of the scapula. The axial CT scan shows a lytic, expansile tumour containing multiple fluid–fluid levels

16.4
Surgical Staging

Accurate surgical staging is a fundamental requisite of all oncological imaging. The staging system regularly used for bone and soft tissue sarcomas is that adopted by the Musculoskeletal Tumor Society (ENNEKING et al. 1980). This assigns one of three grades according to the local extent of the tumour, presence or absence of metastases and the histological grade. Clarification of the first two features of the staging system relies entirely on imaging. The value of a straightforward staging system, such as this, is that it is easily applied, correlates well with prognosis and allows valid comparison of studies of differing treatments and treatment centres. Confirmation or exclusion of metastases is achieved with a chest CT and whole body bone scintigraphy. It is important to recognise that up to half of the pulmonary nodules identified on chest CT are not metastases (PICCI et al. 2001).

While most are familiar with the anatomical compartments in the extremities, the exact anatomy of the compartments about the shoulder remains poorly defined. There are as many as eight different compartments around the shoulder (Table 16.2) but the boundaries and integrity of these compartments as well their potential for tumour containment remains uncertain (CONRAD 1998). Also, this list does not take into account the axillary/brachial nerves and vessels which are contained within their own sheaths and can be involved by extrinsic compression or direct

invasion from aggressive, usually malignant, lesions. The scapula is customarily divided into two zones; the acromial–glenoid complex and the blade–spine portion. This helps provide a functional classification for resections and reconstructions (ENNEKING et al. 1990).

Determination of local tumour extent around the shoulder usually relies on MR imaging. One study of sarcomas at all sites has shown CT to be as good as MR imaging in staging (PANICEK et al. 1997a), although there has been some doubt expressed as to whether the technique and quality of technology used in that particular multicentre study was strictly comparable (STEINBACH 1998). Undoubtedly, there can be difficulties in obtaining good quality images of tumours around the shoulder due to a number of factors. First, the relevant anatomy is displaced from the magnet isocentre in all but the smallest of patients. Second, breathing artefacts may further degrade the images. Third, the shoulder does not readily lend itself to ideal coil design. Dedicated shoulder coils rarely give an adequate field of view to stage large sarcomas and the resolution of the body coil is limited. In the authors' experience, the best compromise it to use a large flexible wrap-around coil. Occasionally, chest wall lesions near the shoulder can be best demonstrated with the patient in an oblique position on a spine coil. Finally, one disadvantage of the shoulder imaging over the lower limb is the absence of images of the contralateral normal side which can sometimes be helpful when looking at subtle changes, normal variants, etc. The MR scan should preferably be performed before the biopsy as the trauma of the procedure may result in haemorrhage and oedema which can exaggerate the true extent of the tumour. The tumour characteristics that should be assessed on MR imaging for the purposes of staging a suspected bone sarcoma are discussed in greater detail in the following sections.

Table 16.2. Anatomical compartments around the shoulder [modified from CONRAD (1998)]

Deltoid	Deltoid muscle
Posterior scapular	Supraspinatus, infraspinatus, teres major and teres minor muscles
Subscapular	Subscapularis muscle
Anterior pectoral	Pectoralis major and minor muscles
Anterior humeral	Biceps and coracobrachialis muscles
Lateral humeral	Brachialis muscle
Posterior humeral	Triceps muscle
Intra-articular	

16.4.1
Extent in Bone

To assess the extent of bone involvement by tumour a T1-weighted sequence should be performed oriented along the long axis of the bone involved (Figs. 16.16, 16.17). This sequence is particularly sensitive to marrow changes. It is necessary to measure the tumour extent from a recognised anatomical reference point which, for the purposes of a bone sarcoma arising around the shoulder, can be the proximal and distal articular cortices of the humerus. Measurement of the extent of a tumour should not be made using the slice positions as indicated on the scanner console or hardcopy as the upper limb is not usually accurately positioned in the line of the main magnet. A gadolinium-chelate should not be used as uptake of the contrast medium may well render the tumour isointense with marrow fat. This problem can be overcome by utilising a contrast-enhanced fat suppressed T1-weighted sequence, but this is an expensive way of achieving the same result. Many benign as well as malignant bone tumours show a variable degree of peritumoral oedema. These include osteoid osteoma, chondroblastoma (Fig. 16.14), Langerhans cell histiocytosis, GCT and osteosarcoma. It appears as a zone of intermediate signal intensity merging imperceptibly with the main tumour. With sarcomas it can be difficult to distinguish where tumour ends and oedema

commences. Arguably, it is prudent to include all altered marrow signal within the measurements of the tumour extent as malignant cells may contaminate the oedematous area beyond the immediate confines of the main tumour. Some researchers have suggested that it is possible on MR imaging to distinguish between tumour tissue and peritumoral oedema using a dynamic contrast-enhanced sequence but it is difficult to believe this technique would pick up isolated nests of malignant cells. It is interesting to speculate whether in the future diffusion weighted MR imaging might help distinguish tumour from oedema. Fortunately, this is not a significant management problem in the majority of patients with a sarcoma arising in the humerus. Increasing the length of a custom-made prosthesis by several centimetres to accommodate the oedematous zone is unlikely to affect the functional outcome. Where precise measurement is critical in determining whether limb salvage surgery is possible then reassessment on the post-chemotherapy scans can be useful as the peritumoral oedema has frequently reduced/resolved in the interim.

16.4.2
Extent in Soft Tissue

If the tumour is confined to bone the cortex will remain intact. Cortical bone appears black on all MR sequences

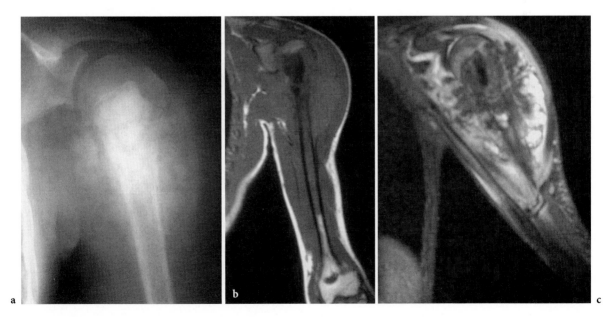

Fig. 16.16a–c. Sclerotic osteosarcoma. AP radiograph (**a**) and coronal T1-weighted image (TR/TE = 520/14) (**b**). The distal limit of the tumour is clearly visible on the coronal image. There is clear definition of the extraosseous component on the coronal STIR image (TR/TE = 4460/27) (**c**). The axillary vessels are closely applied to the medial aspect of the tumour. There is invasion of the axillary recess

as it does not produce a signal. Cortical destruction with loss of the black line is a frequent and characteristic finding of bone malignancy. Not infrequently, however, highly malignant sarcomas such as osteosarcoma and Ewing's sarcoma can penetrate the cortex without frank destruction. In this situation, best demonstrated on axial images, the dark contour of the cortex will persist with permeative appearance analogous to the permeative or moth-eaten pattern on radiographs (Fig. 16.17). It is convention to describe any tumour tissue identified outside the cortex as extraosseous or soft tissue extension. Strictly speaking this is often incorrect as the tumour can remain confined by a largely intact periosteum. Nevertheless, this convention persists and is usually only a source of problems when resolving the findings of MR imaging versus the examination of the pathological specimen. The relatively high water content of most tumours, both bone and soft tissue sarcomas, renders them isointense and therefore indistinguishable from surrounding muscles on T1-weighted images. It is for this reason that to assess soft tissue extension a T2-weighted sequence, with good contrast between tumour and muscle, is required (Figs. 16.16, 16.17). A disadvantage of the widely used fast spin echo (turbo) T2-weighted sequence is slightly reduced spatial resolution and relatively high signal of fat, which may limit the contrast with tumour. This problem can be overcome with the application of fat suppression. Its use in the shoulder can be problematic

as displacement from the magnet isocentre may result in uneven fat suppression. A STIR sequence is an alternative, albeit with a poorer signal-to-noise ratio. The STIR sequence will also tend to overstage the extent of the tumour due to its increased sensitivity to raised water content in a tissue. As in bone the distinction of soft tissue tumour from perineoplastic oedema can be problematic (SHUMAN et al. 1991).

16.4.3
Joint Involvement

It is important to identify shoulder joint invasion by a sarcoma because prior knowledge will prevent the surgeons from opening the joint at operation and thereby potentially contaminating the surgical field with tumour cells (Fig. 16.16). MR imaging is highly sensitive for detecting joint invasion but false positives due to subsynovial rather than true intra-articular spread can lead to overstaging (SCHIMA et al. 1994). This is problematic in the shoulder where inferior extraosseous spread of a humeral or scapular sarcoma will appear to invade the axillary recess where in reality it is frequently displacing it. Of significance is the fact that the absence of a joint effusion has a high negative predictive value for joint invasion (SCHIMA et al. 1994; OZAKI et al. 2002). Joint invasion may occur by one of five mechanisms (OZAKI

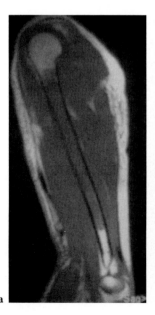 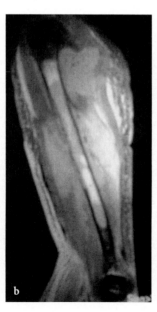 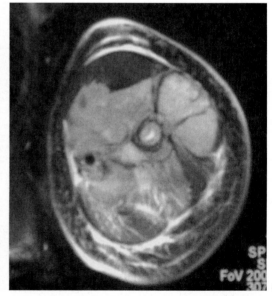

Fig. 16.17a–c. Lymphoma. **a** Sagittal T1-weighted image (TR/TE = 470/14) accurately demonstrating the intramedullary extent of the tumour. The extraosseous component is isointense with the overlying muscles. **b** Sagittal STIR image (TR/TE = 5000/27) demonstrates both the intramedullary and extraosseous components. **c** Axial T2-weighted fat suppressed image (TR/TE = 3860/90) showing permeation of the cortex and a large extraosseous mass. The brachial artery is encased in the medial aspect of the tumour

et al. 2002): (1) Pericapsular extension; (2) tumour extension along the long head of biceps tendon; (3) fracture haematoma from a pathological fracture; (4) direct articular penetration; and (5) subsynovial extension (RUBERT et al. 1999). Pericapsular and direct extension along the long head of the biceps tendon are the commonest routes (MALAWER 1991).

Transarticular spread in the shoulder is rare. Identification of an abnormality on both sides of the shoulder should suggest that the disease process arose de novo in the joint rather than the bone. In older patients it is not uncommon to find an incidental rotator cuff defect. It is important to identify the presence of a tear as this is a potential avenue of tumour spread from the glenohumeral joint into the subacromial/subdeltoid bursa and vice versa.

16.4.4
Neurovascular Involvement

Once a sarcoma has extended beyond the confines of the bone it will tend to grow in the line of least resistance. Around the shoulder this is typically deep to the deltoid muscle and into the axilla (Figs. 16.16, 16.17). MR imaging can demonstrate whether a tumour is close to or in contact with a neurovascular structure in the axilla, but usually cannot distinguish mere contact, adherence or early invasion (PANICEK et al. 1997b). Fortunately, the prevalence of neurovascular involvement in bone sarcomas is less than 4% such that, although the positive predictive value of MR imaging for involvement is poor, the negative predictive value is over 90% (PANICEK et al. 1997b). MR angiography can be used to delineate the relationship of the tumour to vessels (LANG et al. 1995; SWAN et al. 1995), but neither of the authors find it useful routinely.

16.4.5
Skip Metastases and Lymph Node Involvement

The presence of small synchronous foci of tumour, usually osteosarcoma, within the same bone as the primary tumour, or within a bone on the other side of an unaffected joint are called skip metastases. Skip metastases in osteosarcoma have been reported in up to 25% of cases (ENNEKING and KAGAN 1975), although in the authors' experience the true incidence is less than 5%. Also, for some unknown reason which cannot be fully explained by simple relative incidence of the primary sarcomas, skip metastases

in the humerus or across the joint in the glenoid are extremely rare. Lymph node spread in bone and soft tissue sarcomas is uncommon and usually a late manifestation of extensive disease. As at other sites, imaging has difficulty distinguishing metastatic infiltration from reactive hyperplasia (BEARCROFT and DAVIES 1999). The exception is those cases of osteosarcoma with mineralisation, indicating metastatic involvement, which can be easily detected on radiographs or CT and will show increased activity on bone scintigraphy. Rarely, in patients with long-standing prostheses, regional lymphadenopathy may occur due to a foreign body reaction in response to the lymphatic uptake of metal debris (DAVIES et al. 2001), but as this is associated with wear from a prosthetic joint this is not seen around the shoulder. In patients treated by above-elbow amputation, post-traumatic neuromas may mimic lymphadenopathy (BOUTIN et al. 1998).

16.5
Biopsy

With the exception of the "don't-touch-me lesions", verification of the radiological diagnosis will require a biopsy prior to management decisions. As stated above, biopsy should preferably be performed after the appropriate imaging studies. It is well recognised that problems arising from the biopsy occur up to five times more commonly when it is performed at the referring hospital rather than at the specialist treatment centre (MANKIN et al. 1982, 1996). The individual performing the biopsy has to have an idea not only of the likely diagnosis, but also the reconstructive option of limb salvage or tissue coverage following amputation which ensures that the biopsy track is excised in toto with the tumour. One of the more common errors with tumours around the shoulder is to place the biopsy site laterally over the mid-portion of the deltoid (CRAIG and THOMPSON 1987). Subsequent curative limb salvage surgery for a sarcoma of the proximal humerus necessitates sacrifice of the entire deltoid which compromises function and reduces the soft tissue coverage of the prosthesis. There have been numerous discussions in the literature regarding the relative merits of needle versus open biopsy. Suffice it to say that needle biopsy in experienced hands is a cost-effective and less traumatic alternative to open biopsy (STOKER et al. 1991; SKRZNSKI et al. 1996). The expertise required applies as much to the pathologist interpreting the specimen as to the individual responsible for obtaining it. Close liaison within the multidisciplinary team is essential in planning the biopsy and interpreting the results.

16.6
Imaging Follow-up

The imaging follow-up for a patient with a proven sarcoma arising around the shoulder can be divided into short-term (i.e. pre-definitive surgery) and long-term (i.e. post-definitive surgery). In the short-term many patients with a sarcoma will be entered into one of the international adjuvant chemotherapy trials prior to surgery. After a predetermined number of cycles of chemotherapy and immediately before surgery the patient is re-staged with an MR scan of the primary tumour and a CT scan of the chest. This is to ensure that the stage of the tumour has not altered and that the planned surgery is still appropriate. Also, this is an opportunity to use imaging to assess the response of the tumour to the chemotherapy. Histological response to chemotherapy expressed as percentage necrosis is one of the most important prognostic indicators in both osteosarcoma and Ewing's sarcoma. Over the years all types of imaging have been used to estimate the response to chemotherapy.

Postchemotherapeutic radiographic and CT findings do not consistently differentiate the good from the poor responder (SHAPEERO and VANEL 2000). For example, an increase in tumour volume may suggest a poor response but may also represent haemorrhage secondary to necrosis in a responsive tumour (VAN DER WOUDE et al. 1998). Conventional angiography is considered too invasive a procedure for monitoring tumour response to chemotherapy. Although it can identify over 90% of responders it will miss 50% of the poor responders (CARRASCO et al. 1989). It remains to be seen whether MR angiography can fulfil a useful role in this respect (LANG et al. 1995).

If there is a significant extraosseous component to the tumour, Doppler ultrasound can be used to monitor response (VAN DER WOUDE et al. 1995). The technique is operator dependent which may affect reproducibility of results on sequential scanning. Scintigraphy using technetium-99m methylene diphosphonate, thallium-201, gallium-67 and FDG-PET scanning have all been advocated in the estimation of tumour response (SHAPEERO and VANEL 2000). Inherent in all is the limited anatomical resolution and, with PET scanning, limited availability. To date these techniques are largely reserved for research purposes.

Unenhanced MR imaging has a limited role. Increased or unchanged tumour volume and increased peritumoral oedemas after chemotherapy suggest a poor histological response in osteosarcoma and Ewing's sarcoma. Virtual obliteration of the extraosseous component combined with a hypointense rim in Ewing's sarcoma usually indicates a good response. It is, however, impossible to exclude small foci of viable tumour without contrast medium. Standard contrast-enhanced MR imaging is also of limited value as viable tumour, revascularised necrotic tissue, reactive hyperaemia etc. may all enhance. It is for this reason that much of the work on imaging assessment of sarcoma response to chemotherapy over the last 15 years has concentrated on dynamic contrast-enhanced MR imaging. A number of different techniques have been described but all rely on the underlying principle that viable tumour enhances rapidly (i.e. within a few seconds of the contrast medium arriving in the adjacent artery), whereas all other enhancing tissues take much longer. It is possible on the console of most modern scanners to plot a time–intensity curve showing the uptake of the contrast medium. By comparing the curve obtained before commencement of chemotherapy with that obtained after, the tumour response can be estimated. It should be noted that this is a time-consuming and costly exercise with numerous variables that directly influences patient management in very few cases.

In the long-term the patients are closely monitored for evidence of local recurrence (DAVIES and VANEL 1998), metastatic disease (BEARCROFT and DAVIES 1999), and complications of treatment. Local recurrence of a sarcoma is almost inevitable if the original resection margin was not wide. Recurrence may be detected on radiographs as a soft tissue mass with or without bone destruction. Locally recurrent bone sarcoma will usually occur within the soft tissues at the site of the initial surgery as the host bone will have been excised and replaced with a prosthesis (Fig. 16.18). Detection on radiographs is easier if there is evidence of matrix mineralisation. Recurrent tumours with the propensity to mineralise (i.e. osteosarcoma) will usually exhibit focal increased activity on scintigraphy but it is rarely used for this purpose.

MR imaging is the technique of choice in the detection of early recurrence when local control may still be surgically achievable. While ultrasound does have some attractions (CHOI et al. 1991; ALEXANDER et al. 1997), MR imaging will still be required for preoperative evaluation if a recurrence is identified. Depending on the presence or absence of mineralisation, most recurrences will show a high signal intensity mass on T2-weighted or STIR images (Fig. 16.18)

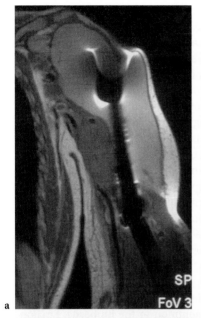
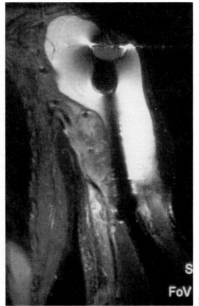

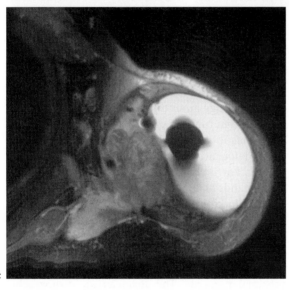

Fig. 16.18a–c. Recurrent osteosarcoma. a Coronal T1-weighted image (TR/TE = 649/14). b Coronal STIR image (TR/TE = 4100/27). c Axial T2-weighted fat suppressed image (TR/TE = 3630/86). Mild image artefact from the titanium proximal humeral prosthesis which is surrounded by a fluid collection containing haemorrhage. There is a 10-cm focus of recurrent tumour lying medially, visible on the STIR and T2-weighted images (b, c)

(VANEL et al. 1994). Diffuse high signal intensity is frequently seen shortly after surgery or can be prolonged following radiation therapy (RICHARDSON et al. 1996). Contrast medium may be required to distinguish enhancing recurrent tumour from seromas, haematomas etc. Dynamic contrast-enhanced MR imaging can be helpful in differentiating small recurrences from other post-operative changes.

It is generally accepted that it is usually the metastatic disease that will eventually kill the patient and not the primary tumour itself. It is for this reason that follow-up imaging is concentrated on the site where metastases are likely to occur, namely the lungs. Chest radiographs are usually considered adequate. Serial chest CT scans are of questionable value in view of the considerable radiation dose involved. The natural history of osteosarcoma has been modified by chemotherapy in that up to 20% of those who develop metastases will first do so in bone prior to there being any evidence of pulmonary metastases. The prognosis for a patient with osseous metastases is so poor that serial follow-up scintigraphy is unlikely to modify the outcome. Scintigraphy is indicated should a patient on follow-up develop bone pain.

It should be recognised that the prolonged medical and surgical management of a patient with a sarcoma is not without risk of complications. Prostheses may be become loose or infected or require replacement if a child has outgrown the extended length of a growing prosthesis. Allografts may also become infected and are prone to fracture. In the long-term follow-up of patients who received radiotherapy, pain or functional impairment within the radiation field should lead to consideration of bone necrosis or radiation-induced sarcoma.

16.7
Bone Tumours

The proximal humerus is the third commonest site of occurrence for most bone tumours after the distal femur and proximal tibia. They can be broadly classified according to their tissue of origin or the tissue they most closely resemble e.g., osseous, cartilaginous, fibrous, lipomatous and an unknown or miscellaneous category.

16.7.1
Benign Bone Tumours

16.7.1.1
Osseous

Benign bone-forming tumours, including surface osteoma and bone island (enostosis) are rare around the shoulder. Multiple bone islands may be seen involving the scapula and glenoid in the dysplasia osteopoikilosis. Approximately 3% of osteoid osteomas arise in the proximal humerus and less than 1% in the scapula. These benign hypervascular tumours are characterised by a small cavity (the nidus), usually in a cortical or subendosteal location, which may or may not contain a small focus of calcification, with a variable amount of surrounding sclerosis (Fig. 16.1). The latter is largely due to mature periosteal new bone formation which is lacking if the lesion is located within the boundaries of a joint. These so-called intracapsular osteoid osteomas may have an atypical presentation with a synovitis (KATZ and THOMAZEAU 1997).

16.7.1.2
Cartilaginous

Benign cartilage tumours of bone can be divided into those that arise within the medulla and those that arise from the surface of bone. Medullary cartilage

tumours are enchondromas, chondroblastoma and chondromyxoid fibroma. Surface cartilage tumours are osteochondroma and periosteal chondroma. Chondromyxoid fibroma is exceptionally rare around the shoulder. It is important to stress that the presence of cartilaginous calcification is helpful in indicating the tissue of origin but does not distinguish benign from malignant cartilage tumours.

Enchondroma is a benign tumour of mature hyaline cartilage accounting for 4% of all primary bone tumours. Approximately 7% occur in the proximal humeral meta-diaphysis and rarely in the scapula or clavicle. The typical radiographic features are a well defined oval or rounded lytic defect, usually central, containing a variable amount of cartilage calcification within the metaphysis or diaphysis (Fig. 16.12). The calcifications tend to be scattered throughout the tumour as opposed to the peripheral linear distribution that is found in medullary infarcts. Bone expansion is not common in the humerus. Enchondromatosis (Ollier's disease) is a condition marked by multiple enchondromas usually involving the metaphyses and meta-diaphyses of the long bones. There is no hereditary or familial tendency and it is usually classified as a bone dysplasia. A monomelic or hemimelic distribution is typical. The spectrum of skeletal change around the shoulder can vary enormously from tiny foci of cartilage, to linear columns of dysplastic unmineralised cartilage to major modelling deformities resulting in marked deformity. If there is any doubt as to the condition, radiographs of the hands and feet will usually clinch the diagnosis. Malignant transformation and the distinction of enchondroma from low grade chondrosarcoma is discussed in Sect. 16.7.2.2.

One of the commonest sites, outside the hands and feet, for a periosteal or juxtacortical chondroma is the proximal humerus. The characteristic radiographic appearance is of a surface lesion causing well defined scalloped erosion of the outer cortex with a peripheral buttress (Fig. 16.19). There may or may not be a peripheral shell and matrix mineralisation. On MR imaging the lobulated cartilage nature of the lesion can be identified (VARMA et al. 1991) although, to the unwary, the hyperintense signal on T2-weighted and STIR images may easily be mistaken for a cystic lesion.

Chondroblastoma is a benign cartilage tumour arising almost exclusively in epiphyses or apophyses with three-quarters less than 20 years of age. Approximately 20% occur in the proximal humeral epiphysis and is the second commonest benign tumour affecting the shoulder after the simple bone cyst. Radiographically, chondroblastoma appears as

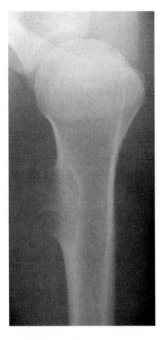

Fig. 16.19. Periosteal chondroma. Well defined erosion of the outer cortex with a fine partial peripheral shell

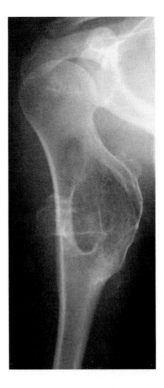

Fig. 16.20. Osteochondroma. Large sessile osteochondroma arising from the medial aspect of the proximal humerus

a well defined lytic lesion within the medulla of the epiphysis (Fig. 16.5). Matrix mineralisation is seen in approximately one quarter of cases. Breaching of the growth plate with metaphyseal involvement occurs in larger lesions with late presentation. A florid inflammatory response is common, similar to osteoid osteoma, typified by surrounding marrow oedema with or without an associated joint effusion. Both are well demonstrated on MR imaging (Fig. 16.14) (OXTOBY and DAVIES 1996). Secondary aneurysmal bone cyst formation may occur in chondroblastoma resulting in blood filled cysts of varying size containing fluid–fluid levels on CT and MR imaging. Rare instances of malignant change in chondroblastoma have been reported.

Osteochondroma is the commonest benign bone tumour. It represents a bony protuberance (exostosis) covered by a hyaline cartilage cap. Approximately 16% arise in the humerus and 5% from the blade of the scapula. It may be single or multiple as in the hereditary form, diaphyseal aclasis. It can be broadbased (sessile) or narrow-based (pedunculated). They arise from the metaphysis and are angulated away from the adjacent joint (Fig. 16.20). An important diagnostic feature is the continuity of the host bone marrow with the marrow of the osteochondroma. The cartilage cap is not visible on radiographs unless it calcifies. The cartilage cap can be readily identified with ultrasound, CT and MR imaging. Complica-

tions of osteochondromas include fracture, pressure on adjacent tendons, nerves and vessels, overlying bursitis and malignant degeneration (MURPHEY et al. 2000), but these are less common around the shoulder than in the pelvis and lower limb. One of the most frequently encountered clinical problems is mechanical obstruction to movement of the scapula from an osteochondroma impinging on the posterior chest wall (Fig. 16.21).

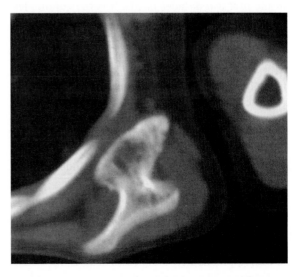

Fig. 16.21. Osteochondroma. Axial CT shows the osteochondroma arising from the inner aspect of the scapula and impinging on the chest wall

16.7.1.3
Fibrous

Less than 4% of the benign fibrous tumours, fibrous cortical defects and non-ossifying fibromas, arise in the proximal humerus. Radiographs show a well defined elliptical, radiolucent defect confined to the cortex in the metaphysis or diametaphysis of the proximal humerus (Fig. 16.6). Fibrous dysplasia may affect any part of the skeleton but is uncommon in its monostotic form around the shoulder, unlike the proximal femur.

16.7.1.4
Lipomatous

Intraosseous lipoma most commonly affects the lower limb bones, particularly the anterior calcaneus. Outside the lower limb the proximal humerus is a recognised site. Radiographs show a well defined lucency within the medulla frequently containing dystrophic calcification. In this situation it may mimic a central chondrosarcoma. The diagnosis can be made with confidence on MR imaging by identifying the predominant fat component of the lesion (NAKATA et al. 2001).

16.7.1.5
Unknown

The simple bone cyst (SBC), also known as a unicameral bone cyst, is a non-neoplastic fluid filled cavity. It is more common in males and is usually detected in the first two decades of life. It is the commonest benign bone tumour affecting the shoulder with approximately 43% cases arising in the proximal humerus. The radiographic appearances are a well defined lytic lesion, centrally located within the metaphysis migrating with time into the diaphysis. A typical, but not pathognomonic sign, is the so-called "fallen fragment" (Fig. 16.4). This represents a fragment of fractured cortex that descends to the dependent portion of the cyst. The differential diagnosis in the proximal humerus include ABC and fibrous dysplasia.

ABC is a non-neoplastic lesion consisting of multiple blood-filled spaces with varying amounts of fibrous, richly vascular connective tissue. Three quarters of cases present in patients under 20 years of age. Approximately 5.5% cases arise in the proximal humerus, 3.5% in the clavicle (Fig. 16.10) and 2% in the scapula (Fig. 16.15). The radiographic features are a well defined multiloculated expansile lesion arising in the metaphysis. If the ABC is growing particularly fast the expanded shell may be thinned or absent (Fig. 16.10). ABC may be a secondary phenomenon occurring in pre-existing bone lesions in which case there may be imaging evidence of the underlying abnormality. Fluid–fluid levels are a typical, but not pathognomonic, feature of ABCs seen on CT and MR imaging (Fig. 16.15). It is necessary for the scan to be perpendicular to the fluid–fluid levels for them to be visible. The important differential diagnosis for an aggressive looking ABC is telangiectatic osteosarcoma. To the unwary, telangiectatic osteosarcoma may resemble an ABC both on imaging (including fluid–fluid levels) and histology. Misdiagnosis can have potentially disastrous consequences as the management of an ABC is curettage and of a telangiectatic osteosarcoma chemotherapy and wide surgical excision.

GCT is a locally aggressive tumour representing approximately 5% of all primary bone tumours and 22% of benign bone tumours. Approximately 5% arise in the proximal humerus. The tumour is considered benign although occasionally it may be multifocal, metastasise to the lungs or undergo malignant transformation. The characteristic radiographic features are an expansile, eccentric, lytic, subarticular lesion which is well defined without marginal sclerosis (Fig. 16.2). The important differential diagnosis, particularly in the older age group, would be a plasmacytoma and expansile metastasis (Fig. 16.3). Treatment of GCT is usually curettage with or without bone grafting or filling of the surgical defect with bone cement. Local recurrence occurs in 20%–30% cases. Dynamic contrast-enhanced MR imaging is of value in distinguishing early intraosseous recurrence from scar tissue.

16.7.2
Malignant Bone Tumours

16.7.2.1
Osseous

Osteosarcoma is the commonest primary malignancy of bone after myeloma. Three quarters of cases are conventional osteosarcoma, also known as high grade intramedullary tumours. Approximately 8% arise in the proximal humerus and less than 1% in either the scapula or clavicle. Peak incidence is in the second decade. The radiographic appearances can vary from purely lytic to purely sclerotic (Fig. 16.16), but most will show a mixed appearance with permeative margins, cortical destruction, soft tissue extension and periosteal new bone formation (Fig. 16.11). The latter may appear lamellated or spiculated and if interrupted will have Codman's angles (Fig. 16.11). Approximately 10% of osteosarcomas are the telangiectatic variety of which 12% arise in the humerus. This tumour is categorised by permeative bone destruction with bony expansion. CT and MR imaging show multiple blood filled cavities with or without fluid–fluid levels. It is the expansion and fluid–fluid levels that may cause diagnostic confusion with an ABC.

Parosteal osteosarcomas is a low grade malignancy and is the commonest of the surface osteosarcomas accounting for approximately 5% of all osteosarcomas. A total of 60% arise on the posterior metaphysis of the distal femur and only 11%–16% in the humerus. Radiographically, it appears as a dense lobulated mass attached to the outer cortex with a thin radiolucent cleft between part of the mass and the cortex as it wraps around the bone (Fig. 16.7). Intramedullary extension visible on CT or MR imaging will be present in approximately one third of cases (Fig. 16.7). Dedifferentiation to high grade osteosarcoma occurs in about 20% cases and should be suspected if there is a large unossified soft tissue component to the tumour. The other forms of surface osteosarcoma, high grade surface and periosteal subtypes, are much less common than parosteal osteosarcoma and rare around the shoulder. Similarly, the low grade intramedullary variant of osteosarcoma is extremely rare in the upper limb.

Secondary osteosarcoma may be seen in Paget's disease and following radiotherapy. In certain series up to one quarter of cases of Paget's sarcoma arise in the humerus. Why the humerus, a bone less commonly affected by uncomplicated Paget's disease, has such a high incidence of malignant transformation is unknown. Rapidly increasing lysis, cortical destruction and a soft tissue mass arising within pagetic bone are all typical features suggestive of malignant transformation (Fig. 16.22). Uncommonly, a focal proliferation of pagetic periosteal new bone may mimic a sarcoma. This so-called pseudosarcoma is remarkably rare in the upper limb (Tins et al. 2001). Approximately 7.5% of radiation sarcomas arise in the proximal humerus (Table 16.1). The most common primary diagnoses are breast carcinoma and lymphoma. The mean latency period for the development of the sarcoma is 15.5 years (Sheppard and Libshitz 2001). The prognosis for a patient developing a secondary osteosarcoma in Paget's disease or previously irradiated bone is much worse than for conventional osteosarcoma.

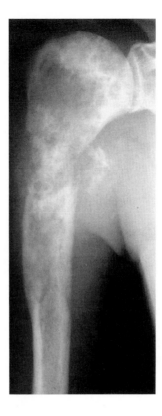

Fig. 16.22. Paget's osteosarcoma. There is lysis with a pathological fracture developing in an area of Paget's disease

16.7.2.2
Cartilaginous

Malignant cartilage tumours, chondrosarcomas, are the third most common primary malignant tumour of bone, after multiple myeloma and osteosarcoma. They can be distinguished from many other primary sarcomas of bone in that they occur in late adulthood rather than childhood or adolescence. As per their benign counterparts, they arise in a central or peripheral location. Approximately 10% of central chondrosarcomas arise in the humerus, more commonly proximally than distally. Chondrosarcoma is the most common primary malignancy of the scapula (Blacksin and Benevenia 2000). Patients with Ollier's disease are at risk of sarcomatous transformation in 5%–30% of cases (Liu et al. 1987). The radiographic appearance of central chondrosarcoma is variable. High grade lesions will appear permeative with cartilage mineralisation, cortical destruction and soft tissue extension. In particularly aggressive tumours dedifferentiation to a higher grade sarcoma (e.g., osteosarcoma or MFH) should be considered. Diagnostic problems are usually encountered with low grade central chondrosarcoma which can be difficult on both radiography and histology to differentiate from an enchondroma. Cartilage tumours of the proximal humeral metaphysis are not an uncommon incidental finding on radiography or MR imaging of the shoulder performed for pain, rotator cuff disease etc. One study concluded that a size greater than 5 cm was the most reliable predictor of chondrosarcoma and that all other morphological features, such as endosteal scalloping, were of little value (GEIRNAERDT et al. 1997). Lesions demonstrating uptake on whole body bone scintigraphy that is less than the anterior iliac spine are unlikely to be malignant (MURPHEY et al. 1998). Although dynamic contrast-enhanced MR imaging has been claimed to be of value in predicting malignancy (GEIRNAERDT et al. 2000) this is not a universally held view (FLEMMING and MURPHEY 2000).

Less than 1% of solitary osteochondromas undergo malignant transformation to a peripheral chondrosarcoma. It is generally accepted that the rate of malignant change in diaphyseal aclasis is higher but probably no more than 1% if one includes all asymptomatic cases of diaphyseal aclasis who do not present for medical treatment (VOUTSINAS and WYNNE-DAVIES 1983). Clinical features that suggest malignant change include pain and increasing size post skeletal fusion. Measurement of the thickness of the cartilage cap using ultrasound, CT or MR imaging can be helpful. A cartilage cap of less than 2 cm is likely to be benign, whereas as the cap exceeds 2 cm in thickness the likelihood of chondrosarcoma increases

(Fig. 16.23). Complications of osteochondromas such as overlying bursitis and pseudoaneurysm formation can mimic malignant change (MURPHEY et al. 2000; LEE et al. 2001). A soft tissue mass due to a bursitis is a common manifestation of an osteochondroma arising from the scapula.

16.7.2.3
Fibrous

Malignant fibrous tumours consist of fibrosarcoma and malignant fibrous histiocytoma (MFH). While they may be distinct histological entities, the imaging features are indistinguishable and are therefore discussed together. Approximately 7.5% occur in the humerus, while 20% arise in pre-existing bone lesions including: Paget's disease, bone infarction, irradiated bone, fibrous dysplasia and non-ossifying fibroma. As with chondrosarcoma, they tend to present in a slightly older age group than most other primary sarcomas of bone with a peak in the fourth decade. Typical radiographic appearances are geographic bone destruction with a wide zone of transition in an eccentric metaphyseal or meta-diaphyseal location. They tend not to extend to the articular margin. Cortical destruction with soft tissue extension is common but periosteal new bone formation is unusual and there is no matrix mineralisation. In the older patient the appearances can be indistinguishable from a metastasis.

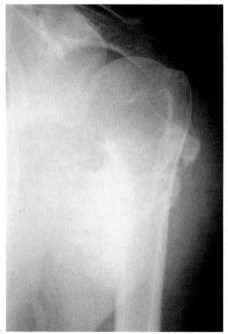

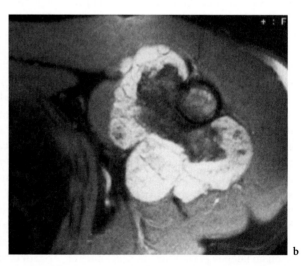

Fig. 16.23a, b. Peripheral chondrosarcoma. AP radiograph (**a**) and axial T2-weighted image with fat suppression (TR/TE = 2886/90) (**b**) showing a large lobulated tumour arising from the surface of the proximal humerus. The dispersal of the soft tissue calcifications and cartilage cap thickness of over 2 cm increases the likelihood that this is a chondrosarcoma and not a simple osteochondroma

16.7.2.4
Unknown

Originally of unknown histogenesis, Ewing's sarcoma and the similar peripheral neuroectodermal tumour (PNET) are now known to be linked to primitive neuroectoderm. Together they are the second commonest malignancy of bone in children and adolescents after osteosarcoma. The classic site in long bones, as illustrated in many texts, is the diaphysis but this occurs in only one third of cases. Approximately 60% arise in the metadiaphysis. Only 5.7% of Ewing's sarcoma arise in the humerus. Approximately 4% in the scapula and less than 1% in the clavicle. The radiographic features are of an aggressive lesion with a permeative or moth-eaten pattern, cortical destruction, and periosteal new bone formation (Fig. 16.8). The latter may show lamellar (onion skin) periosteal reaction with or without Codman's angles. In the humerus, Ewing's sarcomas may resemble the more lytic form of osteosarcoma and other malignant infiltrations seen in childhood such as neuroblastoma metastases. All malignant round cell tumours tend to show prominent soft tissue masses on cross-sectional imaging.

16.7.2.5
Clavicular Tumours

The clavicle is the only long bone to develop by intramembranous ossification. It is largely composed of cortical bone with only a small medullary component. It has been suggested that this might explain why it is relatively uncommon site for metastases. Tumours of the clavicle make up less than 1% of all bony neoplasms. Interestingly, unlike most other sites, tumours of the clavicle are more likely to be malignant than benign. Inflammatory conditions of the clavicle, however, frequently mimic tumours (see Sect. 16.10). In one of the author's (AMD) experience of over 100 tumours and tumour-like lesions of the clavicle the final diagnosis in approximately one third was a tumour, one third infection and one third miscellaneous conditions including arthropathy. Two thirds of the tumours were malignant and one third benign (Fig. 16.10). As a general "rule of thumb", lesions arising in the medial third of the clavicle in children and young adults were more likely to be infective or benign tumours, whereas lesions arising in the lateral third in middle aged or elderly patients were more likely to be tumours, both malignant and benign.

16.8
Soft Tissue Tumours

16.8.1
Benign Soft Tissue Tumours

Depending on the age of presentation, up to 60% of the benign soft tissue tumours arising around the shoulder are lipomas (KRANSDORF 1995a). On CT and MR imaging lipomas appear homogeneous, well circumscribed with low attenuation on CT and high signal intensity on MR imaging (Fig. 16.13). Thin fibrovascular septa may be identified traversing the main mass. If the tumour is sufficiently large and relatively superficial then it may be identified as a low density mass on shoulder radiographs. Small foci of mineralisation and/or ossification may occasionally be seen in long-standing lesions. Parosteal lipomas typically cause localised periosteal new bone formation. Imaging does not reliably distinguish between a simple lipoma and an atypical lipoma, also known as a well differentiated liposarcoma. Such distinction is frequently not critical as the management of both conditions, simple excision, is appropriate for both entities. If the mass does not show moderately uniform fat suppression on a STIR or similar fat suppressed sequence the possibility of an intermediate of high grade liposarcoma should be considered.

Many other benign soft tissue tumours arise around the shoulder with a similar incidence as to elsewhere in the body. However, a couple of benign fibrous conditions merit mention with respect to the shoulder. The first is elastofibroma dorsi which is a rare benign fibrous pseudotumour that is almost always located in the inferior part of the thoracoscapular space elevating the inferior angle of the scapula (NIELSEN et al. 1996). The mass arises on the chest wall deep to the serratus anterior muscle (Fig. 16.24). The site and MR features are considered characteristic of this tumour with intermediate signal intensity interlaced with high signal intensity strands of fat (NAYLOR et al. 1996). Although unusual, marked contrast enhancement has been reported (SCHICK et al. 2000). If case reports are anything to go by, bilateral elastofibromas are not uncommon (HOFFMAN et al. 1996; BRANDSER et al. 1998; HSIEH et al. 1999; TURNA et al. 2002).

The second fibrous tumour is aggressive fibromatosis (extra-abdominal desmoid). They arise most commonly in the lower limb or limb girdle and in the shoulder region. The tumour is benign, but locally aggressive, consisting of spindle-shaped cells with varying amounts of surrounding collagen. Although

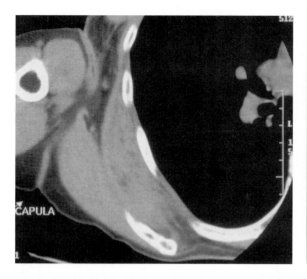

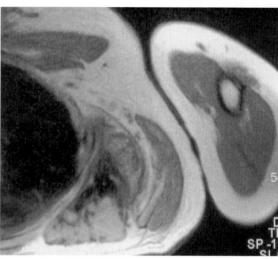

Fig. 16.24. Elastofibroma dorsi. Axial CT showing a diffuse soft tissue mass, containing strands of fat, lying on the posterolateral chest wall, deep to the serratus anterior muscle and scapula

Fig. 16.25. Aggressive fibromatosis. Transverse intermediate weighted image (TR/TE = 3250/14) showing a heterogeneous soft tissue mass lying on the posterolateral chest wall deep to the scapula. The low signal intensity areas are due to collagen

this tumour does not metastasise, it may be multifocal in presentation and there is a local post-surgical recurrence rate of up to 50%. The MR imaging features are variable depending on the collagen content of the lesion. Most appear heterogeneous with foci of low signal intensity on all sequences due to the hypocellular matrix (Fig. 16.25). In this respect, the low signal areas can mimic lesions with haemosiderin deposition or matrix mineralisation. The low signal intensity may be peripheral or central in location (Fig. 16.25) (KRANSDORF et al. 1990; HARTMAN et al. 1992). If the low signal areas predominate the tumour may be difficult to discern on T2-weighted images, particularly if fat suppression is applied. For this reason the authors advocate using a fast dual spin echo sequence as the fibromatosis can often be more conspicuous on the intermediate weighting (proton density) images (Fig. 16.25). Enhancement with a gadolinium chelate can be variable but the low signal intensity areas on the T2-weighted images tend not to enhance.

16.8.2
Malignant Soft Tissue Tumours

The commonest soft tissue sarcomas arising around the shoulder are malignant fibrous histiocytoma, liposarcoma, dermatofibrosarcoma protuberans and malignant peripheral nerve sheath tumour (MPNST) (KRANSDORF 1995b). Most high grade sarcomas show

similar imaging features irrespective of their final histological diagnosis. Similarly, their management, wide surgical excision with or without radiotherapy and chemotherapy, also varies little from tumour to tumour. Typically, on MR imaging soft tissue sarcomas appear well-encapsulated, isointense to muscle on T1-weighted images and heterogeneous with predominately high signal intensity on T2-weighted images. Myxoid tumours can be relatively homogeneous and care should be taken not to confuse these tumours with cysts/ganglia. If there is doubt, enhancement with a gadolinium chelate is advisable. The principle of surgical staging are the same as for a bone tumour carefully noting the anatomical extent of the tumour with close attention to the relationship to the shoulder joint and neurovascular structures in the axilla. Follow-up, looking for local recurrence and the development of metastases is also similar to that applicable to a bone sarcoma (see Sect. 16.6).

16.9
Joint Tumours

In this section the term "tumour" is taken in its literal sense as a swelling or mass. The discussion is therefore not limited just to true neoplasms but includes cystic, metaplastic and proliferative conditions which may present with a mass arising from or adjacent to the knee joint. Polyarticular disorders are not included as they rarely present with an isolated mass. Primary malignant tumours involving the shoulder joint are exceptionally rare and most cases of malignant involvement are due to spread from an adjacent bone or soft tissue sarcoma.

16.9.1
Cysts

Cysts and ganglia are far less common around the shoulder than the knee. The most frequently seen fluid-filled mass around the shoulder is the distended subacromial/subdeltoid bursa. This may be secondary to trauma, a large rotator cuff defect and inflammatory processes such as rheumatoid arthritis or tuberculosis. An unusual but well recognised association with a complete rotator cuff defect and distended subacromial bursa is an acromioclavicular joint cyst (POSTACCHINI et al. 1993). Fluid is forced from the glenohumeral joint through the rotator cuff tear and subacromial bursa into the acromioclavicular joint resulting in a superiorly located cystic mass. Another cyst which can develop as a result of trauma or degeneration is the glenoid labral cyst analogous to the meniscal cyst in the knee (TIRMAN et al. 1994). Fluid is extruded through the labral tear to form a cyst in the paraarticular soft tissues. The incidence of these cysts in one cadaveric study was 1% (TICKER et al. 1998). These so-called paralabral cysts can cause nerve entrapment syndromes depending on their location (CATALANO and FENLIN 1994). The commonest nerve affected is the suprascapular nerve (FRITZ et al. 1992).

16.9.2
Pigmented Villonodular Synovitis

Pigmented villonodular synovitis (PVNS) is an uncommon proliferative disorder of synovium characterised by lipid laden macrophages and recurrent synovial haemorrhage.

It is commonest in the knee and hip but has also been described in most other joints. The intraarticular form may be diffuse or localised. The latter however seems to occur almost exclusively in the knee. Typical imaging features include well defined bone erosions on both sides of the affected joint and dark synovial masses due to repeated bleeding on MR imaging (LLAUGER et al. 1999). PVNS may also arise in the subacromial bursa (KONRATH et al. 1997).

16.9.3
Synovial Chondromatosis

Synovial chondromatosis is a non-neoplastic, proliferative and metaplastic disorder of the synovium. Of the two forms of the condition, secondary synovial chondromatosis, typified by the presence of intra-articular osteocartilaginous loose bodies against a background of disease is common most frequently affecting the knee. In the shoulder the calcified loose bodies tend to aggregate in the subacromial bursa (Fig. 16.26), axillary recess or down the bicipital tendon sheath (HORII et al. 2001). The primary form, in which synovial soft tissue masses are the predominant feature is relatively uncommon. In one of the author's (AMD) personal experience of 20 cases of primary synovial chondromatosis, 11 arose in the knee and only three cases involved the shoulder, of which two affected the acromio-clavicular joint and one the subacromial bursa (WITTKOP et al. 2002). Multiple cartilaginous loose bodies within the subacromial bursa (Fig. 16.26) may resemble rice bodies (see Sect. 16.10). As in the knee, the condition may occasionally be bilateral (OGAWA et al. 1999). There is a rare association between long-standing primary synovial chondromatosis and the development of synovial chondrosarcoma (KENAN et al. 1993b).

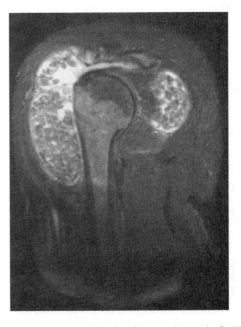

Fig. 16.26. Synovial chondromatosis. Sagittal STIR image (TR/TE = 4284/60) showing multiple small cartilaginous loose bodies within a distended subacromial bursa

16.9.4
Lipoma Arborescens

Lipoma arborescens is a rare intraarticular disorder consisting of villous lipomatous proliferation of the synovium. The term "arborescens" meaning like a tree, refers to the fine frond-like pattern of subsynovial fat readily diagnosed on MR imaging. Although most commonly seen in the knee, it has been reported in the shoulder joint and subacromial bursa (LAORR et al. 1995; DAWSON et al. 1995; NISOLLE et al. 1999).

16.10
Tumour-Like Lesions

What constitutes a tumour mimic depends very much on the expertise of the individual reviewing the imaging. The majority can be classified as normal variants, and inflammatory conditions. Trauma is a much less common cause of tumour mimics around the shoulder than in the lower limb, although post-traumatic osteolysis of the lateral end of the clavicle may simulate a destructive process.

The prudent radiologist will always have close at hand, when reporting, one of the standard reference texts on normal variants which illustrate the wide spectrum of developmental lucencies and irregularities of ossification that can be seen on radiographs of the shoulder girdle. Typical examples of problem normal variants include pseudocyst formation from internal rotation of the humerus, notching of

the medial metaphysis of the proximal humerus in children and prominent deltoid muscle insertions (KEATS and ANDERSON 2001).

Inflammatory conditions include Caffey's disease, SAPHO syndrome (synovitis, acne, palmar/plantar pustulosis, hyperostosis and osteitis) and any infective process around the shoulder. Chronic recurrent multifocal osteomyelitis (CRMO), thought to be in a spectrum of inflammatory disorders including SAPHO syndrome, has a predilection for the clavicle, particularly in children. Typically, the clavicle shows expansion, with mixed medullary lysis and sclerosis, and mature periosteal new bone formation and is often mistaken for a tumour (Fig. 16.27) (JURRIAANS et al. 2001). So-called "rice bodies" may develop in bursae, joints and tendon sheaths with the subacromial bursa the commonest site. Usually associated with inflammation such as rheumatoid or TB, the condition is characterised by massive distension of the bursa with a numerous multiple small radiolucent bodies likened to grains of polished rice (SUGANO et al. 2000; TAKAYAMA et al. 2000). The rice bodies are composed of fibrin and collagen.

Occasionally, the advanced destructive appearance of a neuropathic arthropathy may be mistaken at presentation for a tumour. In the shoulder this is commonly due to undiagnosed syringomyelia. Similar destructive appearances may also be seen with massive osteolysis or Gorham's syndrome (PANS et al. 1999).

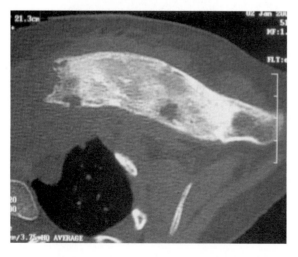

Fig. 16.27. Chronic recurrent multifocal osteomyelitis clavicle. Axial CT showing a predominantly sclerotic lesion with expansion of the diaphysis of the clavicle

References

Alexander AA, Nazarian LN, Feld RI (1997) Superficial soft-tissue masses suggestive of recurrent malignancy: sonographic localization and biopsy. AJR 169:1449–1451

Ardran GM (1951) Bone destruction not demonstrable by radiography. Br J Radiol 24:107–109

Bearcroft PWP, Davies AM (1999) Follow-up of musculoskeletal tumors 2: metastatic disease. Eur Radiol 9:192–200

Blacksin MF, Benevenia J (2000) Neoplasms of the scapula: pictorial essay. AJR 174:1729–1735

Boutin RD, Pathria MN, Resnick D (1998) Disorders in the stumps of amputee patients: MR imaging. AJR 171:497–501

Brandser EA, Goree JC, El Khoury GY (1998) Elastofibroma dorsi: prevalence in an elderly patient population as revealed by CT. AJR 171:977–980

Campanacci M (1999) Bone and soft tissue tumors: clinical features, imaging, pathology and treatment, 2nd edn. Springer, Vienna New York

Carrasco CH, Charnsangavej C, Raymond AK (1989) Osteosarcoma: angiographic assessment of response to preoperative chemotherapy. Radiology 170:839–842

Catalano JB, Fenlin JM (1994) Ganglion cysts about the shoulder girdle in the absence of suprascapular nerve involvement. J Shoulder Elbow Surg 3:34–41

Choi H, Varma DGK, Fornage BD, Kim EE, Johnston DA (1991) Soft-tissue sarcoma: MR imaging vs sonography for detection of local recurrence after surgery. Radiology 157: 353–358

Conrad EU (1998) Tumors and related conditions. In: Rockwood CA, Matsen FS (eds) The shoulder, 2nd edn. Saunders, Philadephia, pp 1127–1169

Craig EV, Thompson RC (1987) Management of tumors of the shoulder girdle. Clin Orthop 223:94–112

Davies AM, Cassar-Pullicino VN (1992) The incidence and significance of fluid-fluid levels on computed tomography of osseous lesions. Br J Radiol 65:193–198

Davies AM, Vanel D (1998) Follow-up of musculoskeletal tumors. 1. Local recurrence. Eur Radiol 8:791–799

Davies AM, Cooper SA, Mangham DC, Grimer RJ (2001) Metal-containing lymph nodes following prosthetic replacement of osseous malignancy: potential role of MR imaging in characterisation. Eur Radiol 11:841–844

Dawson JS, Dowling F, Preston BJ, Neumann L (1995) Lipoma arborescens of the subdeltoid bursa. Br J Radiol 68:197–199

Edelstyn GA, Gillespie PJ, Grebbel FS (1967) The radiological demonstration of osseous metastases: experimental observations. Clin Radiol 18:158–162

Enneking WF, Kagan A (1975) The implications for skip metastases in osteosarcoma. Clin Orthop 111:33–41

Enneking WF, Spanier SS, Goodman MA (1980) A system for the surgical staging of musculoskeletal sarcoma. Clin Orthop 153:106–120

Enneking W, Dunham W, Gebhardt M, Malawer M, Pritchard DA (1990) A system for the classification of skeletal resections. Chir Organi Mov 75 [Suppl 1]:217–240

Fiorella D, Helms CA, Speer KP (2000) Increased T2 signal in the distal clavicle, incidence and clinical implications. Skeletal Radiol 29:697–702

Flemming DJ, Murphey MD (2000) Enchondroma and chondrosarcoma. Semin Musculosletal Radiol 4:59–71

Fritz RC, Helms CA, Steinbach LS, Genant HK (1992) Suprascapular nerve entrapment: evaluation with MR imaging. Radiology 182:437–444

Geirnaerdt MJA, Hermans J, Bloem JL, Kroon HM, Pope TL, Taminiau AHM, Hogendoorn PCW (1997) Usefulness of radiography in differentiating enchondroma from central grade I chondrosarcoma. AJR 169:1097–1104

Geirnaerdt MJA, Hogendoorn PCW, Bloem JL, Taminiau AHM, van der Woude HJ (2000) Cartilaginous tumors: fast contrast-enhanced MR imaging. Radiology 214:539–546

Grimer RJ, Sneath RS (1990) Diagnosing malignant bone tumours: editorial. J Bone Joint Surg (Br) 72:754–756

Hartman TE, Berquist T, Fetsch JF (1992) MR imaging of extraabdominal desmoids: differentiation from other neoplasms. AJR 158:581–585

Hayes CW, Conway WF, Sundaram M (1992) Misleading aggressive MR imaging appearance of some benign musculoskeletal lesions. RadioGraphics 12:1119–1134

Hoffman JK, Klein MH, McInerney VK (1996) Bilateral elastofibroma: a case report and review of the literature. Clin Orthop 325:245–250

Horii M, Tamai M, Kido K, Kusuzaki K, Kubo T, Hirasawa Y (2001) Two cases of synovial chondromatosis of the subacromial bursa J Shoulder Elbow Surg 10:186–189

Hsieh SC, Shih TT, Li YW (1999) Bilateral elastofibroma: two case reports. Clin Imag 23:47–50

Jurriaans E, Singh NP, Finlay K, Friedman L (2001) Imaging

of chronic recurrent multifocal osteomyelitis. Radiol Clin North Am 39:305–327

Katz D, Thomazeau H (1997) Osteoid osteoma of the proximal humereus: two misleading cases. J Shoulder Elbow Surg 6: 559–563

Keats TE, Anderson MW (2001) Atlas of normal roentgen variants that may simulate disease, 7th edn. Mosby, St Louis, p 494

Kenan S, Abdelwahab IF, Klein MJ, Herman G, Lewis MM (1993a) Lesions of juxtacortical origin (surface lesions of bone). Skeletal Radiol 22:337–357

Kenan S, Abdelwahab IF, Klein MJ, Lewis MM (1993b) Case report 817. Skeletal Radiol 22:623–626

Konrath GA, Nahigian K, Kolowich P (1997) Pigmented villonodular synovitis of the subacromial bursa. J Shoulder Elbow Surg 6:400–404

Kransdorf MJ (1995a) Benign soft-tissue tumors in a large referral population: distribution of diagnoses by age, sex and location. AJR 164:395–402

Kransdorf MJ (1995b) Malignant soft-tissue tumors in a large referral population: distribution of diagnoses by age, sex and location. AJR 164:129–134

Kransdorf M, Jelinek J, Moser R, Utz J, Hudson T, Neal J, Berrey B (1990) MR appearance of fibromatosis. Skeletal Radiol 19:495–499

Kricun ME (1983) Radiographic evaluation of solitary bone lesions. Orthop Clin North Am 14:39–64

Lang P, Grampp S, Vahlensieck M, Johnston JO, Honda G, Rosenau W, Matthay KK, Peterfy C, Higgins CB, Genant HK (1995) Primary bone tumors: value of MR angiography for preoperative planning and monitoring response to chemotherapy. AJR 165:135–142

Laorr A, Peterfy CG, Tirman PF, Rabassa AE (1995) Lipoma arborescens of the shoulder: MR imaging findings. Can Assoc Radiol J 46:311–313

Lee KCY, Davies AM, Cassar-Pullicino VCP (2001) Imaging the complications of osteochondromas. Clin Radiol 57:18–28

Liu J, Hudkins PG, Swee RD et al (1987) Bone sarcomas associated with Ollier's disease. Cancer 59:1376–1385

Llauger J, Palmer J, Roson N, Cremades R, Bague S (1999) Pigmented villonodular synovitis and giant cell tumors of tendon sheath: radiologic and pathologic features. AJR 172: 1087–1091

Madewell JE, Ragsdale BD, Sweet DE (1981) Radiologic and pathologic analysis of solitary bone lesions. Part I: Internal margins. Radiol Clin North Am 19:715–748

Malawer MM (1991) Tumors of the shoulder girdle: technique of resection and description of surgical classification. Orthop Clin North Am 22:7–35

Mankin HJ, Lange TA, Spanier SS (1982) The hazards of biopsy in patients with malignant primary bone and soft tissue tumours. J Bone Joint Surg [Am] 64:1121–1127

Mankin HJ, Mankin CJ, Simon MA (1996) The hazards of biopsy revisited. J Bone Joint Surg [Am] 78:656–663

Moser RP, Madewell JE (1987) An approach to primary bone tumors. Radiol Clin North Am 25:1049–1093

Mulder JD, Schütte HE, Kroon HM, Taconis WK (1993) Radiologic atlas of bone tumors. Elsevier, Amsterdam

Murphey MD, Flemming DJ, Boyea SR et al (1998) Enchondroma versus chondrosarcoma in the appendicular skeleton: differentiating features. RadioGraphics 18:1213–1237

Murphey MD, Choi JJ, Kransdorf MJ, Flemming DJ, Gannon FH (2000) Imaging of osteochondroma: variants and complications with radiologic-pathologic correlation. Radio-Graphics 20:1407–1434

Nakata E, Kawai A, Sugiharara S, Naito N, Morimoto Y, Inoue H (2001) Humeral lesion in a 69-year-old woman. Clin Orthop 389:248–250; 253–255

Naylor MF, Nascimento AG, Sherrick AD, McLeod RA (1996) Elastofibroma dorsi: radiologic findings in 12 patients. AJR 167:683–687

Nielsen T, Sneppen O, Myhre-Jensen O, Daugaard S, Norbaek J (1996) Subscapular elastofibroma: a reactive pseudotumor. J Shoulder Elbow Surg 5:209–213

Nissolle JF, Blouard E, Baudraz V, Boutsen Y, de Cloedt P, Esselinckz W (1999) Subacromial-subdeltoid lipoma arborescens associated with a rotator cuff tear. Skeletal Radiol 28:283–285

Ogawa K, Takahashi M, Inokuchi W (1999) Bilateral osteochondromatosis of the subacromial bursae with incomplete rotator cuff tears. J Shoulder Elbow Surg 8:78–81

Oxtoby J, Davies AM (1996) The MRI appearances of chondroblastoma. Clin Radiol 51:22–26

Ozaki T, Putzke M, Rodl R, Winkelman W, Lindner N (2002) Incidence and mechanism of infiltration of sarcomas in the shoulder. Clin Orthop 395:209–215

Panicek DM, Gatsonis CG, Rosenthal DI, Seeger LL, Huvos AG, Moore SG, Caudry DJ, Palmer WE, McNeil BJ (1997a) CT and MR imaging in the local staging of primary malignant musculoskeletal neoplasms: report of the radiology diagnostic oncology group. Radiology 202:237–246

Panicek DM, Hilton S, Schwartz LH (1997b) Assessment of neurovascular involvement by malignant musculoskeletal tumors. Sarcoma 1:61–63

Pans S, Simon JP, Dierickz C (1999) Massive osteolysis of the shoulder (Gorham-Stout syndrome). J Shoulder Elbow Surg 8:281–283

Picci P, Vanel D, Briccoli A, Talle K, Haakenaasen U, Malaguti C, Monti C, Ferrari C, Bacci G, Saeter G, Alvegard TA (2001) Computed tomography of pulmonary metastases from osteosarcoma: the less poor technique. A study of 51 patients with histological correlation. Ann Oncol 12:1601–1604

Postacchini F, Perugia D, Gumina S (1993) Acromioclavicular joint cyst associated with rotator cuff tear. Clin Orthop 294:111–113

Richardson ML, Zink-Brody GC, Patten RM, Koh WJ, Conrad EU (1996) MR characterization of post-irradiation soft tissue edema. Skeletal Radiol 25:537–543

Rosenberg ZS, Lev S, Schmahmann S, Steiner GC, Beltyran J, Present D (1995) Osteosarcoma: subtle, rare and misleading plain film features. Am J Roentgenol 165:1209–1214

Rubert CK, Malawer MM, Kellar KL (1999) Modular endoprosthetic replacement of the proximal humerus: indications, surgical technique, and results. Semin Arthroplasty 10:142–153

Schick S, Zembsch A, Gahleitner A, Wanderbaldinger P, Amann G, Breitenseher M, Trattnig S (2000) Atypical appearance of elastofibroma dorsi on MRI: case reports and review of the literature. J Comput Assist Tomogr 24:288–292

Schima W, Amann G, Stiglbauer R, Windhager R, Kramer J, Nicolakis M, Farres M, Imhof H (1994) Preoperative staging of osteosarcoma: efficacy of MR imaging in detecting joint involvement. Am J Roentgenol 163:1171–1175

Seeger LL, Yao L, Eckardt JJ (1998) Surface lesions of bone. Radiology 206:17–33

Shapeero LG, Vanel D (2000) Imaging evaluation of the response of high-grade osteosarcoma and Ewing sarcoma to chemotherapy with emphasis on dynamic contrast-enhanced MR imaging. Semin Musculoskeletal Radiol 4:137–146

Sheppard DG, Libshitz HI (2001) Post-radiation sarcomas: a review of the clinical and imaging features in 63 cases. Clin Radiol 56:22–29

Shuman WP, Patten RM, Baron RL et al (1991) Comparison of STIR and spin-echo MR imaging at 1.5T in 45 suspected extremity tumours: lesion conspicuity and extent. Radiology 179:247–252

Skrznski MC, Biermann JS, Montag A, Simon MA (1996) Diagnostic accuracy and charge savings of outpatient core needle biopsy compared with open biopsy of musculoskeletal lesions. J Bone Joint Surg [Am] 78:644–649

Steinbach L (1998) CT and MR imaging in the local staging of primary malignant musculoskeletal neoplasms: comment. Sarcoma 2:57–58

Stoker DJ, Cobb JP, Pringle JAS (1991) Needle biopsy of musculoskeletal lesions: a review of 208 procedures. J Bone Joint Surg [Br] 73:498–500

Sugano I, Nagao T, Tajima Y, Ishida Y, Nagao K, Ohno T, Ooishi S (2000) Variation among rice bodies: report of four cases and their clinicopathological features. Skeletal Radiol 29:525–529

Swan JS, Grist TM, Sproat JA, Heiner JP, Wiersma SR, Heisey DM (1995) Musculoskeletal neoplasms: preoperative evaluation with MR angiography. Radiology 194:519–524

Takayama A, Horomoto I, Shirai Y (2000) Subacromial bursitis mimicking a soft tissue tumour. J Shoulder Elbow Surg 9:72–75

Ticker JB, Djurasovic M, Strauch RJ, April EW, Pollock RG, Flatlow EL, Bigliani LU (1998) The incidence of ganglion cysts and other variations in anatomy along the course of the suprascapular nerve. J Shoulder Elbow Surg 7:472–478

Tins BJ, Davies AM, Mangham DC (2001) MR imaging of pseudosarcoma in Paget's disease of bone: a report of 2 cases. Skeletal Radiol 30:161–165

Tirman P, Feller J, Janzen D, Peterfy C, Bergman A (1994) Association of glenoid labral cysts with labral tears and glenohumeral instability: radiologic findings and clinical significance. Radiology 190:653–658

Turna A, Yilmaz MA, Urer N, Bedirham MA, Gurses A (2002) Bilateral elastofibroma dorsi. Ann Thor Surg 73:630–632

Unni KK (1996) Dahlin's bone tumors: general aspects and data on 11,087 cases, 5th edn. Lippincott-Raven, Philadelphia

Van der Woude HJ, Bloem JL, Oostayen JA, Nooy MA, Taminiau AH, Hermans J, Rejnierse M (1995) Treatment of high-grade bone sarcomas with neoadjuvant chemotherapy: the utility of sequential color Doppler sonography in predicting histopathologic response. Am J Roentgenol 165:125–133

Van der Woude, Bloem JL, Hogendoorn PCW (1998) Preoperative evaluation and monitoring chemotherapy in patients with high-grade osteogenic and Ewing's sarcoma, review of current imaging modalities. Skeletal Radiol 27:57–71

Vanel D, Shapeero LG, de Baere T, Gilles R, Tardivon A, Genin J, Guinebretiere JM (1994) MR imaging in the follow-up of malignant and aggressive soft tissue tumors: results of 511 examinations. Radiology 190:263–268

Varma DGK, Kumar R, Carrasco CH, Guo SQ, Richli WR

(1991) MR imaging of periosteal chondroma. J Comput Assist Tomogr 15:1008–1010

Verstraete KL, De Beene Y, Roels H, Dierick A, Uyttendale D, Kunnen M (1994) Benign and malignant musculoskeletal lesions: dynamic contrast-enhanced MR imaging. Radiology 192:835–843

Voutsinas S, Wynne-Davies R (1983) The frequency of malignant change in diaphyseal; aclasis and neurofibromatosis. J Med Genet 20:345–349

Wittkop B, Davies AM, Mangham DC (2002) Primary synovial chondromatosis and synovial chondrosarcoma. Eur Radiol 12:2112–2119

17 Brachial Plexus

H. W. van Es, T. D. Witkamp, M. A. M. Feldberg

CONTENTS

17.1
Introduction

The brachial plexus originates from the last four cervical spinal nerves and the first thoracic spinal nerve. The ventral rami of these spinal nerves intermingle in the neck and in the axilla, where the brachial plexus is closely related to the intervertebral foramina, stellate ganglion, scalene muscles, lung apex, subclavian and axillary artery, subclavian and axillary vein, first rib, and clavicle. Ultrasound (US) (SHEPPARD et al. 1998) and spiral computed tomography (CT) with multiplanar reconstructions (REMY-JARDIN et al. 1997) can depict parts of the brachial plexus in various planes. Due to its inherent contrast differences and its direct multiplanar capabilities, magnetic resonance imaging (MRI) is the imaging method of first choice to visualize the brachial plexus and the surrounding structures in this complex anatomic region.

In this chapter, MRI technique, the anatomy of the brachial plexus, and the various causes of brachial plexopathy will be discussed. These causes include intrinsic and extrinsic tumors, radiation plexopathy, trauma, and demyelinating processes [chronic inflammatory demyelinating polyradiculoneuropathy (CIDP) and multifocal motor neuropathy (MMN)].

17.2
MRI Technique

The brachial plexus can be very well seen with MRI if the nerves are surrounded by fat. On T1- and T2-weighted images the nerves are isointense to muscle. The nerves can be slightly hyperintense if a heavily T2-weighted sequence with fat-suppression is used, for example T2-weighted short tau inversion recovery (STIR) imaging (MARAVILLA et al. 1998). This so-called MR neurography is a promising technique for the evaluation of peripheral nerve disorders, especially with the use of improved surface coils (HAYES et al. 1997).

The brachial plexus is oriented in an oblique coronal plane as it runs from superior-posterior to inferior-anterior. Because of this orientation the best imaging planes are the coronal and sagittal planes. Axial images are used to visualize the roots in the intervertebral foramina. Several imaging strategies have been proposed: axial and coronal views (BILBEY et al. 1994); axial and sagittal views (RAPOPORT et al. 1988); sagittal and coronal views with axial slices only scanned on an as-needed basis (VAN ES et al. 1995a); coronal views with additional axial or sagittal planes (POSNIAK et al. 1993); all planes (SHERRIER and SOSTMAN 1993). The use of oblique coronal images and oblique sagittal images (OBUCHOWSKI and ORTIZ 2000) has also been advocated. An alternative for oblique imaging is a T1-weighted three-dimensional (3D)-volume acquisition (VAN ES et al. 1996) with the availability of thin overlapping slices and multiplanar reconstructions. Our standard protocol includes sagittal spin-echo T1- and T2-weighted images of the affected side, and thin (3 mm, gap 0.3 mm) coronal spin-echo T1-weighted images of both sides. Coronal STIR images, axial spin-echo T1-weighted images

H. W. VAN ES, MD
Department of Radiology, St. Antonius Hospital, Postbus 2500, 3430 EM Nieuwegein, The Netherlands
T. D. WITKAMP, MD; M. A. M. FELDBERG, MD
Department of Radiology, E.01.132, University Medical Center Utrecht, Postbus 85500, 3508 GA Utrecht, The Netherlands

and a sagittal T1-weighted 3D-volume acquisition are scanned on an as-needed basis. For example, STIR imaging in cases of CIDP and MMN, axial images for the evaluation of superior sulcus tumors, and a 3D-volume acquisition in order to optimally visualize the relationship between tumors and the brachial plexus in various directions. Gadolinium is given in cases of tumor. The body coil can be used; however, a suitable surface coil, such as a body-wrap-around coil (VAN Es et al. 1995a), will improve the image quality.

17.3
Anatomy

The lower four cervical roots (C5, C6, C7, and C8) and the first thoracic root (Th1) give rise to the brachial plexus. The ventral and dorsal nerve roots unite at the inner aperture of the intervertebral foramen to form the spinal nerve. The spinal nerve is situated in the intervertebral foramen and divides at the outer aperture into a dorsal and ventral ramus. The dorsal ramus innervates the musculature and the skin of the posterior region of the neck. The *ventral rami* of C5, C6, C7, C8 and Th1 form the proximal extent of the brachial plexus. These ventral rami run inferolaterally and enter the interscalene triangle, which is formed by the anterior and middle scalene muscle (Fig. 17.1a). The subclavian artery also lies within the interscalene triangle; the subclavian vein is located between the anterior scalene muscle and the clavicle. The three *trunks* are formed at the lateral border of the inter-scalene triangle (Fig. 17.1b). The ventral rami of roots C5 and C6 join to become the upper trunk, the ventral ramus of root C7 continues as the middle trunk, and the ventral rami of roots C8 and Th1 unite to become the lower trunk. The dorsal scapular artery, which passes between the upper and middle trunk or middle and lower trunk when originating from the subclavian artery (REINER and KASSER 1996), can often be identified with MRI (Fig. 17.2). Just before, or at the point where, the brachial plexus passes posterior to the clavicle, the *divisions* are formed (Fig. 17.1c). Each of the trunks divides into an anterior and posterior division. Lateral to the first rib's outer border, where the subclavian artery and vein become the axillary artery and vein, the three *cords* are formed. The lateral cord is formed by the anterior divisions from the upper and middle trunks, the medial cord by the anterior division from the lower trunk, and the posterior cord by the posterior divisions from all trunks. In the sagittal plane the lateral cord is located most anteriorly, the

posterior cord most superiorly, and the medial cord most posteriorly in relation to the axillary artery (Fig. 17.1d) (BLAIR et al. 1987; DEMONDION et al. 2000). Just lateral to the pectoralis minor muscle the cords divide into the five *terminal branches*. The median nerve arises from the medial and lateral cords, the ulnar nerve arises from the medial cord, the musculocutaneous nerve arises from the lateral cord, and the axillary nerve and radial nerve arise from the posterior cord (TABER et al. 2000).

17.4
Tumors

17.4.1
Neurogenic Primary Tumors

Neurogenic primary tumors of the brachial plexus are an uncommon but usually well treatable cause of brachial plexopathies (LUSK et al. 1987; SELL and SEMPLE 1987). Neurofibromas and schwannomas are more common than malignant peripheral nerve sheath tumors. Neurofibromas have no capsule and infiltrate the nerve fascicles. Because of the diffuse penetration of tumor into the nerve, it is difficult to resect the tumor without permanent damage to the nerve. The schwannoma is a benign encapsulated eccentric nerve sheath tumor, which arises from Schwann cells and displaces the nerve fascicles instead of infiltrating them. It is usually possible to resect them without sacrificing the nerve or without neurologic damage. With MRI, primary neurogenic tumors of the brachial plexus can be well detected (MUKHERJI et al. 1996; WITTEN-BERG and ADKINS 2000). The MRI characteristics of a neurogenic tumor include: (1) low signal intensity on T1-weighted images, an increased signal intensity on proton-density images, a high signal intensity on T2-weighted images, which can be inhomogeneous, and enhancement after administration of gadolinium; (2) fusiform growth; (3) sharply defined edge; and (4) in many cases the involved nerve can be found entering and leaving the tumor (Fig. 17.3).

17.4.2
Non-neurogenic Primary Tumors

The most common non-neurogenic primary tumor near the brachial plexus is the superior sulcus tumor. Other primary malignant and benign tumors which can extend to the brachial plexus include head and

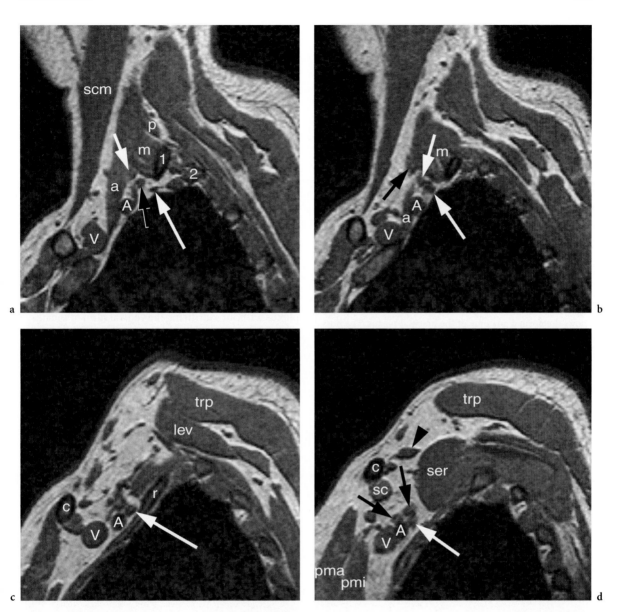

Fig. 17.1a–d. Normal sagittal anatomy (T1-weighted three-dimensional-volume acquisition; slice thickness, 2 mm). **a** The ventral rami of the roots C7 (*short white arrow*), C8 (*black arrow*), and Th1 (*long white arrow*) are in the interscalene triangle, which is formed by the anterior (*a*) and middle (*m*) scalene muscle. *A*, subclavian artery; *V*, subclavian vein; *p*, posterior scalene muscle; *scm*, sternocleidomastoid muscle; *1*, first rib; *2*, second rib. **b** Just lateral to the interscalene triangle the three trunks are seen: the upper (*black arrow*), the middle (*short white arrow*), and the lower (*long white arrow*). **c** The divisions (*arrow*) are formed when the brachial plexus crosses the clavicle (*c*). *r*, First rib; *trp*, trapezius muscle; *lev*, levator scapulae muscle. **d** The three cords: the lateral (*short black arrow*) is positioned anterior, the posterior (*long black arrow*) superior, and the medial (*white arrow*) posterior to the axillary artery (*A*). *V*, axillary vein; *pma*, pectoralis major muscle; *pmi*, pectoralis minor muscle; *sc*, subclavius muscle; *ser*, serratus anterior muscle. [Reprinted with permission from VAN ES et al. (1996)]

neck tumors, sarcoma, lymphoma, bone tumors, aggressive fibromatosis, lipoma, and lymphangioma. MRI plays an important role in the evaluation of these tumors, as it can depict the relationship between the tumor and the brachial plexus in multiple directions. Brachial plexus involvement of tumor appears on MRI as a mass that infiltrates the normal fat surrounding the parts of the brachial plexus and that can abut, displace, infiltrate, or surround the nerves.

According to the TNM classification (MOUNTAIN 1997) *superior sulcus tumors* are by definition at least T3. If there is invasion of the mediastinum or involve-

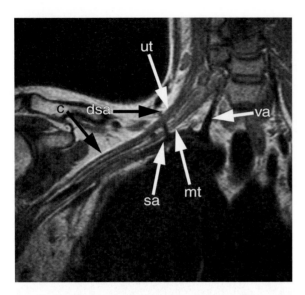

Fig. 17.2. Coronal T1-weighted image (slice thickness, 3 mm) shows the normal anatomy of the brachial plexus. The dorsal scapular artery (*dsa*), which originates from the subclavian artery (*sa*), passes between the upper (*ut*) and middle (*mt*) trunk. *c*, Cords; *va*, vertebral artery. [Reprinted with permission from VAN ES et al. (1995a)]

ment of the heart, great vessels, trachea, esophagus, vertebral body, or carina, or presence of malignant pleural effusion, the tumor becomes T4 and is considered inoperable in most cases. Any lymph node involvement or distant metastases usually preclude

surgery. Curative therapy consists of surgery, which can be preceded by preoperative radiation therapy (PAULSON 1975; SHAW et al. 1961). The purpose of the preoperative radiation therapy is to decrease the extent of disease and to create a pseudocapsule, which increases the resectability. There are two major surgical approaches used for the resection of superior sulcus tumors. The classic posterolateral approach (SHAW et al. 1961) is an en bloc resection of the tumor, the involved ribs, and the nerve roots Th1 and C8 if they are involved. A limitation of this approach is the suboptimal exposure of the structures in the anterior thoracic inlet, such as the brachial plexus and the subclavian vessels. To allow optimal visualization of these vital structures, including the upper part of the brachial plexus, an anterior approach is used (DARTEVELLE et al. 1993). This approach permits subclavian artery reconstruction, and neurolysis of the brachial plexus without sacrificing the ventral rami of the nerve roots above Th1, even if there is upper brachial plexus involvement. Extensive superior sulcus tumors can be treated with a combination of these two approaches. The use of MRI has markedly improved the visualization of the superior sulcus tumors (FREUNDLICH et al. 1996; HEELAN et al. 1989). The sagittal plane shows the cranial extension and the relationship with the subclavian artery (Fig. 17.4a). The coronal plane permits left-to-right comparison, especially for the evaluation of the involvement of the ventral rami of the roots (Fig. 17.4b). Vertebral body destruction and possible

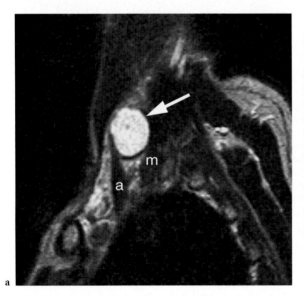

a

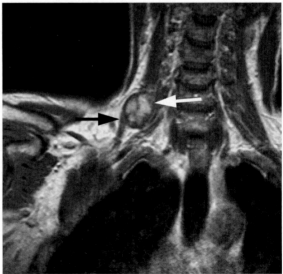

b

Fig. 17.3a, b. Schwannoma of the ventral ramus of root C6. **a** Sagittal T2-weighted image at the level of the interscalene triangle shows the tumor (*arrow*) that causes splaying of the anterior (*a*) and middle (*m*) scalene muscle. **b** Coronal contrast-enhanced T1-weighted image shows the enhancing tumor (*white arrow*). The *black arrow* points to the involved nerve leaving the tumor. [Reprinted with permission from VAN ES et al. (1995b)]

involvement of the nerve roots exiting the foramen are best visualized in the axial plane.

Lymphoma can involve the brachial plexus in two ways. First, the brachial plexus can be compressed or infiltrated by enlarged lymph nodes (Fig. 17.5). Lymphoma of the paravertebral lymph nodes can extend through the intervertebral foramina to extend to the extradural space. Second, neurolymphomatosis can involve the brachial plexus. Neurolymphomatosis is a rare form of lymphoma, which primarily involves the peripheral nerves (DIAZ-ARRASTIA et al. 1992). MRI shows diffuse thickening of the brachial plexus and contrast enhancement (Fig. 17.6) (SWARNKAR et al. 1997; VAN ES 2001).

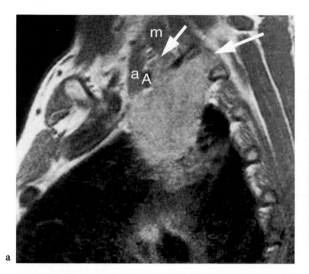
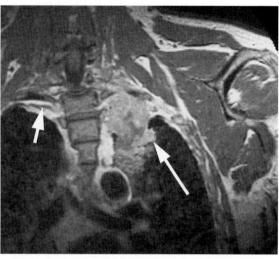

a   b

Fig. 17.4a, b. Superior sulcus tumor (squamous cell carcinoma). **a** Sagittal proton-density image shows the cranial extension of the tumor in the interscalene triangle (*short arrow*) and between the first and second rib (*long arrow*). *A*, subclavian artery; *a*, anterior scalene muscle; *m*, middle scalene muscle. **b** Coronal contrast-enhanced T1-weighted image demonstrates that the tumor (*long arrow*) involves the ventral ramus of root Th1. The *short arrow* points to the right ventral ramus of root Th1. [Reprinted with permission from VAN ES et al. (1995a)]

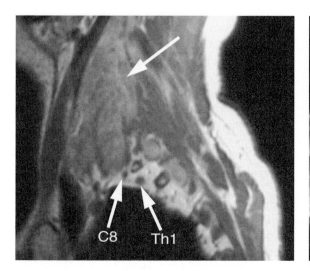
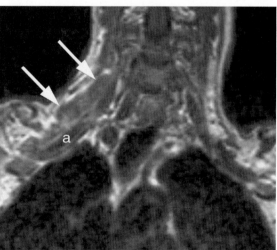

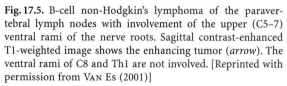

Fig. 17.5. B-cell non-Hodgkin's lymphoma of the paravertebral lymph nodes with involvement of the upper (C5–7) ventral rami of the nerve roots. Sagittal contrast-enhanced T1-weighted image shows the enhancing tumor (*arrow*). The ventral rami of C8 and Th1 are not involved. [Reprinted with permission from VAN ES (2001)]

Fig. 17.6. Neurolymphomatosis of the brachial plexus (B-cell non-Hodgkin's lymphoma). Coronal contrast-enhanced T1-weighted image shows a slightly enhancing diffusely thickened brachial plexus (*arrows*). *a*, Subclavian artery. [Reprinted with permission from VAN ES (2001)]

Aggressive fibromatosis is a benign soft tissue tumor with an infiltrative growth pattern. The axilla and neck are not uncommon sites for aggressive fibromatosis (ENZINGER and WEISS 1988). The tumor primarily arises from the connective tissue of muscle or the aponeurosis. Because of its infiltrative character, which can cause brachial plexus involvement, complete resection is difficult and local recurrence common. The MRI appearance is variable, most tumors show a high signal intensity on the T2-weighted images with scattered foci of low signal intensities and enhance with gadolinium (Fig. 17.7) (GARANT and JUST 1997; KRANSDORF et al. 1990).

17.5
Metastatic Disease and Radiation Plexopathy

The most common lymph node metastases are from breast cancer, lung cancer, and head and neck tumors. Brachial plexopathy in patients with breast cancer can be caused by metastatic tumor or by radiation plexopathy.

Because of its location, radiation-induced damage to the brachial plexus can occur in patients who have had radiation therapy for neoplasms of the mediastinum, breast, lung, or lymph nodes. This was recog-

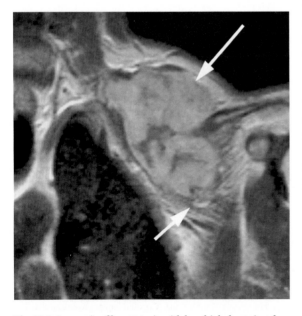

Fig. 17.7. Aggressive fibromatosis with brachial plexus involvement. Coronal contrast-enhanced T1-weighted image shows a large enhancing mass (*long arrow*) with compression of the brachial plexus (*short arrow*)

nized in 1966 by STOLL (STOLL and ANDREWS 1966), who found delayed damage to the brachial plexus in patients treated with radiation therapy after surgery for breast carcinoma. Besides this progressive radiation-induced brachial plexopathy, reversible brachial plexopathy has also been reported. SALNER et al. (1981) reported eight of 565 patients with paresthesias, less commonly with weakness and pain at a median time of 4.5 months after radiation therapy. Complete resolution of all complaints was found in five patients, while in three patients mild paresthesias persisted.

The main problem in diagnosing radiation-induced brachial plexopathy is its differentiation from neoplastic brachial plexopathy. Clinical signs and symptoms may be useful. Horner's syndrome, lower brachial plexus (C7, C8, Th1) involvement, early and severe pain, hand weakness, a radiation dose less than 6000 cGy, and a latency period of more than 1 year are suggestive of tumor infiltration. On the other hand, upper brachial plexus (C5, C6) involvement, doses of more than 6000 cGy, a latency period of less than 1 year, no pain, and lymphedema favor radiation-induced brachial plexopathy (KORI et al. 1981).

MRI can be helpful in the differentiation between tumor and radiation fibrosis (IYER et al. 1996). Tumors (Fig. 17.8) characteristically have a low signal intensity on T1-weighted images, a high signal intensity on T2-weighted images and enhance with gadolinium; however, the signal intensity characteristics can be variable (QAYYUM et al. 2000). Radiation fibrosis usually has a low signal intensity on T1- and T2-weighted images, but can be of high signal intensity on T2-weighted sequences (Fig. 17.9) (THYAGARAJAN et al. 1995; VAN ES et al. 1997a). Radiation fibrosis can also enhance with gadolinium, even 21 years after radiation therapy (VAN ES et al. 1997a). The most reliable distinction between radiation fibrosis and a tumor is the presence of a mass (Fig. 17.8) (LINGAWI et al. 1999; QAYYUM et al. 2000). The use of gadolinium improves sensitivity and accuracy of MRI for recurrent axillary tumor (BRADLEY et al. 2000).

17.6
Trauma

Traumatic lesions to the brachial plexus can be divided into supraganglionic (preganglionic) and infraganglionic (postganglionic) lesions. This subdivision has important therapeutic consequences, as a supraganglionic lesion, which is a nerve root avulsion, cannot be

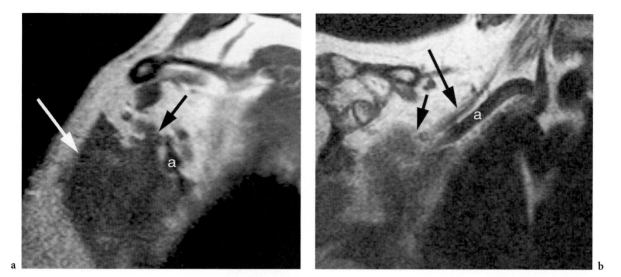

Fig. 17.8a, b. Metastasis of breast carcinoma with brachial plexus involvement. **a** Sagittal T1-weighted image shows a mass (*white arrow*) that is contiguous with the lateral cord (*black arrow*). *a*, Axillary artery. **b** Coronal T1-weighted image confirms the brachial plexus involvement (*short arrow*). Long arrow points to the normal proximal brachial plexus. *a*, Subclavian artery. Findings were confirmed upon surgery, when it was possible to separate the axillary artery and the lateral cord from the tumor. [Reprinted with permission from VAN ES et al. (1995a)]

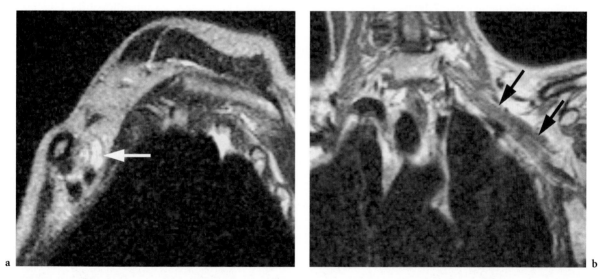

Fig. 17.9a, b. MRI scan 9 months after radiation therapy for breast carcinoma in a patient with a reversible brachial plexopathy. **a** Sagittal T2-weighted image shows an increased signal intensity of the cords (*arrow*). **b** Coronal T1-weighted image shows a slightly swollen brachial plexus (*arrows*). [Reprinted with permission from VAN ES et al. (1997a)]

repaired directly, while the more distal infraganglionic lesions can be restored by local repair.

Nerve root avulsions occur when there is simultaneously traction of the arm and throwing of the head to the opposite side. By far the most common cause in adults is a motorcycle accident. Another important cause is the birth related brachial palsy. Nerve root avulsions are usually accompanied by traumatic meningoceles. However, traumatic meningoceles can exist without nerve root avulsions and nerve root avulsions can occur without traumatic meningoceles (OCHI et al. 1994). It is important to determine the site of the lesion, as this has significant prognostic and therapeutic consequences. Reliable imaging of the presence or absence of nerve root avulsions is most important. CT myelography is considered to be the most reliable investigation for the imaging of the nerve roots (CARVALHO et al. 1997). The main advantage of MRI in trauma patients is the visualization of the extraforaminal part of the brachial plexus. Thickening of the brachial plexus with and without an increased signal intensity on T2-weighted images can be seen (Fig. 17.10), presumably due to edema (RAPOPORT et al. 1988) and fibrosis (MEHTA et al. 1993), respectively. MRI can demonstrate other causes of brachial plexopathy after trauma, such as a hematoma and a clavicle fracture with brachial plexus compression (ENGLAND and TIEL 1999).

17.7
CIDP and MMN

Chronic inflammatory demyelinating polyneuropathy (CIDP) and multifocal motor neuropathy (MMN) can affect the brachial plexus. CIDP is a sensorimotor neuropathy with symmetric weakness and sensory loss in both arms and legs. MMN presents as an asymmetric weakness without sensory loss. CIDP and MMN are probably immune-mediated neuropathies which can respond to high-dose intravenous immunoglobulins (BAROHN et al. 1989; PESTRONK et al. 1988). A biopsy of a patient with MMN showed demyelination and inflammation (OH et al. 1995). MRI can show hypertrophy and an increased signal intensity on T2-weighted images of the brachial plexus (Fig. 17.11) (DUGGINS et al. 1999; VAN ES et al. 1997b).

17.8
Conclusion

MRI is very useful for depicting the anatomy of the brachial plexus, especially in the sagittal and coronal planes. MRI is the imaging method of first choice for the evaluation of superior sulcus tumors, tumors in the supra- and infraclavicular region, as well as for studying brachial plexopathies after radiation therapy. MRI can be helpful in studying trauma, CIDP, and MMN.

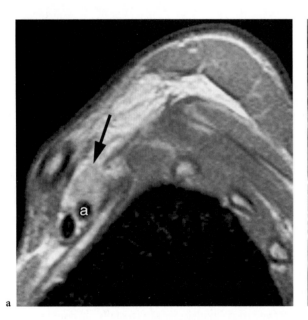
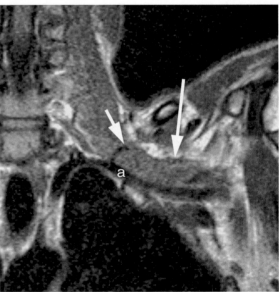

a   b

Fig. 17.10a, b. MRI scan 12 days after a bicycle accident in a patient with a paralyzed arm. **a** Sagittal proton-density image shows that the cords of the brachial plexus have an increased signal intensity (*arrow*). *a*, Subclavian artery. **b** Coronal T1-weighted image shows a diffusely swollen brachial plexus (*long arrow*). The short arrow points to the dorsal scapular artery, which passes through the brachial plexus. Surgery performed 12 weeks later showed rupture of the brachial plexus with neuroma formation. [Reprinted with permission from VAN ES et al. (1995b)]

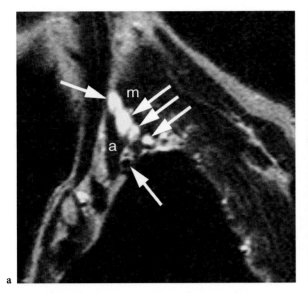

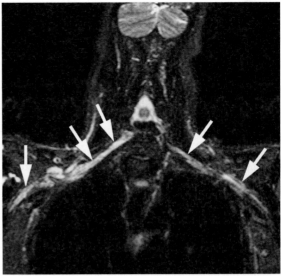

a

b

Fig. 17.11a, b. A patient with multifocal motor neuropathy. **a** Sagittal T2-weighted image shows the thickened ventral rami of the roots (*short arrows*) with an increased signal intensity in the right interscalene triangle. The *long arrow* points to the subclavian artery. *a*, Anterior scalene muscle; *m*, middle scalene muscle. **b** Coronal T2-weighted STIR image shows the increased signal intensity in both the right and left brachial plexus (*arrows*). Note that the right brachial plexus is thicker than the left. [Reprinted with permission from VAN ES et al. (1997b)]

References

Barohn RJ, Kissel JT, Warmolts JR et al (1989) Chronic inflammatory demyelinating polyradiculoneuropathy. Clinical characteristics, course, and recommendations for diagnostic criteria. Arch Neurol 46:878–884

Bilbey JH, Lamond RG, Mattrey RF (1994) MR imaging of disorders of the brachial plexus. J Magn Reson Imaging 4:13–18

Blair DN, Rapoport S, Sostman HD et al (1987) Normal brachial plexus: MR imaging. Radiology 165:763–767

Bradley AJ, Carrington BM, Hammond CL et al (2000) Accuracy of axillary MR imaging in treated breast cancer for distinguishing between recurrent tumour and treatment effects: does intravenous Gd-DTPA enhancement help in cases of diagnostic dilemma? Clin Radiol 55:921–928

Carvalho GA, Nikkhah G, Matthies C et al (1997) Diagnosis of root avulsions in traumatic brachial plexus injuries: value of computerized tomography myelography and magnetic resonance imaging. J Neurosurg 86:69–76

Dartevelle PG, Chapelier AR, Macchiarini P et al (1993) Anterior transcervical-thoracic approach for radical resection of lung tumors invading the thoracic inlet. J Thorac Cardiovasc Surg 105:1025–1034

Demondion X, Boutry N, Drizenko A et al (2000) Thoracic outlet: anatomic correlation with MR imaging. AJR 175:417–422

Diaz-Arrastia R, Younger DS, Hair L et al (1992) Neurolymphomatosis: a clinicopathologic syndrome re-emerges. Neurology 42:1136–1141

Duggins AJ, McLeod JG, Pollard JD et al (1999) Spinal root and plexus hypertrophy in chronic inflammatory demyelinating polyneuropathy. Brain 122:1383–1390

England JD, Tiel RL (1999) AAEM case report 33: costoclavicular mass syndrome. American Association of Electrodiagnostic Medicine. Muscle Nerve 22:412–418

Enzinger FM, Weiss SW (1988) Fibromatoses. In: Enzinger FM, Weiss SW (eds) Soft tissue tumors. Mosby, St Louis, pp 136–163

Freundlich IM, Chasen MH, Varma DGK (1996) Magnetic resonance imaging of pulmonary apical tumors. J Thorac Imag 11:210–222

Garant M, Just N (1997) Aggressive fibromatosis of the neck: MR findings. AJNR 18:1429–1431

Hayes CE, Tsuruda JS, Mathis CM et al (1997) Brachial plexus: MR imaging with a dedicated phased array of surface coils. Radiology 203:286–289

Heelan RT, Demas BE, Caravelli JF et al (1989) Superior sulcus tumors: CT and MR imaging. Radiology 170:637–641

Iyer RB, Fenstermacher MJ, Libshitz HI (1996) MR imaging of the treated brachial plexus. AJR 167:225–229

Kori SH, Foley KM, Posner JB (1981) Brachial plexus lesions in patients with cancer: 100 cases. Neurology 31:45–50

Kransdorf MJ, Jelinek JS, Moser RPJ et al (1990) Magnetic resonance appearance of fibromatosis. A report of 14 cases and review of the literature. Skeletal Radiol 19:495–499

Lingawi SS, Bilbey JH, Munk PL et al (1999) MR imaging of brachial plexopathy in breast cancer patients without palpable recurrence. Skeletal Radiol 28:318–323

Lusk MD, Kline DG, Garcia CA (1987) Tumors of the brachial plexus. Neurosurgery 21:439–453

Maravilla KR, Aagaard BDL, Kliot M (1998) MR neurography. MR imaging of peripheral nerves. MRI Clin North Am 6: 179–194

Mehta VS, Banerji AK, Tripathi RP (1993) Surgical treatment of brachial plexus injuries. Br J Neurosurg 7:491–500

Mountain CF (1997) Revisions in the international system for staging lung cancer. Chest 111:1710–1717

Mukherji SK, Castillo M, Wagle AG (1996) The brachial plexus. Semin Ultrasound CT MRI 17:519–538

Obuchowski AM, Ortiz AO (2000) MR imaging of the thoracic inlet. MRI Clin North Am 8:183–203

Ochi M, Ikuta Y, Watanabe M et al (1994) The diagnostic value of MRI in traumatic brachial plexus injury. J Hand Surg 19B:55–59

Oh SJ, Claussen GC, Odabasi Z et al (1995) Multifocal demyelinating motor neuropathy: pathologic evidence of 'inflammatory demyelinating polyradiculoneuropathy'. Neurology 45:1828–1832

Paulson DL (1975) Carcinomas in the superior pulmonary sulcus. J Thorac Cardiovasc Surg 70:1095–1104

Pestronk A, Cornblath DR, Ilyas AA et al (1988) A treatable multifocal motor neuropathy with antibodies to GM1 ganglioside. Ann Neurol 24:73–78

Posniak HV, Olson MC, Dudiak CM et al (1993) MR imaging of the brachial plexus. AJR 161:373–379

Qayyum A, MacVicar AD, Padhani AR et al (2000) Symptomatic brachial plexopathy following treatment for breast cancer: utility of MR imaging with surface-coil techniques. Radiology 214:837–842

Rapoport S, Blair DN, McCarthy SM et al (1988) Brachial plexus: correlation of MR imaging with CT and pathologic findings. Radiology 167:161–165

Reiner A, Kasser R (1996) Relative frequency of a subclavian vs. a transverse cervical origin for the dorsal scapular artery in humans. Anat Rec 244:265–268

Remy-Jardin M, Doyen J, Remy J et al (1997) Functional anatomy of the thoracic outlet: evaluation with spiral CT. Radiology 205:843–851

Salner AL, Botnick LE, Herzog AG et al (1981) Reversible brachial plexopathy following primary radiation therapy for breast cancer. Cancer Treat Rep 65:797–802

Sell PJ, Semple JC (1987) Primary nerve tumours of the brachial plexus. Br J Surg 74:73–74

Shaw RR, Paulson DL, Kee JLJ (1961) Treatment of the superior sulcus tumor by irradiation followed by resection. Ann Surg 154:29–40

Sheppard DG, Iyer RB, Fenstermacher MJ (1998) Brachial plexus: demonstration at US. Radiology 208:402–406

Sherrier RH, Sostman HD (1993) Magnetic resonance imaging of the brachial plexus. J Thorac Imag 8:27–33

Stoll BA, Andrews JT (1966) Radiation-induced peripheral neuropathy. BMJ 1:834–837

Swarnkar A, Fukui MB, Fink DJ et al (1997) MR imaging of brachial plexopathy in neurolymphomatosis. AJR 169:1189–1190

Taber HT, Maravilla K, Chiou-Tan F et al (2000) Sectional neuroanatomy of the upper limb I: brachial plexus. J Comput Assist Tomogr 24:983–986

Thyagarajan D, Cascino T, Harms G (1995) Magnetic resonance imaging in brachial plexopathy of cancer. Neurology 45:421–427

Van Es HW (2001) MRI of the brachial plexus. Eur Radiol 11:325–336

Van Es HW, Witkamp TD, Feldberg MAM (1995a) MRI of the brachial plexus and its region: anatomy and pathology. Eur Radiol 5:145–151

Van Es HW, Feldberg MAM, Ramos LMP et al (1995b) MRI of the brachial plexus. MedicaMundi 40:84–90

Van Es HW, Witkamp TD, Ramos LMP et al (1996) MR imaging of the brachial plexus using a T1-weighted three-dimensional volume acquisition. Int J Neuroradiol 2:264–273

Van Es HW, Engelen AM, Witkamp TD et al (1997a) Radiation-induced brachial plexopathy: MR imaging. Skeletal Radiol 26:284–288

Van Es HW, van den Berg LH, Franssen H et al (1997b) Magnetic resonance imaging of the brachial plexus in patients with multifocal motor neuropathy. Neurology 48:1218–1224

Wittenberg KH, Adkins MC (2000) MR imaging of nontraumatic brachial plexopathies: frequency and spectrum of findings. Radiographics 20:1023–1032

18 Assessing the Impact of MRI of the Shoulder

P. W. P. Bearcroft

CONTENTS

18.1
Introduction

In the 15 years since magnetic resonance imaging (MRI) was first applied to imaging the shoulder, there has been an explosion of interest in the technique mirrored by a profusion of original articles, review articles, abstracts and case reports in the literature. The other chapters in this book represent a synthesis of this mass of information with a view to summarising the current state of knowledge of MRI of the shoulder. In the various chapters, the preferred imaging approach is outlined together with accurate

P. W. P. BEARCROFT, MB, FRCR
Department of Radiology, Addenbrooke's Hospital NHS Trust, Hills Road, Cambridge, CAMBS CB2 2QQ, UK

statistics for MR imaging in a variety of clinical situations. In essence, these chapters answer the question: "How can MRI produce good anatomically correct images of the shoulder, and do these images allow accurate diagnoses to be made?"

The objective of the current chapter is fundamentally different. Here we assume that our interpretation of the MR images is accurate and we are asking the question: "What evidence is there that performing MRI of the shoulder in patients with shoulder abnormalities makes a difference to either the clinician or to the patient?"

18.2
Background

When the clinical use of MRI commenced in 1980, it was available in only two clinical centres worldwide (STEINER 1985). That number had increased to five by the end of the following year, and the growth since then has been exponential. However, installing, operating and maintaining an MRI system is costly. Enthusiastic original articles and reviews together with powerful industrial marketing fuelled the growth of musculoskeletal applications for MRI. Even in the early days of MRI imaging, it was noticed that the expansion had outpaced the public evidence of efficacy and effectiveness (EHMAN et al. 1988). This in turn led to questions of the value of new diagnostic imaging techniques in general which in turn incited numerous defensive responses (COOPER et al. 1988; SHEPS 1988; KENT and LARSON 1988).

From these exchanges arose the need for a method of health technology assessment (HTA) which can be defined as 'the assessment of the costs, effectiveness and broader impact of all methods used by health professionals to promote health, prevent and treat disease and improve rehabilitation and long term care' (DEPARTMENT OF HEALTH 1991; HEALTH TECHNOLOGY ADVISORY GROUP 1992). The development of an HTA methodology has been worldwide (ABRAMS and

HESSEL 1987; MENON 2000; BANTA and OORTWIJN 2000) and such a methodology incorporates the concepts of *efficacy*, *effectiveness* and *efficiency*.

Efficacy is concerned with whether a technology works (whether it can fulfill the task it is expected to perform); this is initially tested at the design stage in a laboratory setting. Thereafter, in the clinical environment, the technology is optimised and then it can be tested further by conducting accuracy studies, and the technology can be compared to competing systems.

Effectiveness on the other hand, considers whether a technology delivers a benefit to the health care system once the latter has implemented the technology. This is where the effects on patient outcome can be monitored, and where it can be shown that the new technology can favourably influence patient health in routine clinical practice. Effectiveness is sometimes referred to as 'clinical efficacy' (HORII et al. 1997; FINEBERG et al. 1977; KENT and LARSON 1992; THORNBURY 1994). It is relevant that the distinction between efficacy and effectiveness is understood when conducting HTA. Clearly the efficacy of a system must be established before effectiveness is measured (KENT and LARSON 1992).

Efficiency refers more to the concept of resource management and whether, when efficacy and efficiency are taken into consideration, the technology is still the best option in the circumstances and with the resources available. The rate-limiting resource is most frequently money, in which case efficiency equates to cost-effectiveness. Cost-effectiveness, therefore, is an economic concept and it involves an assessment of whether acceptable efficacy and effectiveness are achieved with the most appropriate or optimal combination of resources. The methodology for assessing the cost-effectiveness of MRI has been extensively reviewed (GILLESPIE et al. 1985; GUYATT and DRUMMOND 1985; WEINSTEIN 1985).

18.3
The Radiological Process

For preventative or therapeutic technologies the success of the technology can be measured directly by measuring either the potential for preventing disease or the clinical outcomes of patients that are treated. In a diagnostic technology such as MRI, this is less straightforward as the effects of a diagnostic technology on patient outcome is indirect, reflecting influences resulting from events that include the clinician, the treatments (which may be offered concurrently) and the natural history of the disease. This is particularly true when the technology is used to diagnose a wide range of problems in many different clinical settings (MAISEY and HUTTON 1991; CORMACK et al. 1992)

The ability to improve health is the underlying worth of any medical technology, and is therefore the ultimate objective of performing an MR examination on a patient's shoulder. Several different processes mediate the impact of diagnostic imaging on a patient's outcome and the overall process is summarised in Fig. 18.1.

- Step 1: The images of the shoulder are optimised for the particular MR system. This initially involves fundamental manipulation of a myriad of parameters within the MR system when the machine is installed (i.e. over and above TE, TR, flip angle, FOV, bandwidth, fat saturation etc.), together with the choice of imaging sequences and planes that will be employed. Although several chapters in this book will start with a recommended series of imaging sequences that should be used, it is probably correct to state that no two MR systems in different hospitals anywhere will have exactly the same mix of hardware and software parameters, together with identical imaging methodology in terms of imaging planes and protocols.
- Step 2: The images are interpreted by a trained radiologist. Using concepts and classification systems expounded in this book and others, together with individual training and experience, the radiologist will formulate the report. The accuracy of every radiological examination falls short of 100% and in many applications of MRI of the shoulder an accuracy of 80%–90% would be expected, especially outside of the training centres. There will be inter- and intra-observer variation as with any radiological examination (ROBINSON et al. 1999; LEV et al. 1999).
- Step 3: The textual report is interpreted by the clinician who may also review the images. This is essentially a communication process and it is prone to error and misunderstanding. This is because a radiological report will usually rely on verbal expressions of probability rather than a numerical one. For example the radiologist may incorporate expressions such as "unlikely", "suggests", "probable", "likely", "consistent with" in the report and evidence confirms that there is a difference in the probability ascribed to these expressions between referring clinicians and radiologists which results in a considerable potential for misunderstanding (HOBBY et al. 2000)

Step 4: The clinician alters his differential diagnosis as a result of his interpretation of the radiological report. Unfortunately, from the point of view of demonstrating the effect that the MR report has made, this is not a straightforward process. This is for two reasons. First, it is possible that other non-radiological information is incorporated into the process. This might include results from laboratory tests or from an interval change in the patient's condition. Second, a clinician may choose to ignore all or part of a radiological report's conclusions if he or she feels that they do not fit the clinical picture. This action would probably occur at a subliminal level, but has a mathematical correlate in the form of the statistical principle enshrined in Bayes' theorem (SPIEGELHALTER et al. 2000; MACENEANEY and MALONE 2000): the probability that a patient has a particular condition after a positive radiological test (the post-test probability) will depend on two separate factors equally. First, the accuracy of the radiological test in terms of sensitivity and specificity, and second, the probability that the clinician suspected the patient to have that condition in the first place (the pre-test probability).

Step 5: Based on the clinician's renewed understanding of the patient's diagnosis, a management plan will be decided and exercised. The patients themselves may have an input into this process, especially if an invasive therapeutic procedure is planned. Heterogeneity in both the type of treatment offered and the quality with which it is delivered is to be expected between different clinicians, especially where surgical technique is considered. It is unfortunate that in medicine generally, most treatments offered lack rigorous evidence for their effectiveness.

Step 6: The outcome of the patient will depend upon the management plan of the clinician and the natural history of the disease, and it may take several years before the eventual outcome becomes clear.

Although the underlying objective of any diagnostic imaging technology is to result in a net benefit to the health of the patients which are referred, it is immediately clear from the above and from Fig. 18.1, that the impact of diagnostic imaging on health is mediated through and necessarily masked by other interventions which are out of the hands of the radiologist.

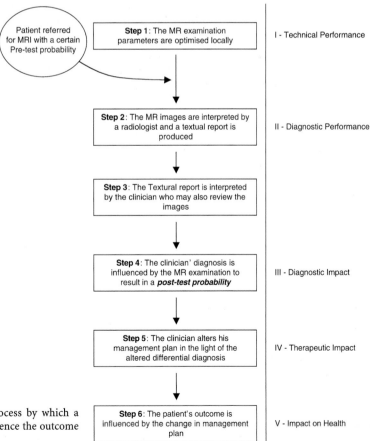

Fig. 18.1. The radiological process. The process by which a radiological evaluation and report can influence the outcome of the patient

18.4
Measuring the Impact of Diagnostic Imaging

In order to address the complexities of evaluating this chain of events a variety of approaches have been applied historically. In general, these forms of assessment have considered the events in terms of the structure, the process and the outcome of the medical intervention. DONABEDIAN (1966) first described this assessment methodology in 1966. In the context of MRI of the shoulder for example, the structure would consist of the MRI resources available at a particular institution, the process would involve the steps taken to ensure optimal patient care in terms of referral for MRI and interpretation of the examination, and the outcome is the benefit to the patient as a result of the MR examination. This type of assessment is now widely accepted and used by the health profession to assess the benefits of imaging technology (ROYAL COLLEGE OF PHYSICIANS 1989).

The question of the impact of imaging on patient outcome is particularly important in the context of increasing demands and costs for healthcare in the western world which threatens to outstrip the funds available. Over 30 years ago the medical profession was prompted to consider the "economic" as well as the medical consequences of their decisions (FUCHS 1968), and also to evaluate the clinical usefulness of radiological examinations (LUSTED 1968). After the introduction of CT during the early 1970s, much debate was generated surrounding the impact of such a health technology and the evaluation of diagnostic imaging. As a result of this, the assessment by DONABEDIAN (1966) was further refined to analyse diagnostic imaging in particular. This led FINEBERG

et al. (1977) to suggest the hierarchical system or four 'levels of efficacy'. These were 'technical output', 'diagnostic information', which tackled the question of diagnostic accuracy of the imaging and its impact on clinical diagnostic confidence, 'therapeutic impact' and 'patient outcome'. This original system was further refined into five levels by MACKENZIE and DIXON in 1995 to form the more widely accepted version for use in the assessment of diagnostic imaging (Fig. 18.2) (KENT and LARSON 1992; THORNBURY 1994; MAISEY and HUTTON 1991; SANFORD SCHWARTZ 1985).

The concept of five hierarchical stages can also be applied to HTA where technical and diagnostic performances are related to the assessment of efficacy. Diagnostic and therapeutic impact and the patient outcome are related to effectiveness. However, the framework does not address efficiency which is nevertheless an important component of HTA. The hierarchy simplifies analysis of efficiency; each level produces an output that can be compared with other imaging investigations analysed in the same way. If it can be shown that another imaging investigation performs equally well at every level, and costs less, then it would be the investigation of choice. In reality, comparison of techniques side by side is rarely straightforward and more comprehensive analysis of costs and benefits to the patient are usually needed.

Evaluations of effectiveness of musculoskeletal MRI have included the knee (MACKENZIE et al. 1996), spine (DIXON et al. 1991), shoulder (BLANCHARD et al. 1997, 1999a,b; SHER et al. 1998; ZANETTI et al. 1999) and wrist (HOBBY et al. 2001). It is the intention of the next sections to address the question of effectiveness and efficacy of magnetic resonance imaging of the shoulder.

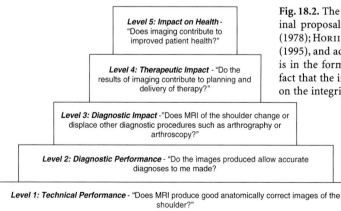

Level 5: Impact on Health - "Does imaging contribute to improved patient health?"

Level 4: Therapeutic Impact - "Do the results of imaging contribute to planning and delivery of therapy?"

Level 3: Diagnostic Impact - "Does MRI of the shoulder change or displace other diagnostic procedures such as arthrography or arthroscopy?"

Level 2: Diagnostic Performance - "Do the images produced allow accurate diagnoses to me made?

Level 1: Technical Performance - "Does MRI produce good anatomically correct images of the shoulder?"

Fig. 18.2. The five-stage evaluative framework [based on original proposals by DONABEDIAN (1966) and FINEBERG et al. (1978); HORII et al. (1997), modified by MACKENZIE and DIXON (1995), and adapted for MRI of the shoulder]. The framework is in the form of a pyramid stressing the importance of the fact that the integrity of each level of the framework depends on the integrity and validity of the levels below

18.5
An Evaluative Framework for MRI of the Shoulder

The five levels generally accepted for the evaluation of diagnostic imaging are listed in Fig. 18.2. An important feature of the framework is that it is a hierarchy, and for a technique to be effective at a particular level, it must first be shown to be effective at the levels below. Put colloquially, "MRI must be shown to be accurate before it is likely to make a difference". A sixth level has been suggested, namely "impact on society" which serves to detect whether an imaging technology has benefited a population, or society at large. The levels of the hierarchy are elaborated below.

18.4.1
Level 1–Technical Performance

Technical Performance corresponds to Step 1 in the radiological process outlined in Fig. 18.1. It can be reworded as "Does MRI of the shoulder reliably result in good quality images that are anatomically representative?" and "Is it possible to use MRI to accurately differentiate the various anatomical structures of the shoulder?" The choice of imaging parameters and surface coil or of the slice orientation for example comes under the umbrella of technical performance. Papers that address such issues comprised the majority of original articles in the literature in the 1980s (BEAR-CROFT et al. 2000) and initial cadaveric studies were fundamental to the demonstration of the technique's ability to delineate anatomical detail accurately.

18.4.2
Level 2–Diagnostic Performance

The diagnostic accuracy of an imaging technique is also fundamental to its usefulness. It corresponds to step 2 of the radiological process in Fig. 18.1 and it is assessed by comparing MRI findings with those of an alternative "gold standard" technique with derivation of accuracy statistics including sensitivity, specificity, predictive value, ROC curves, as well as inter- and intra-observer variability. Colloquially, therefore, diagnostic performance answers the question "Does MRI of the shoulder allow accurate diagnoses to be made?" and whether it does will be influenced the parameters chosen above at level 1 of the hierarchy. Clearly, if the technique is not accurate or if there is wide variability in any interpretation of the findings between different

radiologists, then this will have a significant impact on the ability of the technology to influence higher levels of the hierarchy favourably. Papers that addressed questions of diagnostic performance predominated in the 1990s (BEARCROFT et al. 2000). They came in various forms including case reports of the MR appearances of a variety of conditions, formal assessments of one or more of the accuracy statistics and papers combining diagnostic and technical performance by comparing the accuracy statistics for differing imaging approaches and parameters.

18.4.3
Level 3–Diagnostic Impact

The principal route by which a diagnostic imaging technique can influence the patient's outcome is by changing the clinician's diagnostic thinking, thereby changing the clinician's therapeutic approach to the patient. That change may manifest in one of several ways. Predominantly, the imaging may alter the diagnosis that the clinician holds. Alternatively it may alter the confidence with which a clinician's diagnosis is retained, or it may increase or decrease the number of differential diagnoses. Corresponding to step 4 in the radiological process in Fig. 18.1, the diagnostic impact therefore reflects the influence of MRI on the clinician's differential diagnosis and diagnostic confidence. It is assessed, therefore, by measuring both the clinical diagnosis and diagnostic confidence before, and again after, the information from imaging is available. A separate aspect of diagnostic impact is the ability of MRI to displace other diagnostic technologies (e.g. arthrography, arthroscopy, ultrasound).

18.4.4
Level 4–Therapeutic Impact

The therapeutic impact concerns whether the imaging technique can contribute to planning and delivery of the patient's treatment. Indeed, an alteration in the clinicians differential diagnosis is only of value if it leads to a change in management or provides prognostic information (KELSEY FRY 1984). Therefore, the therapeutic impact is considered a separate level in the evaluative hierarchy since imaging could influence diagnostic thinking without affecting the planning or delivery of treatment. It corresponds to step 5 of the radiological process as outlined in Fig. 18.1 and is measured by assessing how the patient's proposed treatment is affected or altered by the imaging. This is achieved in practice by documenting the management plan prior to imaging in terms of the proposed management if imaging was unavailable or denied. To some extent, this is artificial as treatment plans would not usually be finalised until all of the relevant data, including the results of imaging, had been obtained. Nevertheless, the pre-treatment plans are compared to the post-treatment plans and differences highlighted and counted across the study population. Arguably the most relevant changes in treatment would involve a change to or from interventional treatment, such as surgery, or a change in the type of performed procedure which the patient is to undergo (e.g. open surgery versus arthroscopic surgery).

18.4.5
Level 5–Impact on Health

The impact on the health of a patient is a crucial part of the assessment of any health technology. It represents the ultimate aim of any health care process and is the driving force behind medical practice and the development of diagnostic technology (KENT and LARSON 1992). An all-embracing definition of health is missing but the World Health Organisation gives us a useful contribution: ".. a state of complete physical, mental and social well-being ...". In common with other diagnostic technologies, MRI does not have any immediate therapeutic benefits to the patient and therefore it is difficult to see how a change in health can be documented. An exception would be when a normal examination is sufficient to allay a patient's fear in relation to symptoms. A comparison of health status immediately before and immediately after imaging is unlikely to yield any significant differences, as an improvement in physical, mental or social-well being is not a product of diagnostic technology such as MRI. Indeed, MRI may not be used in isolation and may be one of several tests being used, and establishing the particular contribution that MRI has made to the overall process is impossible. In particular, any effect on the health is almost certainly mediated through the clinician's response to the MRI result (the diagnostic and therapeutic impact) rather than through the MRI itself. Only one paper has previously demonstrated a positive benefit to the patient's health from MRI, and this is in relation to MRI of the knee (MACKENZIE et al. 1996).

The assessment of the quality of the patient's life and the ability of that patient to function normally within society lies at the centre of the most qualitative determinants of health. There are several shoulder function tests available to assess the physical aspects of shoulder

problems [e.g. The Constant Shoulder Score (CONSTANT and MURLEY 1987), Shoulder Pain and Disability Index (SPADI) (ROACH et al. 1991), the Simple Shoulder Test (LIPPITT et al. 1993), the Modified American shoulder and Elbow Surgeons shoulder patient self-evaluation form (RICHARDS et al. 1994), and the Shoulder Severity Index (PATTE 1987)]. These physical aspects assume an important significance as patients who experience pain in their daily activities, or who have difficulty with sleep and mobility, are likely as a result to return lower mental and social functioning scores also. There are a number of methods available for assessing the impact of illness on general well-being, and therefore health, and these include questionnaires such as the Short Form 36 (SF36), Rosser Index and Euroquol indices. These studies concentrate on both the physical and emotional aspects of the quality of the life, including social interaction and self esteem. The philosophy and methodology for the assessment of health-related quality of life has been extensively reviewed both in general terms (FITZ-PATRICK 1991; WALKER and ROSSER 1993) and in the specific context of MRI (MACKENZIE et al. 1994)

18.4.6
Level 6–Impact on the Health of Society

There is a further level of impact which has not traditionally been considered in the evaluative framework, and that relates to the effect of imaging technology on the health of a population of patients served by a nation's health system. It would be desirable to show that the health of a nation had been improved for example by the widespread investment in imaging technology in general. As the scope of such an assessment is wider than specifically MRI of the shoulder, the subject will not be covered further in this chapter, but the results of such assessments will be important in the long-term planning of the delivery of health services for a society, especially when the state is responsible for the costs of installing and running expensive imaging facilities.

18.6
Effectiveness of Shoulder MRI

18.6.1
The Published Evidence

Of the many hundreds of papers written about MRI of the shoulder, only five so far address the question of effectiveness of magnetic resonance imaging (BEAR-CROFT et al. 2000). Four of these are concerned with conventional MRI (BLANCHARD et al. 1997, 1999a,b; SHER et al. 1998) and the fifth is concerned with MR arthrography (ZANETTI et al. 1999). Considering the four conventional MRI papers first, it is useful to consider the variations between the study designs of these four papers in an attempt to explain any differences in the results and conclusions between them. Indeed, studying the differences in results between these papers may help to allow us to predict how the effectiveness of MRI of the shoulder may differ from one clinical setting to another.

18.6.2
Methodologies Employed

The background information relating to the five papers is summarised in Table 18.1 in the chronological order in which they were published.

In *paper I* (BLANCHARD et al. 1997) referrals were accepted from a wide range of clinicians including rheumatologists and orthopaedic surgeons, and the referral base was not limited to the hospital where the examinations were performed. Furthermore, a wide variety of diagnoses were considered. In addition, all patients were requested to fill in a quality-of-life questionnaire in the form of a SF-36 form, both before the examination, immediately afterwards and again 6 months later. *Paper II* (BLANCHARD et al. 1999a) focused on a group of rheumatologists and there was no limit on the number of admissible pre-test diagnoses. In *paper III* (BLANCHARD et al. 1999b) the referrals were limited to those coming from a single dedicated orthopaedic shoulder surgeon and the diagnoses were limited to the single diagnosis of whether or not there was a full thickness rotator cuff tear present. All three papers shared the same basic methodology. Clinicians

were required to fill in a detailed assessment sheet prior to referring the patient for MRI. This questionnaire incorporated the diagnosis or diagnoses which the clinician was suspecting, together with a scale from 0% to 100% on which the clinician was required to indicate the degree of certainty with which each diagnosis was considered likely [VAS Visual Analogue Scale; STREINER and NORMAN 1995]. The proposed management plan was also indicated. After the MR examination was completed, the clinician was required to assimilate the results of imaging and then to fill in an identical follow-up questionnaire without reference to the initial form. Differences in the responses were then quantified and ascribed to the effect of the MR examination. In papers I and II, the follow-up form was filled in when the patient returned to the clinic and this may have introduced noise to the resulting data as other influences may have had an effect on the way that the form was filled in by the clinician. In paper III, all patients underwent conventional arthrography and MR examinations of the shoulder and the surgeon was required to fill out a questionnaire after the results of each individual examination was revealed to him. The order in which the results from arthrography and MRI were revealed to him was randomised so that the relative impact of these two techniques can be compared. Furthermore, the process took place before the next clinic appointment so that no other influences would be affecting any change in diagnosis and management plans.

In *paper IV* (SHER et al. 1998) a different study methodology was applied and MRI referrals were considered from the practice of two orthopaedic surgeons. In these patients MRI had already been performed before the surgeon saw the patient, and therefore the surgeon was able to develop a differential diagnosis and management plan prior to the results of imaging being known. The surgeon then read the results of imaging and immediately quantified how the result had influenced his diagnostic thinking and management plan.

Table 18.1. Summary of the methodology used in the papers that consider the effectiveness of shoulder MRI

Paper (Reference)	Technique	Source of referrals	Hierarchical levels (KENT and LARSON 1992) addressed	Patients (n)	Diagnoses considered
I (BLANCHARD et al. 1997a)	MRI	Various	3/4/5	86	Various
II (BLANCHARD et al. 1999a)	MRI	Rheumatologists only	3/4	53	Various
III (BLANCHARD et al. 1999b)	MRI	Orthopaedic shoulder surgeons only	3/4	117	FTRCT only
IV (SHER et al. 1998)	MRI	Orthopaedic shoulder surgeons only	3/4	100	Various
V (ZANETTI et al. 1999)	MR arthrography	Orthopaedic shoulder surgeons only	3/4	73	Various

FTRCT: full thickness rotator cuff tear

In addition, the surgeon decided before reading the imaging results whether he would have requested an MRI in that situation and therefore divided the patients into two groups depending on whether he felt MRI was required. In this study, therefore, it is also possible to selectively determine the therapeutic and diagnostic impact for the two groups separately.

Paper V (ZANETTI et al. 1999) addressed the question of the clinical impact of MR arthrography of the shoulder, and is unique in this respect. It focused on a group of orthopaedic surgeons, and allowed a wide range of diagnoses related to impingement: patients with instability were not included in the study population and therefore direct comparison with the other four papers that used conventional MR is possible. A similar methodology to papers I and II was adopted with the clinician being required to document the differential diagnosis and management plan before imaging and again afterwards at the next outpatient clinic appointment.

18.6.3
Results–Therapeutic and Diagnostic Impact

The overall results are summarised in Table 18.2. In *paper I* (BLANCHARD et al. 1997) the MR examination altered the working diagnosis in 34% of patients and in the remainder, where the pre-test diagnosis was retained, the certainty with which the diagnosis was held was increased in 66% of patients ($p < 0.001$). The management plans were changed for 61% of patients, but interestingly an equal number of patients changed from surgical to non-surgical and from non-surgical to surgical procedures, and therefore the overall number of operations was not significantly altered. The presumption is that the surgery would have been better targeted to those patients who would benefit most from it.

In *paper II* (BLANCHARD et al. 1999a) MRI demonstrated a change in diagnosis in 68% of individuals with a shift in certainty of diagnoses in those in whom the pre-test diagnosis was retained by 21%. Management plans were changed in 51% of patients with 37% of patients receiving more invasive therapy as a result of imaging and 14% receiving less invasive treatment.

In *paper III* (BLANCHARD et al. 1999b) the diagnosis held by the surgeon was changed in 30% of individuals and this led to a change in management plan in 36% of individuals. Further subdivisions of these groups were not made in the paper.

In *paper IV* (SHER et al. 1998), in those patients in whom the orthopaedic surgeon would have required an MRI the diagnosis changed in 23% and the management changed in 15%. Conversely, in those patients in whom the orthopaedic surgeon would not have requested MRI, but instead the MRI had been requested by the primary care physician, the corresponding values were lower with a 9% change in diagnosis and 3% change in management plan.

Paper V (ZANETTI et al. 1999) documented a change in diagnosis in 47% of patients and showed that the treatment plan was altered in 49% of patients. A total of 64% of these had more invasive therapeutic procedures than initially planned, and 13 patients underwent more conservative therapy.

18.6.4
Results–Impact on the Patient's Health

Only paper I (BLANCHARD et al. 1997) attempted to quantify the impact of MRI imaging on the health of the individual patients as measured by an SF-36 form. There were slight improvements in scores for six of the eight SF-36 scales, but none of these assumed statistical significance at the 5% level. Furthermore, there was no significant change in the group as a whole.

An interesting observation of paper I, however, is that the SF-36 was able to differentiate the patients with shoulder problems from the normal population

Table 18.2. Summary of the results from the papers that consider the effectiveness of shoulder MRI

Paper (Reference)	Patients (n)	Diagnostic impact	Therapeutic impact*
I (BLANCHARD et al. 1997a)	86	New diagnosis 34%; shift confidence 66%	61%
II (BLANCHARD et al. 1999a)	53	New diagnosis 68%; shift confidence 7%	52%
III (BLANCHARD et al. 1999b)	117	New diagnosis 30%	36%
IV (SHER et al. 1998)	100	New diagnosis 23%	15%
V (ZANETTI et al. 1999)	73	New diagnosis 47%	49%

* Proportion of patients in whom management was changed

in ways that are likely to be related to the shoulder symptoms. Compared to a healthy sample of individuals surveyed by JENKINSON et al. (1993a,b) the patients in the study group had significantly poorer scores in each of the eight scales than the SF-36 addressees (Table 18.3). Furthermore, the self-reported health status of patients with shoulder problems was significantly worse than those with knee problems (MACK-ENZIE 1996) which is an indication, perhaps, of the disability associated with shoulder pain.

18.6.5
Discussion of Results

What is striking about the results of these five papers is the evidence that, in all five studies, MRI was shown to have a positive impact on the clinician's diagnosis and the management of the patient. Nevertheless, there was wide variation in the degree of that impact when it was quantified. In particular, the impact varied depending on whether referrals arose from multiple general clinicians rather that dedicated shoulder surgeons, and on the number on indications for referral that were considered. It is clear therefore that the clinical impact of MRI of the shoulder in particular and, by extrapolation, the impact of other radiological tests, will depend on several factors. These include the experience of the referring clinician or clinicians, the case mix of patients referred and the range of allowable diagnoses, together with the way that the diagnostic therapeutic impact is measured.

18.6.5.1
Referring Clinician

The ability of the referring clinician to diagnose specific shoulder abnormalities accurately will significantly affect the measured effectiveness of MRI of the shoulder. This is intuitive. If a clinician was always 100% accurate in his or her diagnosis then imaging would have little impact on the clinician's diagnosis of the patient's management. Conversely, a clinician whose diagnosis was almost always wrong will report a large impact of imaging on his diagnostic thinking. In only one study was the accuracy of the clinician quantified. In paper III (BLANCHARD et al. 1999b), the clinician was a single dedicated shoulder surgeon. In this case, the surgeon was accurate in diagnosing a full thickness rotator cuff tear in 73% of individuals. This accuracy could be considered excellent and indeed compares well with the accuracy of various

Table 18.3. The eight scales that make up the SF-36 test instrument to measure the health of an individual patient

Scale
Physical functioning
Role limitation due to physical problems
Pain
General health
Energy and vitality
Social functioning
Role limitation due to emotional problems
Mental health

radiological tests including the accuracy of shoulder MRI in some series (YEU et al. 1994; IMHOFF and HODLER 1996; EVANCHO et al. 1988). Nevertheless, even in this situation the surgeon reported that the MRI provided confirmatory evidence and helpful information about the anatomy likely to be encountered during the subsequent intervention, the nature of which was influenced by the MRI findings in 36% of cases. Where referrals from a wide variety of clinicians using different referral paradigms were studied, the overall shift in confidence of the therapeutic plans is greatest. Conversely, a closed knit group of orthopaedic surgeons working to the same diagnostic and referral criteria in close co-operation with their radiological colleagues will result in an apparently reduced diagnostic and therapeutic impact. Although it is gratifying that all papers indicate a positive impact on both the clinical diagnosis and therapeutic plans, the actual quantification of the effectiveness of MRI of the shoulder will depend on the institution were it is measured. Arguably, the most common referral situation will be analogous to paper I, where a wide range of surgeons and physicians are referring the patients and a variety of clinical diagnoses is being considered. It is satisfying that, in this situation, the therapeutic and diagnostic impact of shoulder MRI is greatest.

In the fourth study there is indirect information about the effectiveness of MRI in patients who are referred from clinicians with arguably poorer clinical skills. In those patients in whom the surgeon would not have asked for an MRI, but who had already been referred for an MRI anyway prior to the surgical appointment, the therapeutic and diagnostic impact of MRI was the lowest.

The implications of this are important. In situations where MRI is a limited resource then it may not be best targeted at patients referred from clinicians who either have a very high diagnostic accuracy or who have a very low diagnostic accuracy. In the first situation, the MRI will not often alter the clinician's diagnosis, and therefore the measured diagnostic and therapeutic impact will be low. In the second situation, although the measured effectiveness would be high, it may be more cost-effective to refer the patients to a specialist with a higher diagnostic accuracy and reserve the MRI for the individuals in whom there remains a degree of uncertainty.

18.6.5.2
Casemix

A further complicating factor is the casemix of the patients referred. In the same way that sensitivity and specificity values (level 2 of the evaluative framework in Fig. 18.2) depend upon the prevalence of disease in the studied population, the same argument might apply for measurements of the effectiveness (levels 3–5 in Fig. 18.2). With only five papers in the literature, all from tertiary referral hospitals, it is difficult as yet to test this contention. Indirect evidence comes from the fourth study where there is a group of patients for whom the orthopaedic surgeon would not have required an MRI examination. One would expect the group as a whole to have a low probability of disease, and accordingly the measured impact on diagnosis and treatment was low. Intuitively, if the incidence of a particular disease is low, and it is unlikely that any particular patient will have that disease, then it is expected that the therapeutic and diagnostic impact of MRI in that context would also be low.

18.6.5.3
Impact on Health

As has been indicated previously, the ability to improve the health of a patient (or of a population of patients) must be recognised as the ultimate worth of any medical technology (MACKENZIE et al. 1994; MACKENZIE and DIXON 1995). Nevertheless only one out of these five papers attempted to evaluate the impact of MRI of the shoulder on the patient's health or outcome. Arguably, the study methodology makes it unlikely that a small improvement in health would have been detected, and therefore the methodology deserves further comment.

In paper I (BLANCHARD et al. 1997), the investigators used the short self-administered test SF-36 comprising 36 question items which combine to give health in the context of eight health scales. The questions are designed to investigate both physical and emotional well-being in terms of physical function, surgical functioning, pain, role limitation, emotional

well being, energy and vitality. The SF-36 has been shown to discriminate a sample of patients from the normal population and also to differentiate patients according to different physical problems. Simplicity is essential with this type of test to make it reliable and in addition it has to be completed quickly and has to appear in an easy-to-understand format employing tick boxes, yes or no responses and one-word answers. The test has been shown to possess good repeatability implying that it can be used in longitudinal studies to see whether a patient has improved on medication or investigation. In this paper, the test was applied before, immediately after and 6 months after MRI of the shoulder. However, the SF-36 does not control for other outcomes, and it is arguably a relatively blunt instrument. Therefore, it may be unrealistic to expect to detect a small change in health status with a small heterogeneous sample size with the SF-36 form. As indicated above, with one exception (MACKENZIE et al. 1996), attempts to prove that health status can be directly improved because of MRI have been fruitless (MACKENZIE et al. 1994). Therefore, although paper I did not demonstrate an improvement in health status it should be noted that the number of patients is relatively small and any change in health status would have to be large to have been detectable on such a small sample size. In addition, the natural history of patients with chronic shoulder problems is not known and it could be argued that health status scores could be going down gradually and that a static score represents possible improvement. Finally, the study was observational in nature, and arguably a randomised control trial would be required before it could be concluded that MRI did not have an impact on the patient's health.

Despite these provisos, paper I documented a reduction in the SF-36 scored in all eight scales in patients with shoulder disability when compared to the normal population. In the physical well-being aspects of health (physical functioning, pain and role limitation due to physical problems) this would be expected. But poorer scores were also documented in scales relating to the emotional well-being aspects of health. This probably reflects the fact that the majority of patients had problems that had been present for more than 3 months before the MRI referral, and also that physical pain and limitation affects social functioning and has negative emotional ramifications. Furthermore, the fact that the health status of patients with shoulder problems was significantly worse than those with knee problems is an indication, perhaps, that the disability associated with shoulder pain is worse than that associated with knee pain.

18.6.5.4
Comparison With Other Imaging Techniques

One of the criticisms aimed at radiologists is that they were too quick to jump on the "MR bandwagon" when investigating patients with a wide variety of conditions (COOPER et al. 1988; SHEPS 1988; KENT and LARSON 1988) as MRI applications for a wide variety of diseases outpaced the published evidence of the effectiveness, or even the efficacy of the technique. As far as shoulder impingement was concerned, MRI rapidly displaced conventional arthrography. This is in spite of the fact that the latter is a technique with a long pedigree, which is accurate in determining whether or not a patient has sustained a full thickness rotator cuff tear. Such a tear is detected when contrast that was injected into the joint passes through the tear into the subacromial–subdeltoid bursa. Accuracy values in excess of 85%–90% are expected (BANTA and OORTWIJN 2000; EVANCHO et al. 1988), particularly if interval tears are not included in the accuracy results (BLANCHARD et al. 1998). Coincidentally, the pivotal question often posed by the orthopaedic surgeons in patients with impingement is whether or not the rotator cuff is torn. Often the symptoms are bad enough to require an arthroscopic subacromial decompression, but if a full thickness tear is confirmed then an open repair would be the preferred procedure. It is interesting, therefore, in this context, that in the third study (BLANCHARD et al. 1999b) all patients received both conventional arthrography and MRI and the order in which the information was presented to the surgeon was randomised. The important observation here is that, as far as full thickness rotator cuff tears are concerned, there was no significant difference between the diagnostic and therapeutic impacts of conventional arthrography and MRI. Of course, MRI gives other information not available on an arthrogram, and avoids ionising radiation and an intra-articular injection although this did not translate into a difference in effectiveness in this context.

It could be argued that, where two diagnostic tests have equal effectiveness, it may be worth considering the technique which the patients consider more agreeable. In this context the expectation would be that patients would prefer MR to arthrography. However, this has not been shown to be the case (BLANCHARD et al. 1997). Indeed, in patients who have had both MRI and arthrography, there is no statistically significant evidence that they prefer one technique over the other. It may be that the patient/doctor contact, which is more intense in the case of an arthrogram, is a positive factor that is not offset by the minor irritation and discomfort of the injection.

Paper V addresses the effectiveness of MR arthrography for patients referred with signs attributable to shoulder impingement and a comparison with the other four papers is revealing. The referring clinicians were from an orthopaedic team that specialises in shoulder surgery and therefore the results are best compared to papers III and IV where the experience of the referring clinicians is comparable. The effectiveness in terms of diagnostic impact and therapeutic impact was greater for MR arthrography than for conventional MRI, although the comparison is being made on the basis of a single paper. It would be interesting to determine whether such a difference was repeated in future studies of the effectiveness of MR arthrography.

Medical imaging is a dynamic field and new techniques are evolving. As far as impingement is concerned, ultrasound is developing into a robust and inexpensive technique to assess the rotator cuff, with excellent accuracy in experienced hands. What has not yet been addressed is a comparison of effectiveness of MRI compared to ultrasound. If it were shown that ultrasound can deliver the same results with regard to diagnostic and therapeutic impact as MRI, then there would be motivation to transfer patients away from MRI into the ultrasound department.

18.7
Conclusion

The overall effectiveness of any radiological technique is as important as its accuracy, and is arguably more so. It is a prerequisite for any assessment of cost-effectiveness of the technique. With MRI of the shoulder, the effectiveness, in terms of the positive impact on the clinician's diagnosis and treatment is proven, although quantification of that benefit shows wide variation between the studies depending upon patient casemix and the referring clinician's diagnostic acumen. In the most common context of general rheumatologists and orthopaedic surgeons referring a wide range of patients, the therapeutic and diagnostic impact of shoulder MRI is greatest. Nevertheless, even in the case of an experienced and dedicated shoulder surgeon, MRI makes a positive and significant contribution to the clinician's diagnostic thinking and management plans. Variability in the measured results of diagnostic and therapeutic impact between institutions will have important implications for cost-effectiveness analyses as it may not be appropriate to apply a cost-effectiveness analysis performed at a tertiary referral centre to other institutions. It is clear that patients with shoulder problems who have been referred for MRI have significant morbidity as measured by a standard health assessment instrument, and that the degree of morbidity is greater than for patients referred for MRI of the knee. Although it has not been possible to demonstrate a direct benefit of MRI on the health of the referred patients, this lack of evidence is probably related to the study design.

References

Abrams HL; Hessel S (1987) Health technology assessment: problems and challenges AJR Am J Roentgenol 149: 1127–1132

Banta D, Oortwijn W (2000) Health technology assessment and health care in the European Union. Int J Technol Assess Health Care Spring 16:626–635

Bearcroft PWP, Blanchard TK, Dixon AK, Constant CR (2000) Literature review: An assessment of the effectiveness of magnetic resonance imaging of the shoulder. Skeletal Radiol 29:673–679

Blanchard TK, Mackenzie R, Bearcroft PWP, Gray A, Lomas DJ, Constant CR, Dixon AK (1997a) Magnetic resonance imaging of the shoulder: assessment of effectiveness. Clin Radiol 52:363–368

Blanchard TK, Bearcroft PW, Dixon AK, Lomas DJ, Teale A, Constant CR, Hazleman BL (1997b) Magnetic resonance imaging or arthrography of the shoulder: which do patients prefer? Br J Radiol 70:786–790

Blanchard TK, Constant CR, Bearcroft PWP, Marshall TJ, Dixon AK (1998) Imaging of the rotator cuff: an arthrographic pitfall. Eur Radiol 8:817–820

Blanchard TK, Bearcroft PWP, Maibaum A, Hazleman BL, Sharma S, Dixon AK (1999a) Magnetic resonance or arthrography for shoulder problems: a randomised study. Eur J Radiol 30:5–10

Blanchard TK, Bearcroft PWP, Constant CR, Griffin DR, Dixon AK (1999b) Diagnostic and therapeutic impact of MRI and arthrography in the investigation of full-thickness rotator cuff tears. Eur Radiol 9:638–642

Constant CR, Murley AH (1987) A clinical method of functional assessment of the shoulder. Clin Orthop 214:160–164

Cooper PS, Chalmers TC, McCally M, Barrier F, Sachs HS (1988) The poor quality of early evaluations of magnetic resonance imaging. JAMA 259:3277–3280

Cormack J, Evill CA, Langlois S, Le P, Sage MR, Tordoff A (1992) Evaluating the clinical efficacy of diagnostic imaging procedures. Eur J Radiol 16:1–9

Department of Health (1991) Research for health: a research and development strategy for the NHS. Department of Health, London

Dixon AK, Southern JP, Teale A et al (1991) Magnetic resonance imaging of the head and spine: effective for the clinician or the patient? BMJ 302:79–82

Donabedian A (1966) Evaluating the quality of medical care. Milbank Memorial Fund Q 44:166–206

Ehman RL, Berquist TH, McCleod RA (1988) MR imaging of the musculoskeletal system: a five year appraisal. Radiology 166:313–320

Evancho AM, Stiles RJ, Fajman WA et al (1988) MR imaging diagnosis of rotator cuff tears. AJR 151:751–754

Fineberg HV (1978) Evaluation of computed tomography: achievement and challenge. AJR 131:1–4

Fineberg HV, Bauman R, Sosman M (1977) Computerized cranial tomography. Effect on diagnostic and therapeutic plans. JAMA 238:224–227

Fitzpatrick R (1991) Surveys of patient satisfaction II. Designing a questionnaire and conducting a study. Br Med J 302: 1129–1132

Fuchs VR (1968) The growing demand for medical care. N Engl J Med 279:190–195

Gillespie KN, Elixhauser A, Reker DM et al (1985) Cost-benefit and cost-effectiveness of magnetic resonance imaging. Int J Technol Assess Health Care 1:537–550

Guyatt, G Drummond M (1985) Guidelines for the clinical and economic assessment of health technologies: the case for magnetic resonance. Int J Technol Assess Health Care 1:551–566

Health Technology Advisory Group (1992) Assessing the effect of health technologies. Department of Health, London

Hobby JL, Tom BDM, Todd, C, Bearcroft PWP, Dixon AK (2000) Communication of doubt and certainty in radiological reports. Br J Radiol 73:999–1001

Hobby JL, Dixon AK, Bearcroft PWP, Tom BDM, Lomas DJ, Rushton N, Matthewson MH (2001) MR imaging of the wrist: effect on clinical diagnosis and patient care. Radiology 220:589–93

Horii M, Kubo T, Naruse S, Hirasawa Y (1997) Relationship between pulse sequences and signal intensity of joint fluid in the gradient-echo MR imaging. Magn Reson Imaging 15:597–603

Imhoff A, Hodler J (1996) Correlation of MR imaging, CT arthrography, and arthroscopy of the shoulder. Bull Hosp Jt Dis 54:146–152

Jenkinson C, Coulter A, Wright L (1993a) Short form 36 (SF-36) health survey questionnaire: normative data for adults of working age. BMJ 306:1437–1440

Jenkinson C, Coulter A, Wright L (1993b) Quality of life measurements in health care: a review of measures and population norms for the UK SF-36. Health Services Unit, Oxford

Kelsey Fry I (1984) Who needs high technology? Br J Radiol 294:954–956

Kent DL, Larson EB (1988) Magnetic resonance of the brain and spine: Is clinical efficacy established after the first decade? Ann Intern Med 108:402–424

Kent D, Larson E (1992) Disease, level of impact, and quality of research methods. Three dimensions of clinical efficacy assessment applied to magnetic resonance imaging. Invest Radiol 27:245–254

Lev MH, Rhea JT, Bramsom RT (1999) Avoidance of variability and error in Radiology. Lancet 374:272

Lippitt SB, Harryman DT, Matsen FA (1993) A practical tool for the evaluation of function: the Simple Shoulder Test. In: Matsen FA, Fu FH, Hawkins RJ (eds) The shoulder: a balance of mobility and stability. American Academy of Orthopaedic Surgeons, Rosemont, Illinois, pp 501–518

Lusted LB (1968) Introduction to medical decision making. Thomas, Springfield

Maceneaney PM, Malone DE (2000) The meaning of diagnostic test results: a spreadsheet for swift data analysis. Clin Radiol 55:227–235

Mackenzie R, Hollingworth W, Dixon AK (1994) Quality of life assessments in the evaluation of magnetic resonance imaging. Qual Life Res 3:29–37

Mackenzie R, Dixon AK (1995) Measuring the effects of imaging: an evaluative framework. Clin Radiol 50:513–518

Mackenzie R, Dixon AK, Keene GS, Hollingworth W, Lomas DJ, Villar RN (1996) Magnetic resonance imaging of the knee: assessment of effectiveness. Clin Radiol 51:245–50

Mackenzie R (1996) Assessment of the clinical value of magnetic resonance imaging of the knee. PhD thesis. University of Cambridge, Cambridge

Maisey M, Hutton J (1991) Guidelines for the evaluation of radiological technologies. British Institute of Radiology, London

Menon D (2000) An assessment of health technology assessment in Canada. Can J Public Health 91:120

Misamore GW, Woodward C (1991) Evaluation of degenerative lesions of the rotator cuff. A comparison of arthrography and ultrasonography. J Bone Joint Surg (Am) 73:704–706

Patte D (1987) Directions for the use of the index severity for painful and/or chronically disabled shoulders. The First Open Congress of the European Society of Surgery of the Shoulder and Elbow, Paris, pp 36–41

Richards RR, An KN, Bigliani LU et al (1994) A standardized method for the assessment of shoulder function. J Shoulder Elbow Surg 3:347–352

Roach KE, Budiman-Mak E, Songsiridej N, Lertratanakul Y (1991) Development of a shoulder pain and disability index. Arthritis Care Res 4:143–149

Robinson PJ, Wilson D, Coral A, Murphy A, Verow P (1999) Variation between experienced observers in the interpretation of accident and emergency radiographs. Br J Radiol 72:323–330

Royal College of Physicians (1989) Medical audit: a first report. What, why and how? Royal College of Physicians, London

Sanford Schwartz J (1985) Evaluating diagnostic technologies. In: Institute of Medicine (ed) Assessing medical technologies. National Academy Press, Washington DC, pp 80–89

Sheps SB (1988) Technological imperatives and paradoxes. JAMA 259:3312–3313

Sher JS, Ianotti JP, Williams GR et al (1998) The effect of shoulder magnetic resonance on clinical decision making. J Shoulder Elbow Surg 7:205–209

Spiegelhalter DJ, Myles JP, Jones DR, Abraams KR (2000) Bayesian methods in health technology assessment: a review. Health Technol Assess 4:34

Steiner RE (1985) Magnetic resonance imaging: its impact upon diagnostic radiology. AJR 145:883–893

Streiner DL, Norman GR (1995) Health measurement scales. A practical guide to their development and use, 2nd edn. Oxford University Press, Oxford UK, P 32

Thornbury J (1994) Clinical efficacy of diagnostic imaging: love it or leave it. AJR 162:1–8

Walker SR, Rosser RM (eds) (1993) Quality of life assessment: key issues in the 1990s. Kluwer Academic Publishers, London

Weinstein MC (1985) Methodologic considerations in planning clinical trials of cost effectiveness of magnetic resonance. Int J Technol Assess Health Care 1:567–581

Yeu K, Jiang C, Shih T (1994) Correlation between MRI and operative findings of the rotator cuff tear. J Formos Med Assoc 93:134–139

Zanetti M, Jost B, Lustenberger A, Hodler J (1999) Clinical impact of MR arthrography of the shoulder. Acta Radiol 40:296–302

19 Future Developments in Shoulder Imaging

D. Weishaupt, S. Wildermuth, N. Teodorovic

19.1 Introduction

Recent advances in hard- and software have made nearly isotropic or isotropic computed tomography (CT) and magnetic resonance (MR) imaging data a regular part of clinical routine. Combined with sophisticated algorithms and high-performance computing, cross-sectional CT and MR imaging data sets may be processed to display three-dimensional (3D) representations of selected structures (Calhoun et al. 1999; Pretorius and Fishman 1999). Availability of 3D rendering techniques enhances the potential of post-processing techniques and opens up an entire generation of new diagnostic opportunities. Apart from routine maximum intensity projections (MIP), surface shaded displays, and 3D volume rendering, other, more elaborate, methods may be used. Based on the acquisition of a 3D volume data set, virtual-reality applications, such as virtual endoscopy, surgical planning, soft tissue modeling, and real-time tissue interaction, have become possible.

Virtual endoscopy has gained increasing interest in various fields of radiology (Vining 1996; Wilder-

muth and Debatin 1999). This form of virtual-reality image processing is capable of rendering endoluminal views, i.e., intraarticular views of joints similar to those obtained during arthroscopy (Applegate 1998; Weishaupt et al. 1999).

Kinematic imaging of joints is evolving in musculoskeletal radiology. Since open-configuration MR systems allow dynamic imaging of the shoulder joint over a wide range of motion, direct insight into glenohumeral biomechanics has become possible (Beaulieu et al. 1999).

This chapter describes principles and potential applications of newer shoulder imaging techniques, including virtual-reality techniques and kinematic imaging. Special attention is directed towards 3D rendering techniques. Potential challenges confronting the entire generation of these new imaging techniques are critically discussed.

19.2 Three-Dimensional Rendering Techniques

Three-dimensional rendering techniques are based on either two-dimensional (2D) or 3D acquisition and manipulate the resultant 2D images into a 3D display. All 3D rendering techniques attempt to display 3D spatial relationships in a two-dimensional image. The quality of 3D displays is directly influenced by the quality of the underlying source data. The following three characteristics determine the suitability of data sets of 3D rendering techniques:

- Pristine imaging quality with minimal motion artifacts for distinct edge detection
- Isotropic or nearly isotropic spatial resolution for full exploitation of 3D postprocessing possibilities
- High-contrast resolution for easy data segmentation

Both CT and MR data sets fulfill these requirements, with CT being superior due to inherent higher spatial resolution. In particular, the advent of multislice

D. Weishaupt, MD; S. Wildermuth, MD;
N. Teodorovic, RT
Institute of Diagnostic Radiology, University Hospital,
Rämistrasse 100, CH-8091 Zurich, Switzerland

spiral CT, with its ability to achieve true volumetric imaging, will have an enormous impact on medical virtual-reality applications, setting new standards for virtual reality applications. Three-dimensional post-processing of MR data is best accomplished by using ultrafast spoiled 3D gradient-recalled echo sequences (WILDERMUTH and DEBATIN 1999). The combination of MR arthrography with a dilute gadolinum chelate, a high contrast between the intraarticular fluid and the bony and soft-tissue structures is the basis of virtual intraarticular imaging.

To prepare images for 3D rendering techniques, all images must undergo segmentation that includes integrating two-dimensional CT data and eliminating noise to define the region of interest. The process of segmentation is potentially risky for certain clinical applications of such techniques (SHAHIDI et al. 1998).

19.2.1
Multiplanar Reconstruction

Multiplanar reconstruction (MPR) is the simplest method for visualizing structures that lie along the non-acquired orthogonal orientations of a 3D data set (Fig. 19.1). MPR is accomplished by rearranging the order of voxels in the volume image and can be done interactively when the volume is entirely stored in the memory of the computer. MPR is a very fast and interactive algorithm, suitable for representing several imaging planes at once, and permits reconstruction of even curved sections. Implementation of MPR techniques on powerful workstations allows for

a real-time interactive display of these images. MPRs are usually based on CT data sets. Image quality of MPRs have been significantly increased by the advent of multislice CT. Because multislice CT allows acquisition of isotropic data sets and minimizes stair-step artifacts high-quality MPRs can be obtained.

19.2.2
Maximum Intensity Projections

In MIPs each voxel along a line from the viewer's eye through the volume of the data is evaluated, and the maximum voxel value is selected on the basis of maximum signal intensity. The utility of MIP in shoulder imaging is limited. MIPs are considered most useful in MR and CT angiography.

19.2.3
Surface Rendering (Shaded Surface Display)

Shaded surface display (SSD) extracts the object of interest out of the volume by means of thresholding. SSD algorithms take the first voxel encountered along a projection ray that exceeds a user-defined threshold value and define the position and attenuation value of that voxel as the surface. During object projection it is possible to introduce different perspectives, simulating various positions of the observer relative to the surface of the object. Shaded surface displays provide a comprehensive assessment 3D impression of a structure by displaying its surface. However, SSDs

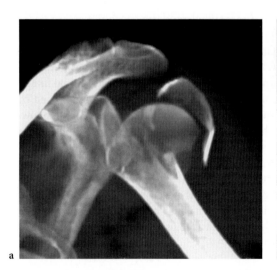 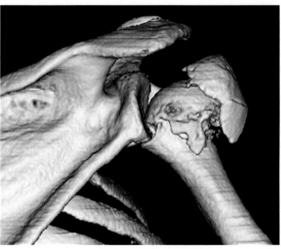

a   b

Fig. 19.1a, b. A 25-year-old patient with a Neer four-part fracture following a fall during snowboarding. **a** Multiplanar reconstruction of multislice spiral computed tomography (CT) data from an anterior view. **b** Posterior view of a coronal oblique volume-rendered multislice spiral CT image

do not maintain information regarding the internal properties of structures.

SSDs are mainly used for communication with referring clinicians whenever the abnormality cannot be correctly assessed based on axial images alone, or to facilitate preoperative planning of fractures. Since SSDs focus on a specific surface, they are generally very useful for virtual endoscopy applications. Their disadvantage is their propensity to artifacts, since image quality is strongly dependent on the chosen threshold range for the definition of the displayed 3D object.

19.2.4
Volume Rendering

In volume rendering (VR), parallel projection rays are cast through the entire image volume and not just its surface elements (Fig. 19.1). Contrary to SSD, in VR the contributions of each voxel along a line of sight from the viewer's eye through the data set are added up. In addition, VR uses an opacity function to connect each signal intensity with an opacity value to create the image. This process is repeated many times in order to determine each pixel value in the displayed image. Hence, VR displays visual images from the entire volume data, enabling the viewer to reveal the entire internal structure and information of the 3D data (Fig. 19.2). VR images may be viewed in any plane and in a range of opacities from transparent to opaque.

Unlike other projection techniques, such as SSD and MIP, VR does not distort the object and has no tendency to stair-step artifacts. This favours its use in combination with multislice CT data sets, which enables the acquisition of isotropic voxels. However, because VR incorporates the entire information of the data set into the resulting image, VR requires considerably more computer power than other rendering algorithms.

19.2.5
Virtual Endoscopy

Virtual endoscopy (VE) is a term to describe computer-simulated endoscopy procedures derived from high-resolution 3D CT or MR data sets. VE provides simulated endoscopic views of patient-specific organs and can be performed using surface- or volume-rendering algorithms. VE is a typical application of virtual reality (ROBB 2000). The virtual-reality paradigm allows the observer to act in synthetic, computer-generated worlds (SATAVA 1995). In contrast to conventional visualization systems, the user

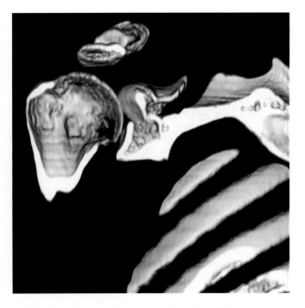

Fig. 19.2. A 33-year-old patient with a glenoid fracture. Cutaway anterior volume-rendered multislice spiral computed tomography image best shows the full extent of the glenoid fracture

may become an active part of the scene, virtually blending into its surroundings.

VE has been applied to a number of organic systems including rendering of endoscopic views of vessels, trachea, and bronchial tree, as well as of colon, urinary bladder, biliary tree, spinal canal, and stomach (WILDERMUTH and DEBATIN 1999). Similarly, feasibility of virtual arthroscopy based on 3D MR arthrographic data sets has been shown (APPLEGATE 1998; WEISHAUPT et al. 1999). The technique is based on MR arthrography in conjunction with the acquisition of a fast spoiled 3D gradient-recalled echo sequence (Fig. 19.3). The intraarticular injection of T1-shortening paramagnetic contrast agent permits joint distension and provides high contrast-to-noise ratio between the intraarticular and/or periarticular soft-tissue structures and the intraarticular fluid. By virtually placing the observer within the articular space, a truly arthroscopic illusion is created. Virtual MR arthroscopy represents an easy add-on to any conventional MR arthrographic study. Since the process of segmentation requires a high contrast between the intraarticular fluid and the intraarticular and periarticular structures, the concentration of the intraarticular gadolinium should be slightly higher than the usually administered concentration. However, the increase in contrast concentration of the administered gadolinium does not affect the quality of the other sequences.

Beyond being noninvasive, virtual arthroscopy

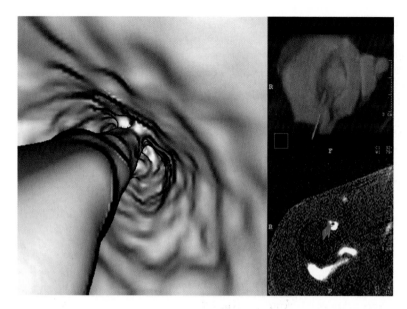

Fig. 19.3. Three-dimensional shoulder magnetic resonance arthrogram from an intraarticular perspective (virtual arthroscopy), looking superior to inferior along the long head of the bicipital tendon. The virtual observer's position is simulated within the shoulder joint and is marked by an *arrow* on the corresponding source image (*bottom right*). This position permits the observer to look downward into the bicipital groove and the tendon sheath of the long head of the biceps tendon

allows unobstructed virtual movement and camera control, permitting any desirable vantage point. The joint distension resulting from the presence of the intraarticular contrast permits an animated flight through the joint to negotiate even narrow intraarticular structures. Although the virtual arthroscopy appears not to increase the amount of diagnostic information contained within the 2D source data, it is important to recall that the main advantage of postprocessing is to merely facilitate the extraction of the diagnostic relevant information. Virtual arthroscopy may foster improved understanding of the complex relationships and common variants in the shoulder joint (APPLEGATE 1998). Because VE provides quantitatively exact geometric and densitometric information, it may be useful for preoperative planning. Recent developments in color mapping of mucosal layers (SCHREYER et al. 2000) may also be applied to synovial layers in order to differentiate between normal, thickened, or inflamed synovium.

19.3
Surgical Planning and Surgical Simulation

Currently, the orthopaedic shoulder surgeon can take advantage of many inherent features of advanced postprocessing of 3D volume data sets to adequately tailor

treatment to suit the patient's needs. The creation of orthogonal and oblique multiplanar reformatted images permits the orthopaedic surgeon to visualize the articular structure in full context, rather than only in the plane of acquisition. In addition, postprocessing of a 3D data set provides the ability to create images necessary for direct quantitative analysis. Fractures of the scapula are often subtle on plain radiographs, but volume-rendered CT images are very sensitive in the detection and characterization of such fractures (THOMPSON et al. 1985). In the evaluation of three- and four-part fractures of the proximal humerus, the superiority of spiral CT with multiplanar reconstruction over plain radiography has been demonstrated (JURIK and ALBRECHTSEN 1994). VR or SSD permits exact location of the different fracture fragments and the assessment of their degree of rotation-critical factors in determining whether a proximal humeral head fracture should be managed surgically.

Most of the currently used surgical planning applications are based on complex polygonal surface models, whereas marching cube models are used for extraction isosurfaces from segmentation results. Using multiple object segmentation techniques and rendering techniques, the humeral head can be defined as a separated object and the remaining scapula and glenoid fossa may be simulated independently (Fig. 19.4).

Modern 3D imaging may become enormously helpful in planning surgical procedures. So far, surgical planning and surgical simulation are limited to

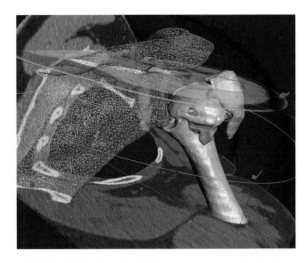

Fig. 19.4. Advanced rendering techniques allow definition of bony and soft-tissue structures as separated objects

ment intuitively, using all five senses: sight, sound, touch/haptics, smell and taste.

Simulation of soft tissue, including skin deformation, cutting characteristics of different organs, and bleeding after cutting, is another crucial task for virtual-reality techniques. Different prototype systems for surgical simulation address this issue (Fig. 19.5). A recently developed system has shown that a real-time virtual simulation system for rat dissection, including soft-tissue deformation, force feedback, and variable gravity, is feasible (WILDERMUTH et al. 2001).

Augmented reality (AR) is another approach that will be of interest for future interventional and surgical techniques. AR superimposes computer-gener-

rigid bony tissue and standard implants. However, in order to simulate a real environment for surgical procedures it is necessary to simulate the soft-tissue conditions overlaying the bony structures. Simulation of soft tissues is a challenging task and is feasible by using CT data only or in combination with a skin digitizer. The quality of soft-tissue simulation has been significantly improved by the use of multislice CT data sets. Compared to conventional CT, the higher temporal and spatial resolution of multislice CT permits fast thin collimation scanning over a large scanning range with minimal motion-related artifacts. Thin collimation data sets in conjunction with perfect timing of vessel contrast produces optimal raw data for soft-tissue reconstruction.

Development of real-time working and interactive systems is of paramount importance for future acceptance and practicability of virtual-reality techniques in surgical planning and surgical simulating systems. Virtual-reality techniques currently under development combine human–computer interfaces, graphics, sensor technology, high-end computing, and networking. Virtual-reality simulation tries, through the use of head-mounted displays and tracking of hand-and-instrument motion that uses a data glove or other interactive devices, to create realistic simulation of interaction in an artificial environment (AKAY 1996). Realistic interactive surgical environments must be capable of correctly interpreting the motion of both the human hand and virtual objects. This requires mathematical modelling of deformable and solid objects. Hence, the aim of virtual-reality models is to create human–computer interfaces which interact with the virtual environ-

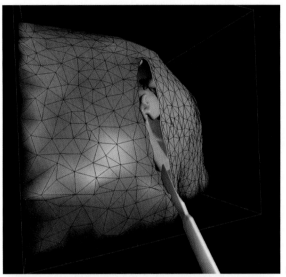

a

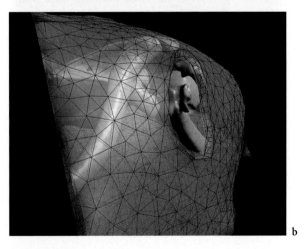

b

Fig. 19.5a, b. Based on the multislice computed tomography data set, a high-resolution, polygon surface model was generated with the resulting mesh visible on the skin. The model allows for interactive simulation such as virtual dissection of the skin. The natural behavior of the soft tissues during dissection is simulated by this model

ated images on the user's own visual perception of the real world or provides a completely computer-generated environment. Such systems can be used to provide additional visual input by labeling certain structures or by superimposing imaging data of different modalities onto, e.g., the surgeon's or interventionalist's perception of reality. The most widely known AR interface is the head-mounted display.

19.4
Kinematic Imaging

MR imaging, using conventional closed-magnet design, provides detailed information of anatomy and pathology. To establish a direct correlation of imaging findings with the specific patient's symptoms is difficult. Because of the design of MR magnets, the shoulder is almost always imaged in the neutral position of the humeral head with regard to the glenoid fossa. Imaging in positions other than the neutral position of the shoulder is limited.

Open-configuration MR systems with both horizontal and vertical access to the patient allow for shoulder imaging in an upright sitting position over a wide range of joint motion (Fig. 19.6). BEAULIEU et al. (1999) have established imaging protocols for kinematic MR imaging of the shoulder. Using this technique, MR imaging during slow but continuous motion, initiated and maintained by the subject without the use of a positioning device or restraint, is possible. The authors demonstrate that during abduction and adduction and internal and external

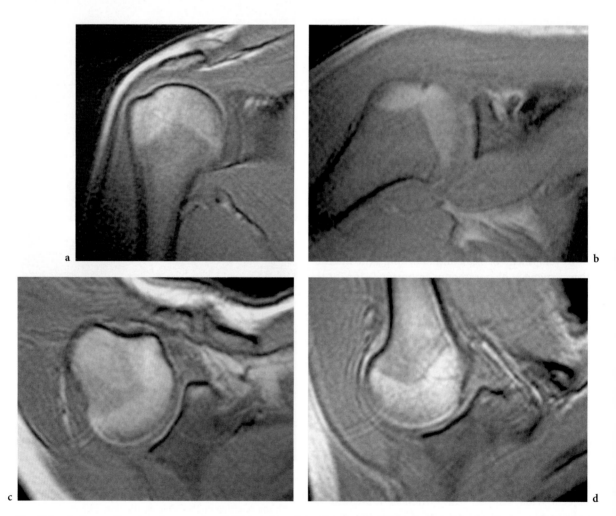

Fig. 19.6a–d. Kinematic magnetic resonance (MR) imaging of the glenohumeral joint during abduction in an asymptomatic volunteer. The kinematic MR imaging examination was conducted obtaining oblique coronal images acquired at various incremental positions of abduction. The study revealed a normal humeral-glenoid relationship

rotation the humeral head remains precisely centered on the glenoid fossa in asymptomatic subjects. In addition, feasibility of MR imaging during actual physical manipulation of the shoulder by a physician has been demonstrated (HODGE et al. 2001). Kinematic shoulder MR imaging opens up new possibilities in joint imaging. If combined with high-quality static MR imaging of anatomic components, a comprehensive diagnostic imaging evaluation of the shoulder joint will soon become possible.

19.5
Conclusion

The rapid development of CT, MR and other imaging modalities has resulted in exciting new applications and possibilities of shoulder imaging. Three-dimensional techniques are currently a major area of clinical and research interest. Three-dimensional volume techniques including surface and volume rendering can help the radiologist to more effectively interpret imaging studies and to facilitate communication with the clinician. They have the ability to demonstrate the complicated spatial information about the relative positions of fracture fragments in complex shoulder trauma cases, a feature that is of great use to the orthopedic surgeon. In addition, 3D rendering techniques provide new applications such as virtual endoscopy, which is considered as a powerful tool for exploring 3D data sets.

The rapid development of information technology and computer graphics will result in new tools for surgical training, planning, and procedures. High-performance human–computer interfaces permit the interaction between computer-generated images and the real world. New designs of magnets for kinematic MR imaging allow new insights into biomechanical mechanisms and into the relationship between the osseous and the soft-tissue components of the shoulder joint during a wide range of motion.

References

Akay M (1996) Virtual reality. IEEE Eng Med Biol Mag 15:14

Applegate GR (1998) Three-dimensional MR arthrography of the shoulder: an intraarticular perspective. AJR 171:239–241

Beaulieu CR, Hodge DK, Bergmann AG, Butts K, Daniel BL, Napper CL, Darrow RD, Dumoulin CL, Herkens RJ (1999) Glenohumeral relationships during physiological shoulder motion and stress testing: initial experience with open MR imaging and active imaging-plane registration. Radiology 212:699–705

Callhoun PS, Kuszyk BS, Heath DG, Carley JC, Fishman EK (1999) Three-dimensional volume rendering of spiral CT data: theory and methods. Radiographics 19:745–764

Hodge DK, Beaulieu CF, Thabit GH, Gold GE, Bergmann AG, Butts RK, Dillingham MF, Herfkens RJ (2001) Dynamic MR imaging and stress testing in glenohumeral instability: comparison with normal shoulders and clinical/surgical findings. J Magn Reson Imaging 13:748–756

Jurik AG, Albrechtsen J (1994) The use of computed tomography with two- and three-dimensional reconstructions in the diagnosis of three- and four-part fractures of the proximal humerus. Clin Radiol 49:800–804

Pretorius SC, Fishman EK (1999) Volume-rendered three-dimensional spiral CT: musculoskeletal applications. Radiographics 19:1143–1160

Robb RA (2000) Virtual endoscopy: development and evaluation using the visible human datasets. Comput Med Imaging Graph 24:133–154

Satava RM (1995) Medical applications for virtual reality. J Med Syst 19:275–280

Schreyer AG, Fielding JR, Warfield SK, Lee JH, Loughlin KR, Dumanli H, Jolesz FA, Kikinis R (2000) Virtual CT cystoscopy: color mapping of bladder wall thickness. Invest Radiol 35:331–334

Shahidi R, Tombropuolos R, Grzeszczuk RP (1998) Clinical applications of three-dimensional rendering of medical data sets. Proc IEEE 86:555–568

Thompson DA, Flynn TC, Miller PW, Fischer RP (1985) The significance of scapular fractures. J Trauma 25:974–977

Vining DJ (1996) Virtual endoscopy: is it reality? Radiology 200:30–31

Weishaupt D, Wildermuth S, Schmid MR, Hilfiker PR, Hodler J, Debatin JF (1999) Virtual arthroscopy based on 3D MR datasets–new insights into joint morphology. J Magn Reson Imaging 9:757–760

Wildermuth S, Debatin JF (1999) Virtual endoscopy in abdominal MR imaging. MRI Clin North Am 7:349–364

Wildermuth S, Bruyns C, Montgomery K, Weishaupt D, Marincek B (2001) A virtual reality environment for animal dissections based on multidetector CT datasets. Eur Radiol 11 [Suppl]:372

Subject Index

List of Contributors

VINCENT BAUDREZ, MD
Department of Radiology
University Hospital de Mont-Godinne
Catholic University of Louvain
5530 Yvoir
Belgium

PHILIP W.P. BEARCROFT, MB, FRCR
Department of Radiology Box 219
Addenbrooke's NHS Trust
Hills Road
Cambridge CB2 2QQ
UK

THOMAS H. BERQUIST, MD, FACR
Diagnostic Radiology
Mayo Clinic
4500 San Pablo Road
Jacksonville, FL 32224
USA

STEFANO BIANCHI, MD
Division of Radiodiagnosis and Interventional Radiology
Hopital Cantonal Universitaire de Geneve
24 rue Micheli-du-Crest
1211 Geneva 4
Switzerland

ALAIN BLUM, MD
Professor of Radiology
Service d'Imagerie Guilloz
Hopital Central , CHU Nancy
29 Avenue du Maréchal de Lattre de Tassigny
54035 Nancy Cedex
France

YANNICK CARRILLON, MD
Clinique Saint Jean
30 rue Bataille
69008 Lyon
France

VICTOR N. CASSAR-PULLICINO, MD, FRCR
Consultant and Clinical Director
Department of Diagnostic Radiology
Robert Jones & Agnes Hunt Orthopaedic Hospital
Oswestry, Shropshire SY10 7AG
UK

CHRISTINE B. CHUNG, MD
Osteoradiology Section (114), Radiology Department
Veterans Affairs San Diego Healthcare System
University of California, San Diego
3350 La Jolla Village Drive
San Diego, CA 92161
USA

A. MARK DAVIES, MD
Consultant Radiologist
MRI Centre
Royal Orthopaedic Hospital
Birmingham B31 2AP
UK

LORENZO E. DERCHI, MD
Istituto di Radiologia
Università di Genova
Largo R Benzi 8
16100 Genoa
Italy

JEAN FASEL, MD
Professor, Division of Anatomy
Department of Morphology
University Medical Center
Rue M. Servet 1
1211 Geneva 4
Switzerland

M.A.M. FELDBERG, MD
Department of Radiology, E.01.132
University Medical Center Utrecht
Postbus 85500
3508 GA Utrecht
The Netherlands

JEAN F. GARCIA, MD
Department of Radiology
Hopital Cantonal Universitaire de Geneve
24 rue Micheli-du-Crest
1211 Geneva 4
Switzerland

JÜRG HODLER, MD, MBA
Department of Radiology
Orthopedic University Hospital Balgrist
Forchstrasse 340
8008 Zurich
Switzerland

KARL JOHNSON, MD
Radiology Department
Birmingham Children's Hospital
Steelhouse Lane
Birmingham B13 9SZ
UK

ALAIN KELLER, MD
Department of Radiology
Hopital Cantonal Universitaire de Geneve
24 rue Micheli-du-Crest
1211 Geneva 4
Switzerland

PHILIP LANG, MD, MBA
Department of Radiology
Brigham and Woman's Hospital
75 Francis Street, ASB I, Floor L1, Room 003E
Boston, MA 02115
USA

NITTAYA LEKTRAKUL, MD
Osteoradiology Section (114), Radiology Department
Veterans Affairs San Diego Healthcare System
University of California, San Diego
3350 La Jolla Village Drive
San Diego, CA 92161
USA

CARLO MARTINOLI, MD
Istituto di Radiologia
Cattedra "R" di Radiologia
Università di Genova
Largo Rosanna Benzi, 8
16100 Genova
Italy

LARS NEUMANN, FRCS
Consultant Orthopaedic Surgeon
Nottingham Shoulder and Elbow Unit
City Hospital
Nottingham NG5 1PB
UK

WILFRED PEH, MBBS, MD, FRCPG, FRCPE, FRCR
Senior Consultant, Department of Diagnostic Radiology
Singapore General Hospital
Singapore 169608
Singapore

NICOLÓ PRATO, MD
Division of Radiodiagnosis
Ospedale San Carlo
Piazzale Gianasso
16158 Genova
Italy

BRYAN J. PRESTON, MB, BS, FRCR
Consultant Radiologist, Department of Imaging
University Hospital
Queens Medical Centre
Nottingham NG7 2UH
UK

SWEE-TIAN QUEK, MBBS, FRCR
Consultant, Department of Diagnostic Radiology
National Cancer Centre
Singapore 1696010
Singapore

JEAN-JACQUES RAILHAC, MD
Professor of Radiology
Service Central de radiologie et d'Imagerie Médicale
Hôpital Purpan
31059 Toulouse Cédex
France

DONALD RESNICK, MD
Osteoradiology Section (114), Radiology Department
Veterans Affairs San Diego Healthcare System
University of California, San Diego
3350 La Jolla Village Drive
San Diego, CA 92161
USA

BERNARD ROGER, MD
Service de Radiologie ostéo-articulaire
Hôpital Pitié Salpêtrière
Bd. de l'Hôpital
75013 Paris Cédex
France

AXEL STÄBLER, MD
Institute for Radiologic Diagnostic
Klinikum Grosshadern
Ludwig-Maximilians University
Marchioninistrasse 15
81377 Munich
Germany

THIERRY TAVERNIER, MD
Clinique de la Sauvegarde
Avenue Ben Gourion
69261 Lyon
France

NINOSLAV TEODOROVIC, MD
Institute of Diagnostic Radiology
University Hospital
Raemistrasse 100
8091 Zurich
Switzerland

BERNHARD TINS, MD
Department of Diagnostic Radiology
Robert Jones & Agnes Hunt Orthopaedic Hospital
Oswestry, Shropshire SY10 7AG
UK

BRUNO C. VANDE BERG, MD, PhD
Department of Radiology and Medical Imaging
University Hospital St. Luc
Avenue Hippocrate 10
1200 Brussels
Belgium

DANIEL VANEL, MD
Department of Radiology
Institut Gustave Roussy
39 rue Camille Desmoulins
94805 Villejuif
France

H. WOUTER VAN ES, MD
Department of Radiology
St. Antonius Hospital
Postbus 2500
3430 EM Nieuwegein
The Netherlands

DOMINIK WEISHAUPT, MD
Institute of Diagnostic Radiology
University Hospital
Raemistrasse 100
8091 Zurich
Switzerland

SIMON WILDERMUTH, MD
Institute of Diagnostic Radiology
University Hospital
Raemistrasse 100
8091 Zurich
Switzerland

T.D. WITKAMP, MD
Department of Radiology, E.01.132
University Medical Center Utrecht
Postbus 85500
3508 GA Utrecht
The Netherlands

B. WOLLMAN
Department of Radiology
Stanford University, California
USA

H. YOSHIOKA, MD
Department of Radiology
Brigham and Woman's Hospital
75 Francis Street, ASB I, Floor L1, Room 003E
Boston, MA 02115
USA

MARCO ZANETTI, MD
Department of Radiology
Orthopedic University Hospital Balgrist
Forchstrasse 340
8008 Zurich
Switzerland

MICHAEL B. ZLATKIN, MD, FRCP (C)
President, National Musculoskeletal Imaging
13798 NW 4th Street, Suite 305
Sunrise, FL 33325
USA

and

Voluntary Professor of Radiology
University of Miami School of Medicine
Miami, FL
USA

MEDICAL RADIOLOGY Diagnostic Imaging and Radiation Oncology

Titles in the series already published

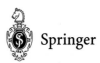
Springer

MEDICAL RADIOLOGY   Diagnostic Imaging and Radiation Oncology

Titles in the series already published

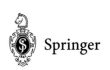

Springer